Martin Abel
August 1981
New York

Medical Mystery

Dr. Jonas is editor and co-author of
Health Care Delivery in the United States
and author of
Quality Control of Ambulatory Care: A Task for Health Departments

Medical Mystery

The Training of Doctors in the United States

Steven Jonas, M.D.

W · W · NORTON & COMPANY
NEW YORK/LONDON

Published simultaneously in Canada by George J. McLeod Limited, Toronto. Printed in the United States of America.

First Edition

Library of Congress Cataloging in Publication Data

Jonas, Steven.
Medical mystery: the training of doctors in the United States.

Bibliography: p.
Includes index.
1. Medical education—United States. 2. Medical care—United States. I. Title. [DNLM: 1. Education, Medical—United States. 2. Delivery of health care—United States. W18.3 J76m]
R745.J65 1978 362.1'0973 78–16909
ISBN 0–393–06437–9

1 2 3 4 5 6 7 8 9 0

Grateful acknowledgment is made for permission to quote from the following:

Light in Dark Corners by Russell Baker. © 1977 by The New York Times Company. Editorials by Dr. Franz Ingelfinger. Reprinted by permission from the *New England Journal of Medicine,* vol. 294, p. 442, 1976 and vol. 295, p. 565, 1976. *Medical and Dental Education in the United States and Canada* by Abraham Flexner. Reprinted by permission from The Carnegie Foundation for the Advancement of Teaching. *A New Paradigm for Medical Education* by Dr. Lawrence Weed. Reprinted by permission of the Josiah Macy, Jr. Foundation. *Toward Defining the End Product of Medical Education* by Robert Kane, F. Ross Woolley, and Rosalie Kane. Reprinted by permission from the *Journal of Medical Education* and the authors. *Guide to the Development of Skills in Problem Based Learning and Clinical (Diagnostic) Reasoning* by Dr. Howard S. Barrows and Robyn M. Tamblyn. Reprinted by permission of the authors. *The "McMaster Philosophy": An Approach to Medical Education* by Dr. Victor Neufeld and Dr. Howard Barrows. Reprinted by permission from the *Journal of Medical Education* and the authors. "Who Killed Cock Robin?", table: "Changes in Mortality (1900–1940)" by C.-E.A. Winslow. Reprinted by permission from the *American Journal of Public Health,* vol. 34, p. 658, 1944. "Functions and Structure of a Medical School," from *Accreditation of Schools of Medicine: Policy Documents and Guidelines.* Reprinted by permission of American Medical Association. "Doctors" by Anne Sexton in *The Awful Rowing Toward God.* Copyright © 1975 by Loring Conant, Jr. Reprinted by permission of Houghton Mifflin Company. "My Faith in Doctors," by Piet Hein, *Harvard Medical Alumni Bulletin,* Nov./Dec., 1976, p. 12. Reprinted by permission of author.

For my children, Jacob Henry and Lillian Sara.

I have tried to faithfully record the past and describe the present; my children are my passage to the future.

And so the Hippocratic physicians and their followers studied how a man should live in order to maintain his health. And they came to the conclusion that it was impossible for a man to remain in perfect health unless he organized his entire life for such a purpose.

—*Henry Sigerist*
Medicine and Human Welfare

CONTENTS

Foreword

Landing Ship, Tank (LST) was the designation of one of the United States Navy's least popular classes of vessels in World War II. LSTs were essential for amphibious operations—our landings in the Pacific, Africa, and Europe would have been impossible without them—but they suffered a serious flaw. They were so big and clumsy that their crews claimed the acronym stood for "Large Stationary Target."

A generation later the nation has another Large Stationary Target: its health care system. It is essential—our society and our economy would be crippled without it—but it is so mammouth and unwieldy that few can resist taking a shot at it. It can absorb a lot of punishment, but the torpedoes are getting more destructive. Some of the most dangerous are being launched by well-meaning people who seem intent on stopping the system dead in the water, pumps straining to keep it awash.

To continue this nautical analogy, in World War II there were not enough trained professionals to navigate all the Navy's ships, but, with skilled instructors, intelligent laymen quickly learned how. Our health care system is also navigated by the laymen (tripling the production of doctors in thirty years is one example of the system's response to the public hand on its helm), but its erratic course in recent decades betrays the public's superficial understanding of the system and its societal role. An informed citizenry is needed to set a true and steady course for our health care system.

This book, by an expert who knows the ship of health care from bridge to keel, imparts in non-technical language the knowledge concerned citizens must have if they are to make badly needed course corrections and maneuver their venerable vessel into waters where it can be overhauled. The book will be useful to any intelligent person but particularly valuable to citizens already involved in navigation—members of Health Systems Agency boards, trustees of hospitals, officials of federal, state and local governments, insurance executives, and those responsible for industrial health care benefits. Health professionals, who are woefully ignorant of the reasons why the confused system in which they work is the way it is, will profit from this book too. Its smooth style and simple language offer a welcome respite from the technical literature they customarily read.

Although the language is not technical, this book is no primer. Its readers will finish it with a sophisticated understanding of the place of the scientific method in effective medical practice and of the place of health care in the social fabric. The complexities, contradictions, and confusion that obscure these two basic precepts are stripped away as the author skillfully unravels the threads of history and explains how things in today's tangled health care system that seem utterly illogical are derived from origins that were once logical.

The book is dedicated to reform of the health care system, but it is not of the torpedo genre that seems so popular (and sells so well) today. To shoot from a distance without concern for alternatives if the target sinks may be emotionally satisfying to author and reader, but it is a sterile exercise. Far more difficult to write (and demanding to read) is a book that is conservative in the best, literal sense of that word. This one examines all aspects of the health care system, selects those that should be conserved, and offers feasible, reasonable alternatives to those that are so easy to castigate but so hard to change.

Focusing on the centrality of doctors to our health care system, Dr. Jonas posits that a significantly new health care system will require the creation of significantly new doctors. He demystifies the "mystery" of his title by explaining, as only an insider can, how doctors have learned to do what they do from their traditional, disease-oriented professional education. To create "significantly new doctors," he thinks a complete reversal in educational emphasis is essential. His alternative—*health*-oriented professional education—has the sound ring of logic. And, unlike those large stationary targets of yesteryear, it has a positive acronym: HOPE.

JOHN GORDON FREYMANN, M.D.,
President,
National Fund for Medical Education

Acknowledgments

A number of people have assisted me in the preparation and writing of this book. First, thanks must go to my literary agent, Sheri Safran. Without her encouragement and help, this book never would have been. Next, I must thank my editor at Norton, Eric Swenson, for giving a chance to an author unknown to the general public and for offering most helpful advice in the preparation of the manuscript, in amongst a lot of talk about our mutual passion, sailing. I hope that this book will justify Eric's faith in me. My very good friend, David Banta, read the manuscript all the way through as it was being written. His tough, insightful criticism was invaluable.

John Gordon Freymann and Stephen Stowe offered valuable advice on Chapter 8. Wendy Waddell did the same for Chapter 11.

I would like to thank my friend and former student Michael Taylor, for his help in developing the HOPE and DOPE acronyms.

The production of the book was made possible in part by the generous support of my father, Harold J. Jonas. With many thanks I acknowledge his assistance.

The typing of the manuscript was done principally by Eugenia DiGirolano. I thank her for her help. To my copy editor at Norton,

Sue J. Lowe, who did an outstanding job, I would also like to give my thanks.

There are two books to which I am particularly indebted. One is *The American Health Care System* (Huntington, N.Y.: Krieger Publishing Co., 1977), by John Gordon Freymann, who has kindly written the foreword to this book. The other is *American Medicine and the Public Interest,* by Rosemary Stevens (New Haven: Yale University Press, 1971). These are both monumental works of medical history. However, they are not simply descriptive history books. They are books which attempt to use past history as a guide both to understanding the present and to making correct policy for the future. This is a young tradition in medical history, having been inaugurated in the 1930s by the late, great Henry Sigerist.

I would like especially to acknowledge the publisher of *Health Care Delivery in the United States,* Ursula Springer, and my co-authors of that book: David Banta, Carol McCarthy, Nancy Barhydt, Ruth Hanft, Lorrin Koran, Michael Enright, and Barbara Rimer. Ursula, Dave, Carol, Mike, and Barbara have given me permission to use specific portions of that book in this one. But all of the co-authors and Ursula together made *Health Care Delivery* possible in the first place. Without *Health Care Delivery,* I doubt there would have been *Medical Mystery.*

I owe them all my thanks.

Prologue: The Parable of the Bakers

Once upon a time there was a kingdom between the seas. The land was rich and bountiful, the people intelligent and hardworking—a people who valued their health almost above all else. Their King had once said: "[T]he health of our people is, inescapably, the foundation for the fulfillment of all our aspirations."[1] Now it happened that bread was very important to the health and welfare of the people of the kingdom. But there was something special about the bread industry. Although many different kinds of people were involved along the way in making and selling the bread—from the farmers who grew the grain to the keepers of the stores which sold the finished product—there was one group of people who exerted an unusual degree of control over the whole bread making and delivery system. They were called the Bakers. A few rare kinds of bread were sold by others, but most non-Bakers who tried to sell bread were charged with "selling bread without a license."

Although the kingdom originally established the laws licensing the Bakers, the Bakers themselves actually controlled the licensing process: To get a Baker's license, a person had to go to a school controlled by the Bakers (meeting requirements for entrance set by the Bakers), take courses selected by the Bakers, pass examinations devised by the Bakers, and have supervised work experience as required by the Bakers. Once a person earned his Baker's license, only other Bakers could decide if any of his actions warrented removal of it. In practice this happened rarely. To lose his license, a Baker had to make or sell pretty bad bread indeed. And it happened that the whole process was controlled by the Bakers' Guild and its relative, the Guild of Bakers' Schools.

At first, the Bakers seemed to be very concerned about the quality of what they were doing. But as the years passed, they came to be much more concerned about maintaining their monopoly and restricting competition. They came to regard the license as a property right, not as a privilege enabling them to help people who needed bread. Often the courts of the kingdom upheld that view. The number of schools for Bakers, which had been quite high, was vastly reduced. This action improved the quality of the remaining schools, but it reduced the Baker population ratio. Bakers, because of their license-based monopoly, became increasingly rich and powerful.

They began to learn how to make different kinds of breads, and, even more important for the development of their occupation, they began to learn how to make cakes and exotic pastries, only a few of which met the basic health needs of the people. Increasing numbers of up and coming Bakers were attracted to cake-making because of its higher income potential and because it was thought to be more "interesting" than bread-making. Besides, it was oftentimes easier to be a cake-maker, making the same kind of cake over and over again, than it was to be a bread-maker and have to know how to make many varieties of bread. Thus the age of the specialist Baker was born.

At the same time that the Bakers were establishing a virtual monopoly over the making and selling of bread, cakes, and pastries, they were radically changing the schools for training Bakers. The controls were exerted both directly and through the laws for licensing individual Bakers. Large corporations and private foundations were induced to give generous sums of money to the favorite schools of the Bakers' Guild. Although the number of graduates fell, the quality of instruction improved significantly. Bakers were trained to make and sell the best kind of bread and cakes and the kingdom benefitted.

The rulers of the kingdom initially had some direct control over the Bakers' schools. However, they gradually gave up that authority, convinced that the Bakers could do a better job of it themselves. This situation led to several difficulties. Insulated from any direct responsibility to the rulers of the kingdom, or to the people, the Bakers' schools gradually came to define their needs, and programs in their own terms, rather than in terms of the needs of the people. The people needed good, ordinary bread, distributed widely, at a price they could afford. But the Bakers' schools became increasingly concerned with research into bread-making: what happened with this yeast, or that batter, where did they come from, what were they really made of. Sometimes this research was very useful in making a new kind of bread, but sometimes researchers worked with yeast and batters that never had been or ever would be used in any kind of bread. Moreover, the schools came to do more and more research in cakes and pastries, spending more and more time and energy training cake-bakers than bread-bakers. They concentrated increasingly on research and specialization.

Now, strangely enough, in this particular kingdom people knew little about the content of bread, and even less about what went into cake. Although they usually knew when they needed baked goods they usually didn't know how much or what kind they should buy. More often than not it was the Baker rather than the buyer who decided what was needed—bread, or cake, or pastry, how much of each, and what kind. Further, the Bakers were talking to the people less and less. In olden times, the Bakers used to discuss bread and cake with the people, explaining why they should have this sort or that. But as the Bakers' Guild grew more powerful and more secure in its monopoly, as more Bakers became cake-makers rather than bread-makers, and as the Bakers' schools became more interested in research and in training cake-makers, so the Bakers' facility and interest in talking to their buyers and explaining the pros and cons of this or that bread or cake fell. The Bakers often rationalized their behavior by saying that the people couldn't understand about bread and cake because it was too complicated, and anyway they weren't interested. Thus a "Bakers' Mystique" developed.

The rulers were becoming very concerned about all of this. They were spending a lot of money on the Bakers' schools and didn't seem to be getting the product the buyers really needed. For a long time, certain people had been complaining about the bread and the Bakers' system: it was too expensive, costs were rising too rapidly, the Bakers were geographically unevenly distributed, more and more Bakers were cake- and pastry-makers, who concentrated in localities where people could afford to buy cake. So they approached the Bakers' schools, at first quietly and respectfully. After all, the kingdom's Bakers' schools were the best in the world, or so their leaders said. "The people aren't getting enough bread," the rulers would say. "Let 'em eat cake," would come back the reply (the speaker saying to himself, "Haven't I heard that somewhere before?") "Your research should really be directed towards making better bread," the rulers would say. "We know what we are doing. Just give us the money," the schools' leaders would say gruffly. The people would say, "Why can't you explain about bread and cake before you make us buy it, and eat it?" The leaders of the Bakers' schools would reply, "Who needs a Baker who can communicate? All they have to know is how to make good bread and cake, and sell it."

Then another issue was raised. The people and the rulers became increasingly aware that other things were important for health, too, even more important than what Bakers did. The history of the kingdom showed that over the years improved general nutrition, pure water supply and sanitary sewage disposal, and immunization against infectious diseases all had a greater influence on general health levels than what the Bakers did—contrary to what the Bakers said. Furthermore, it was being shown that cigarette smoking, environmental pollution, overeating, and lack of exercise had important negative influences on the peoples' health. Thus increasingly was heard throughout the kingdom: "You cannot live by bread alone—and cake isn't the answer either."

But the Bakers knew little about this and seemed to care less. They were selling plenty of bread, cakes, and pastries, and that was fine with them. This attitude was not surprising since virtually no attention was paid to such matters in the Bakers' schools. And thus we come to modern times.

(Ordinarily a parable would present a resolution of the contradictions at about this point, and the moral of the story would be revealed. However, this parable, based as it is on the history and present state of medicine and medical education in the United States, cannot offer a resolution. The contradictions in the real system on which the parable is based have existed for many years. My intention is to illuminate those contradictions and to suggest some ways for resolving them in a manner satisfactory to at least a majority, if not all, of the parties concerned. I hope to happily conclude my parable in the not too distant future. But for now a conclusion simply cannot be written.)

SECTION *I*

Health and Health Care: Problems for the American People

1

Introduction

Many difficulties impede the delivery of health care services in the United States:

rising costs
financial barriers to care
overspecialization of physicians
geographic maldistribution of facilities and manpower
unnecessary hospitalization and surgery
uneveness in availability, accessibility, and acceptability of services
defects in quality and in quality control
poor communication between providers and patients
emphasis on curative medicine at the expense of preventive medicine

These problems have been with us for a long time. Contrary to a prevalent view, the system is not in "crisis." Rather it has a serious, chronic illness. It is my thesis that the medical education system in this country directly and indirectly creates obstacles to adequate health care delivery. I intend to substantiate that thesis and to offer some solutions to the problem. For those readers who may not be familiar with the term, the health care delivery system is the legal, administrative, and organizational framework within which personnel, institutions, and financing methods combine to provide to the people services based on our body of knowledge concerning the maintenance of health and the curing of disease.

The Basic Argument

Doctors are the keystone of the health care delivery system in the United States. The functioning of the whole system revolves around what doctors do, regardless of the fact that they make up less than 10 percent of the health care workforce. There are a variety of non-doctor health care professionals who give certain kinds of carefully defined and restricted services to patients: nurses, optometrists, podiatrists, speech pathologists, clinical psychologists, chiropractors, and physical and occupational therapists. Although in most states these professionals are allowed by law to provide certain services to patients, independent of doctors' orders, in many cases, patients receive these services only on doctors' orders. Doctors admit patients to hospitals and order what is to be done to them once they are in. The fact that "admit" and "order" are words of command is no accident.

Finally, most of the huge sum we spend each year on health services is spent, directly or indirectly, at the instance of doctors. Patients buy health insurance, but doctors decide how the patient should spend his health insurance benefits. Pharmaceutical companies make drugs and pharmacists sell them. But only a doctor or dentist can prescribe the supposedly more powerful or more potentially dangerous drugs, not classified by the government as "over-the-counter." A patient chooses to visit a doctor's office. But the doctor recommends how many return visits the patient will make, and if the patient is to see other doctors. Doctors, not patients, decide when surgery is in order. Doctors have these powers of determining expenditure levels not only in private practice, but also in government-operated direct service programs, in county hospitals, state mental hospitals, Veterans' Administration programs, and local health department services, to name a few.

I agree that there should be a trained person to have the responsibility and authority to engage in what we generally call medical decision-making. But often when people talk about the "health care crisis," and discuss rising costs, or too many hospital beds, or geographic maldistribution of personnel, or a "two-class system of care," the fact of the centrality of the doctor to the system is lost sight of. My point is that if there are problems in our health care delivery system, and it seems abundantly clear that there are, to begin solving them we must start by analyzing what the doctor does and how he or she is trained to do it.

Medical schools obviously have a very strong influence over the nature of medical practice: through their admissions procedures, they choose the people who will be future doctors—and then train them. To understand medical practice, one must understand medical education; how and why it has developed the way it has and what it does now.

The major problems in medical education in the United States today are, as I will demonstrate: lack of concern or involvement with disease prevention, focussing instead on acute care; overspecialization; stress on research and rare diseases, rather than on common problems; denigration of the importance of chronic disease; stress on hospital practice rather than ambulatory practice; training doctors to remember rather than to think; lack of attention paid to the problems of geographic distribution; little concern with team practice and the proper utilization of other kinds of health professionals; overemphasis on the basic medical sciences and fundamental errors in the way basic medical sciences are taught; lack of concern with and teaching of knowledge concerning practice organization; and poor training in doctor-patient communication and care.

In the face of all of this, the medical education system has established for itself the same kind of "mystique" in relation to problems of the health care delivery system that Dr. Marvin Belsky and Leonard Gross have described for the individual physician in relationship to individual patients in their book *Beyond the Medical Mystique:*[1] "We're terrific; we know what we're doing; just pay us and don't bother us."

To receive medical service—the product of medical education that is unsatisfactory in so many ways—the American people expend a great deal of tax money. Thus they are really entitled to know what is going on and to have a voice in policy formation and implementation. But the medical education system has managed to keep itself fairly well shielded from public view, while being relatively unresponsive to public need. Reform is urgently required in the medical education system—especially urgent because the physician training process takes so long. Even if a thorough reform could be accomplished in the next five years, it would be another eight years after that before the first graduates of the new system would enter practice. Nevertheless, if a medical education system which can train doctors who are truly responsive to the needs of the people is to be developed, reform must begin sometime. I hope that this book will be of some assistance in achieving that end.

In the notes found at the back of the book and divided by chapters, are references to the major source materials used plus specific references for quoted statements, data, or particularly controversial points. Also in the Notes are specific references to relevant bibliographic material from a textbook which I edited and co-authored, *Health Care Delivery in the United States* (New York: Springer Publishing Co., 1977). Readers may want to refer to Appendix I, "Sources of Data," in the textbook for a brief description of, and how to easily locate, the major sources of data on the U. S. health care delivery system.

I have derived the material for this book from many sources. I have drawn on my own experiences as a medical student, a public health physician, and a medical educator, as well as on parts of the voluminous literature on health care delivery and medical education. I have herein used certain portions of the textbook as noted, with the kind permission of the publisher. In writing and editing the textbook, I learned a great deal about how our health care delviery system works, and in a sense that book led naturally to this one. I suggest that interested readers of this book who do not find in the notes all of the references they might like to have about one point or another refer to the relevant chapters of the textbook, where a great many references to the literature on the U. S. health care delivery system are provided.

A Digest of the Contents

Medical Mystery has four sections. Section I, "Health and Health Care: Problems for the American People," begins with this chapter. In Chapter 2, I commence the book's argument by discussing health, disease, and illness. After offering some of the many existing definitions of these basic human conditions, I describe how we measure them. I then consider the factors which have brought about the improvements, observed over the last three centuries, in health levels in the Western World. The results of this analysis demonstrate that if health is to be the principal concern of a health care delivery system, then its principal functions should be the maintenance of health and prevention of illness, with treatment of disease being important but secondary. I then go on to discuss the nature of prevention, how it is achieved, and the current controversy over "life-style," its influence on health and how it can be changed. In this context, I consider the multiple goals of the health care delivery system as it now operates, and the contradictions among those goals. The rest of the book is really about the potential role of the medical education system in resolving those contradictions. In Chapter 3, I review the present problems of our health care delivery system, and point out that it is not in "crisis," as is so often stated, but rather that most of its serious difficulties have been with us for many years.

Section II, "U.S. Health Care Delivery System: Current Status," includes Chapters 4 through 6. In Chapter 4, I describe the role of government in the health care delivery system and the financing mechanisms. Chapter 5 is devoted to considering the personnel and institutional inputs to the system. (Readers knowledgeable about the U.S. health care delivery system will be able to skim or skip entirely Chapters 4 and 5.) In Chapter 6, I describe quality control mechanisms, and explain how the licensing system gives the physician his dominant position.

Section III, "Medical Education: Historical Development and

Present Status," includes Chapters 7 through 11. Chapter 7 traces the history of medical education in our country from its beginnings in colonial times to 1910, the date of publication of the single most influential document ever written on medical education in this country, the Flexner Report. The Flexner Report and events associated with it form the great watershed in the development of American medical education. Chapter 8 is devoted to the Report and some considerable reinterpretation of it, that is, compared with conventional interpretations.

Chapter 9 examines developments during the period 1910–45, generally "Years of Consolidation." Since World War II, medical schools have undergone tremendous growth in research operations and in the number of graduates produced annually. These Years of Expansion are treated in Chapter 10. Finally, in this section, Chapter 11 describes the current status of U.S. medical education: numbers of schools, graduates, faculty, and other basic data; admissions policies and procedures; curriculum, the basic pattern and its major variations; the relative importance of admissions policies and curriculum in determining outcome; the balance, and imbalance, between the teaching, research, and service roles of medical schools; the role of specialization in medical education; costs; the structure and function of the Association of American Medical Colleges; and finally, regulation and quality control in medical education.

The fourth and final Section, "Problems and Solutions," includes Chapters 12 and 13. In Chapter 12, I examine the problems of the U.S. health care delivery system as described in Chapters 2 through 6 in the context of the U.S. medical education system as it is described in Chapters 7 through 11. I discuss those problems in the health care delivery system for which the medical schools can be held principally responsible, as well as those for which they cannot be. I then go on to consider the principal proposed solutions to the problems of the health care delivery system. I conclude that it is of critical importance to change the manner in which we train our physicians.

I consider the three prevailing attitudes toward the problems of doctors and their training. The first, held by important segments of the medical education leadership, is to do nothing. Most of these people deny that any of the problems of the health care delivery system have anything to do with the medical education system, whether or not those problems have anything to do with doctors. The second is that the physician should be written off as a lost cause. His present status should be generally left untouched, but he should be worked around, in personnel, institutions, and financing mechanisms to deal with the identified problems. The third view, held by me and others, is that change must begin at the beginning. If doctors are the center of the system, creating a significantly new health care delivery system requires that we create significantly new doctors. I provide an outline for a new health care delivery system designed to deal with existing problems, and describe the basic characteristics of the doctor who will work in it. The principal characteristic of both the new system and the new physicians is that the disease-orientation of the present will in the future give way to health-orientation.

Finally, in Chapter 13, I give my prescription for medical education reform. The overall plan is described as the HOPE system: Health-Oriented Physician Education. It is to replace the present DOPE system: Disease-Oriented Physician Education. HOPE has five major components: the philosophical basis of medical practice is to be grounded in health maintenance and disease prevention; the active practice of healthy living is to be part of medical education for all who are involved in it; problem-based learning, the active use of the scientific method, is to be the principal tool for education; computer-assistance, to replace rote memory, becomes a fundamental technique of both learning and practice; and finally, for the first time, a profession of medical educator is created.

To conclude, I propose how all of this change can be achieved. The process is a complicated one, of course. It will take a long time, and will not be accomplished over night. After all, the process of "Flexnerian Reform" which is customarily dated 1910, the year the Flexner Report was published, took many years to complete. Actually the process took about forty years from 1890, with the earliest glimmerings of it appearing about thirty years before that. We must not grow impatient for change, but neither must we say, "Oh, change takes so long, why bother to start." It was not only Mao Tse-Tung who said: "A journey of a thousand miles begins with but a single step." When one sits down to begin writing a book, the first page is always blank.

A Personal Note to My Friends—and Others—in the Medical Profession

This book has a critical tone. Some will think it highly critical. And it is. But it is critical of a *system,* not of individuals. I describe many problems with doctors and the way they practice, with the health care delivery system and the way it operates, with the medical education system and the way it functions. By and large these problems are created by history and people working in a particular historical and social context. For the most part, they are not caused by evil individuals. Some practicing physicians are insensitive to patient needs and work primarily to meet their own personal needs—for self-satisfaction, prestige, or money. Some medical educators do precisely the same thing, in the medical education context. But by and large people do not function badly because they are bad *people.* They function badly because they are the product of and work in a bad *system.* If placed in a different system, with different goals and motivating forces, I am certain that most physicians and medical educators could function very well, in relation to the needs of the people of our country.

This is why I am so concerned with history. We must understand how our system came to be what it is today. If nothing else, this book is intended to demonstrate the utility of history as a guide to making policy. To achieve positive change is not simply a matter of replacing "bad" people with "good" ones, or of replacing "professional" control with "community" control. If we put good people in a bad system, the good people will turn bad soon enough. If all major decisions are made by amateurs, the outcome will be just as unacceptable, if in a different way, as the outcome of a system where all major decision are made only by professionals. Believe me, I have seen it happen often.

Real change often appears to be much more painful than it really is. I think that in this book I demonstrate objectively, by professional and scientific standards that we, the medical profession, are not doing a particularly good job in delivering health services to the people of our country. But that does not mean that I think that you, Doctor *A,* or you, Professor *B,* are mean or evil.

It does mean that I think that we are all caught up in a bad system that prevents us from practicing medicine of really good quality. It does mean that if we, as a profession, can recognize the deficiencies of the system, then, by working together with the people we serve, we can develop a system which will liberate ourselves, our students, and our patients, and help the American people achieve levels of healthy living previously unknown in history.

2

Health, Disease, Illness, and the Health Care Delivery System

When health is absent, wisdom cannot reveal itself, art cannot become manifest, strength cannot fight, wealth becomes useless, and intelligence cannot be applied.

—*Herophilus, Ancient Greek*

The failure of the awesome power of the federal government to . . . [enforce] Prohibition suggests that, despite their efforts, the medical proselytizers will fail to get Americans to stop smoking, drinking, and ereating and to get more exercise. Medical zealots, enough is enough! Let the rest of us enjoy ourselves!

—*Jack R. Harnes, M.D.*

Improvement in the health status of the American people will depend, in great measure, on the design and application of programs which place major emphasis on the preventive aspects of human disease. The nature of our health problems dictates that application of known methodologies in prevention and health maintenance can cause a substantial improvement in our nation's health statistics.

—Preventive Medicine, U.S.A.

There is a age-old philosophical distinction between the concept of *health* and that of *disease*. The medical historian Henry Sigerist has pointed out that " [the majority of] ancient Greek physicians had an explanation for health. Health, they believed, was a condition of perfect equilibrium. When the forces or humors or whatever constituted the human body were perfectly balanced, man was healthy. Disturbed balance resulted in disease. This is still the best general explanation we have."[1] However, the Greek cult of Asklepios concentrated its attention on disease and miracle cures, and, with the rise of Christianity, this approach continued. Later, scientific medicine began to develop, but the idea of miracle cures persisted, as it does in present day medicine. It is a seductive dream: the idea that cures can compensate for the abuses of the individual and society, correcting at a stroke the effects of smoking or of breathing polluted air or of eating saturated fats over a period of years, has been perpetuated. Dr. John Gordon Freymann points out that the mechanistic philosophy of René Descartes has contributed significantly to this approach, which postulates that "for every disease there is a single specific cause."[2]

Webster's Unabridged Dictionary reflects the conflict over whether health is a positive or negative state: the definition begins, "physical and mental well-being" but continues, "freedom from defect, pain, or disease." Health statistics, of course, are actually disease statistics, and health care is often disease care. The World Health Organization defines health as a "state of complete physical, mental, and social well-being, and not merely the absence of disease or infirmity." Such scholars as Rene Dubos have criticized this definition as being utopian. In it, health is certainly not measurable. Nonetheless, its concept of health is as a positive rather than a neutral state. That is significant.

The concept of health as a positive state appears in the thinking of non-Western cultures. Sidney Kark, the South African/Israeli epidemiologist, quotes a Hindu physician:

> To the Hindu, health is harmony; [harmony is] being at peace with the Self, the community, God and the cosmos.[3]

Kark, quoting Adair and Deuschle, also cited the Navajo concept of health:

> [When there is] balance between the individual and his total physical and social environment, as well as . . . balance between the supernatural and man . . . good health is the result; an upset in this equilibrium causes disease.

Note the similarity between the concepts of the Hindu, the Navajo, and the ancient Greeks quoted above.

Turning to concepts of *disease,* Rudolf Virchow, the great nineteenth-century German scientist who was the father of the medical discipline, pathology, and a philosophic follower of Cartesian mechanism, said:

> Disease will always have to be considered an altered vital state of larger or smaller numbers of cells or cell-territories, and, whether the cause of the disease circulates in the blood or arrives directly at the cells, our evaluation of the relationship of the primary causes to the cells will not change.[4]

Interestingly enough, as we shall see in Chapter 12, although Virchow had a very cellular concept of disease, he understood well its social relationships, as well as the social role of medicine.

In modern times, disease has come to be defined more ambiguously. Webster's suggests "uneasiness or distress," and more sweepingly, "any departure from health." Blakiston's *New Gould Medical Dictionary* terms disease "a failure of the adaptive mechanisms of an organism to counteract adequately the stimuli and stresses to which it is subject, resulting in a disturbance in function or structure of some part of the body," which is really an elaboration of Sigerist's definition: "Disease is nothing else but the sum total of abnormal reactions of the organism or of its parts to abnormal stimuli."[5]

Illness is another matter. Disease is a biomedical concept. Illness is a state of being, as Eric Cassell has said, "a *feeling* of unfitness" (my italics). Cassell goes on to say "let us use the word 'illness' to stand for what the patient feels when he goes to the doctor and 'disease' for what he has on the way home from the doctor's office. Disease, then, is something an organ has; illness is something a man has."[6] Animals are diseased; people are ill. In our language, the opposite of "health" is "ill-health," not "dis-health." People are ill, not simply diseased. Illness has social and psychological as well as biomedical components.

Measuring Health and Disease

Prized though the state of health may be, whether to the ancient Greeks or to Lyndon Baines Johnson, we find it something which is as difficult to measure as it is to define. Although a great deal of work to develop useful health status indicators is being undertaken by various scholars, the data collected on a routine basis in this country measure the extent of disease, not health. One can only infer, by looking at indicators of disease, a population's state of health.

Mortality

The most definitive measure of disease is death. Death, or mortality, rates (that is, the number of deaths for a given population for a given time period) are collected routinely by public health authorities.[7] Death rates are published by cause of death and certain other descriptors, such as age and sex. Death itself is usually a well-defined state, although the case of Karen Ann Quinlan teaches us that that is not always so. However, it is not possible in every case to determine the precise cause of death, so there is a certain inexactitude even in disease-specific death rates. In 1976, the ten leading specific killers in our country were:

Heart disease
Cancer
Stroke
Accidents (almost half of the total caused by motor vehicles)
Influenza and pneumonia (mainly pneumonia)
Diabetes mellitus
Cirrhosis of the liver
Bronchitis, emphysema, and asthma (mainly emphysema)
Suicide
"Certain causes of mortality in early infancy"

(Homicide was the eleventh leading cause of death.) However, mortality rates in no way completely define the disease profile of a population.

Morbidity

There are many prominent diseases in our country which, while they do not ordinarily kill, cause a great deal of pain and limitation of activity. Morbidity, sickness or illness, is counted in a variety of ways. They are all less exact than counting of deaths. When one tries to measure morbidity by asking people for information, one has to take into account the feeling aspects of illness: the same physical disability can make one person feel ill, but not another. In deriving morbidity information from provider sources, one has to remember that diagnosis is not a precise art or science.

We collect morbidity data in a variety of ways in our country.[8] The National Health Survey, an ongoing, home interview program of the U.S. Department of Health, Education, and Welfare (USDHEW) found that for 1975 the most common acute illnesses were upper respiratory conditions, reported by 28 percent of the population, influenza (22 percent), and injuries (17 percent). Acute conditions were associated with over 960 days of restricted activity per 100 persons per year. It was also found that 14.3 percent of the population experienced limitation in all activity owing to chronic conditions. The major chronic problems causing limitations in activity are heart conditions, arthritis and rheumatism, impairments of lower extremities and hips, impairments of back or spine, cerebrovascular disease and paralysis, complete or partial. Some of these conditions are causes of death, but most are not.

USDHEW also collects morbidity information from providers. The *Hospital Discharge Survey* collects diagnoses at time of release from hospital.[9] In 1975, almost 80 percent of hospital discharges from nonfederal, short stay hospitals were accounted for by six diagnostic groups:

diseases of the circulatory system, 13 percent
diseases of the digestive system, 13 percent
complications of pregnancy, childbirth, and the puerperium (time of mother's life immediately following labor and delivery), 12 percent
diseases of the genitourinary system, 10 percent
diseases of the respiratory system, 10 percent
accidents, poisonings, and violence, 10 percent

The six most common specific hospital discharge diagnoses are: malignant neoplasms; ischemic heart disease;* fractures, all sites; diseases of the urinary system; pneumonia; and enlargement of tonsils and adenoids; and all other heart and hypertensive disease. Two of the top six are major killers, but the others are not.

Finally, the USDHEW collects information from physicians on what kinds of patient problems they are seeing in their offices.[10] Table 2.1. shows the twenty most common complaints as reported by patients to physicians in 1973–74. The vast majority of these complaints do not represent serious illness. Table 2.2 shows the fifteen most frequent diagnoses made by physicians. In the latter list, killer diseases appear only in the fourth, eighth, and fifteenth places on the list. Thus we see that illness and disease can be, and are, characterized in many ways. No matter how we do it, however, we are still not measuring health, only its obverse, ill-health.

Changes in Population Health Levels over Time

In the last three centuries, the population of the Western World has, by and large, become healthier. However, since we cannot measure health, we know that fact only indirectly. But in any case, knowing the factors that have accounted for that improvement can guide us in setting health and health care policies for the future. Henry Sigerist and Thomas McKeown along with his collegues in England have provided us with the basis for understanding these events.[11] They use the science of epidemiology, the study of the distribution of disease and health in populations.

The earliest indication, albeit indirect, we have of the improving health in Western Europe and Great Britain is the acceleration in the rate of population growth which began around 1700 A.D. and continued into the present era. Although national population censuses were not undertaken in the eighteenth century, there is a great deal of indirect evidence, political, sociological, and historical, for population growth. There is also evidence, including some birth statistics from mid-eighteenth-century Sweden, that the population increase was due to a declining death rate, not an increas-

*Malignant neoplasms are most often cancers; ischemic heart disease is the kind of heart disease which often leads to angina pectoris and heart attacks.

Table 2.1. **Number, percent, and cumulative percent of office visits to office-based physicians by the twenty most common patient problems, complaints, or symptoms: United States, May 1973–April 1974.**

[Symptomatic groupings and code number inclusions are based on a symptom classification developed for use in the NAMCS.]

Rank	Twenty most common patient problems, complaints, or symptoms		Number of visits in thousands	Percent of visits	Cumulative percent
1	Progress visits	980,985	75,673	11.7	11.7
2	Other problems, NEC	990	37,126	5.8	17.5
3	Physical exam	900,901	26,117	4.0	21.5
4	Pain, etc.—lower extremity	400	25,944	4.0	25.6
5	Pregnancy exam	905	25,942	4.0	29.6
6	Throat soreness	520	20,726	3.2	32.8
7	Pain, etc.—upper extremity	405	18,956	2.9	35.7
8	Pain, etc.—back region	415	18,824	2.9	38.7
9	Cough	311	18,347	2.8	41.5
10	Abdominal pain	540	16,418	2.5	44.0
11	Cold	312	13,460	2.1	46.1
12	Gynecological exam	904	13,154	2.0	48.2
13	Visit for medication	910	13,103	2.0	50.2
14	None	997	13,043	2.0	52.2
15	Headache	056	12,314	1.9	54.1
16	Fatigue	004	11,768	1.8	56.0
17	Pain in chest	322	11,350	1.8	57.7
18	Well baby exam	906	10,699	1.7	59.4
19	Fever	002	9,822	1.5	60.9
20	Allergic skin reaction	112	9,458	1.5	62.4
	All other symptoms		242,650	37.6	100.0

Source: *Monthly Vital Statistics Report,* July 14, 1975, Supplement (2), table 7.

ing birth rate. The latter actually fell as the death rate went down, although obviously the birth rate fell more slowly than did the death rate. Great Britain began officially counting births and deaths in 1838, so we know for certain the relationship between the two rates after that date.

Having established the fact that population growth was accounted for by declining death rates, the next question is, what was the decline due to? Knowing the state of medical knowledge dur-

Table 2.2. **Number, percent, and cumulative percent of office visits to office-based physicians by the 15 most frequent principal diagnoses classified by ICDA category: United States, May 1973–April 1974.**

[Diagnostic groupings and code number inclusions are based on the Eighth Revision, International Classification of Diseases, Adapted for Use in the United States, 1965.]

Rank	Principal diagnosis classified		Number of visits in thousands	Percent of visits	Cumulative percent
1	Medical or special examinations	Y00	39,613	6.1	6.1
2	Medical and surgical aftercare	Y10	32,345	5.0	11.2
3	Prenatal care	Y06	25,359	3.9	15.1
4	Essential benign hypertension	401	22,752	3.5	18.6
5	Acute respiratory infection	465	21,514	3.3	22.0
6	Neuroses	300	16,570	2.6	24.5
7	Observation, without need for further medical care	793	15,893	2.5	27.0
8	Chronic ischemic heart disease	412	15,487	2.4	29.4
9	Hay fever	507	12,166	1.9	31.3
10	Otitis media	381	10,523	1.6	32.9
11	Acute pharyngitis	462	10,415	1.6	34.5
12	Obesity	277	10,136	1.6	36.1
13	Refractive errors	370	9,175	1.4	37.5
14	Other eczema and dermatitis	692	9,152	1.4	38.9
15	Diabetes	250	8,904	1.4	40.3
	All other diagnoses		384,889	59.7	100.0

Source: *Monthly Vital Statistics Report,* July 14, 1975, Supplement (2), table 4.

ing the eighteenth and nineteenth centuries (it was quite low), the death rate decline certainly cannot be attributed to that factor. Conceivably, the bacteria and other agents causing the major infectious diseases—the principal killers—could have changed in character and become milder, an event known to have occurred in the past in the case of certain individual diseases. However, for this to have been the principal cause of the declining death rates, a whole series of infectious agents would have had to have changed in severity at the same time, an unlikely event.

The major factor which McKeown and his colleagues have been

able to identify in accounting for the increasing growth of population (which, because it is related to a declining death rate indirectly indicates that health levels were improving), is nothing other than improved nutrition! Technological changes which began in British agriculture in the seventeenth century led to an approximate doubling of the available food supply during the eighteenth century. These changes, coupled with improvements of the distribution system (primarily canals in the eighteenth century), led simply to more calories being available per person, as well as better quality food. During the eighteenth century in Great Britain, the food supply approximately doubled, and so did the population. The supposition is that improved nutrition made people more able to naturally resist the ravages of the common infectious diseases which were the major killers, particularly diseases like tuberculosis, pneumonia, and influenza. This argument is made by inference and indirection, but it has not been successfully challenged. Thus, improved nutrition is the most important factor historically in improving health levels.

During the nineteenth century, health levels continued to improve. In Great Britain, from 1838 on, births and deaths were counted, and thus more precise information became available. Population growth continued unabated through the nineteenth century, literally fed by improved nutrition. Urbanization, with its crowding and lack of hygiene, presumably had a negative effect on health in some ways, but, as health continued to improve, was apparently beneficial in other ways. It appears that in cities, even crowded, dirty ones, general living conditions were better than they had been in the country.

The fall in the tuberculosis death rate during the time before specific antibiotic therapy became available also supports this thesis. The incidence of TB is not affected by specific hygienic measures such as pure water supply and sanitary sewage disposal, but is related to general living conditions and nutrition. Although many treatments for TB were developed from the mid-nineteenth century onwards, from prolonged rest to radical surgery, no treatment measure was widely enough applied to have had an effect on TB incidence in the population as a whole until streptomycin, an antibiotic, was discovered in 1948, to be followed soon by other more effective, less toxic drugs. Nevertheless, Sigerist pointed out that "in 1857 in the State of Massachusetts, 450 persons out of every 100,000 died of tuberculosis. From then on the death rate dropped constantly. It was down to 250 in 1890, 114 in 1920, and was 35.6 in 1938."[12] New York City had a similar experience. By year, the death rates per 100,000 population were, respectively: 1870, 396.1; 1890, 361.9; 1910, 210.5; 1930, 73.1; 1950, 29.4; and 1970, 4.9.[13] The rate fell by almost half during 1870–1910, a time when the city was being inundated by poor, TB-prone immigrants from southern and eastern Europe! Living conditions and nutrition were improving enough to provide for this decrease.

Sanitary Reform

The next great leap forward in health levels following the nutrition revolution came in the last quarter of the nineteenth century, when the second most important factor in improving health levels, historically, made its appearance. The introduction of pure water supply, sanitary sewage disposal, food and milk inspection, and all of the other measures known collectively as "the hygiene movement" quickly led to a further reduction in mortality rates, particularly in waterborne infectious diseases such as typhoid fever and cholera. Control of the gastro-intestinal infectious diseases especially effected a reduction in infant mortality rates, since GI infections were such major killers of children under five. It is the reduction in the infant mortality rate which has been principally responsible for the growth in life expectancy which we have observed in the last seventy-five years or so.

Life Expectancy and the Reduction in the Infant Mortality Rate

Life expectancy is the number of years a person can expect to live from birth. Life expectancy is a probability of survival. It is calculated from the actual number of years lived by a group of people born in a given year. Put another way, life expectancy is a prediction based on past experience of what future experience will be. It assumes that no presently unknown or unpredicted causes of death will appear, such as new, unstoppable infectious diseases, virulent cancers, or nuclear holocaust.

Life expectancy is not to be confused with longevity. Life expectancy is a probability of survival, a prediction that the probability is that the *average* person *X,* born in year *Y,* will live to age *Z.* Longevity is an empirical observation of the number of years considered to constitute "old age" at a given time, regardless of how many or how few "old people" there are. Although life expectancy has increased greatly since Biblical times, longevity has not. Then, even though there were relatively few of them, an old person was "three score and ten years." Today, although there are many elderly people, "three score and ten" is still considered "old." In fact, by our customs, laws, and regulations, we now officially declare sixty-five to seventy years as the beginning of "old age."

Since 1900, life expectancy has increased principally because of the reduction in the infant mortality rate resulting from the sanitary revolution. Formally, the infant mortality rate is the number of deaths among persons under one year of age during a given time period, usually a calendar year, per 1000 live births in the same time period. A reduction in the infant mortality rate leads to an increase in life expectancy by permitting more people to survive that critical first year when all human beings are so vulnerable to disease. Since life expectancy is nothing more than a probability of survival from birth, the more people who are available to live to an old age, the greater will the *average* life expectancy from birth of any *one* person be.

Tables 2.3., 2.4., and 2.5. will perhaps illustrate this point more clearly. Table 2.3. shows the life expectancy from birth rising as the infant mortality rate falls in the United States between 1900 and 1970. Table 2.4. shows that while in 1970 the mortality rate for the one-to-four age group as a whole was only 4 percent of what it was in 1900, the mortality rates in 1970 for the age groups over fifty-five were still more than 60 percent of what they were in 1900. Finally, table 2.5. compares the changes in expectancy of additional years of life at given ages, between 1900 and 1971. Life expectancy from birth increased almost 45 percent. Additional life expectancy at all other ages increased in most cases no more than 25 percent.

Thus, infant mortality reduction is critical to life expectancy increase in our country in this century, an important measure of

Table 2.3. **Mortality Rate, Infant Mortality Rate, and Life Expectancy From Birth, United States, 1900–1970.**

	Crude Mortality Rate (per 1,000 Population)	Infant Mortality Rate* (per 1,000 Live Births)	Life Expectancy From Birth (in Years)
1900	17.2	(99.9)	47.3
1920	13.0	85.9	54.1
1940	10.8	47.0	62.9
1960	9.5	26.0	69.7
1970	9.4	19.8	71.0

*Data available only from 1915.

Sources: Data for 1900–1960 derived from Grove, R.D. and Hetzel, A. M.: Vital Statistics Rates in the United States, 1940–1960, National Center for Health Statistics, U.S. Dept. of Health, Education, and Welfare, 1968, tables 38, 51, and 53. Data for 1970 derived from Statistical Abstract of the United States, 1971, Bureau of the Census, U.S. Dept. of Commerce, 1971, tables 57 and 69, and Statistical Abstract, 1974, table 82.

Table 2.4. **Age-Specific Mortality Rates, United States, 1900 and 1970.**

Age-Group (Years)	Age-Specific Mortality Rate (per 1,000 Population) 1900	1970	1970 Rate as % of 1900 Rate
1–4	19.8	0.8	4.0
5–14	3.9	0.4	10.3
15–24	5.9	1.3	22.0
25–34	8.2	1.6	19.5
35–44	10.2	3.1	30.4
45–54	15.0	7.3	48.7
55–64	27.2	16.6	61.0
65–74	56.4	35.8	63.5
75–84	123.3	80.0	64.9
85 plus	260.9	163.4	62.6

Source: Data derived from Statistical Abstract of the United States, 1974, Bureau of the Census, U.S. Dept. of Commerce, 1974, table 83.

Table 2.5. Average Remaining Lifetime in Years at Specified Ages, United States, 1900 and 1971, and Percentage Change Between 1900 and 1971.

Age in Years	Life Expectancy 1900	Life Expectancy 1971	Years Difference	Percent Change
0	49.2	71.0	21.8	44.3
5	55.0	67.6	12.6	22.9
15	46.8	57.9	11.1	23.7
25	39.1	48.8	9.5	24.3
35	31.9	39.3	7.4	23.2
45	24.8	30.3	5.5	22.2
55	17.9	22.1	4.2	23.5
65	11.9	15.1	3.2	26.9
75	7.1	9.1*	2.0*	28.2*
85	4.0	4.8*	0.8*	20.0*

*Figures for 1968

Sources: Data derived from Statistical Abstract of the United States, 1971, Bureau of the Census, U.S. Dept. of Commerce, 1971, and Statistical Abstract, 1974.

health. Reduction in the infant mortality rate is primarily related to improved sanitary conditions, which sharply reduced infant infectious diseases, although continually improving nutrition for both pregnant women and children, improved pre-natal care, and improved obstetrical techniques are related as well. Data from New York City again make this point clear. Deaths per 100,000 children under five years of age from diarrheal disease per year were as follows: 1870, 3380; 1890, 2060; 1910, 1167; 1930, 157; 1950, 14; 1970, 7. As in tuberculosis, specific antibiotic therapy for childhood diarrheal diseases was not available until 1950 or so. What accomplished this miracle, which led to accelerating population growth indicating improving health levels, was the revolution in water supply sanitation and food hygiene—public health measures.

Immunology and Communicable Disease Control

Before the bacteriological revolution initiated by the discoveries of Pasteur, Koch, and others in the last third of the nineteenth century, the only artificial means man had to present any communicable disease was smallpox vaccination, discovered accidently by Jenner in the eighteenth century. However, the reasons for the effectiveness of vaccination were not understood; it was not a universal practice and, according to McKeown, made only a small contribution to the reduction of mortality in nineteenth-century England. In the early part of the twentieth century, however, smallpox vaccination became widely available. Effective vaccines also became available for whooping cough, tetanus, diphtheria, and yellow fever. Immunization was the first effective preventive measure which could be applied directly to individuals.

The next, and last, great step forward was the introduction of antibiotics during and since World War II. Antibiotics have allowed us to control bacterial pneumonia as a cause of death, to continue the reduction in the incidence of tuberculosis, and to further the reduction in rheumatic heart disease. Unfortunately, however, the other "miracles of modern medicine," such as highly advanced surgery, great hospital technology, laboratory and x-ray equipment of amazing complexity and ability have done little to affect health, at least *to the extent we can measure it.* This is not to say that advanced surgical techniques or sophisticated laboratory analysis may not be of great value, to the extent of saving life for a time, of many individuals. But the results of these advances have not, at least to date, been shown to have had much effect on death rates, life expectancy, and health of the population as a whole.

Leonard Hayflick has put all of this succinctly:

> Despite the common impression that the triumphs of modern medicine have lengthened the human lifespan, this supposition is not supported by either vital statistics or biologic evidence. What has happened is that the ability to prevent or treat the ills of early years has been improved and, therefore, that more people are reaching what appears to be an immutable, upper age limit. Thus, life expectancy has increased, but the human life span has remained virtually unchanged since recorded history. Medical achievements have simply allowed more people to reach the limit of what appears to be a fixed life span.[14]

Hayflick points out that significant further improvements in life expectancy can be achieved only by reduction of heart disease, cancer, and stroke—conditions which have not yet been very amenable to the treatment modalities currently available. Behind all of this is the phenomenon of natural cell-aging in the absence of disease. It is a phenomenon which we understand poorly, but it is cell-aging which primarily determines longevity while it is disease which determines life expectancy.

Changes in Disease-Specific Death Rates over Time

Perhaps the importance of disease in determining life expectancy can be better understood if we compare the ten leading causes of death in 1900 with those in 1975, see table 2.6. In 1900, the ten leading causes of death were influenza and pneumonia; tuberculosis; gastroenteritis; heart disease; stroke; accidents; chronic nephritis; malignant neoplasm; diseases of early infancy; and diphtheria. In 1975, the ten leading

Table 2.6. The Ten Major Causes of Mortality, United States, 1900 and 1976, Rates per 100,000 Population and Rank in Frequency.

1900		Disease	1976	
Rank	Rate		Rate	Rank
	1719.1	*All Causes*	917.8	
1	202.2	Influenza and Pneumonia	34.3	5
2	194.4	Tuberculosis	1.7	19
3	142.7	Gastroenteritis	0.9	21
4	137.4	Diseases of the heart	472.1	1
5	106.9	Cerebrovascular Diseases	91.0	3
6	81.0	Chronic nephritis	(1)	
7	72.3	All accidents	45.2	4
8	64.0	Cancer and other malignant neoplasm	174.7	2
9	62.6	Certain diseases of early infancy	11.1	10
10	40.3	Diphtheria	0.0	—
25	11.0	Diabetes Mellitus	17.1	6
19	12.5	Cirrhosis of the Liver	14.4	7
15	22.9	Bronchitis, emphysema, and asthma	12.3	8
26	10.2	Suicide	12.1	9

Sources: *The Facts of Life and Death.* National Center for Health Statistics (Washington, D.C.: USDHEW, 1965), table 15; Grove, R.D. and Hetzel, A.M. *Vital Statistics Rates in the United States, 1940–1960* NCHS (Washington, D.C.: USDHEW, 1968), table 65; *Monthly Vital Statistics Report,* 25, (8), , Oct. 27, 1976, table 6.

(1) No comparable classification.

causes were heart disease; cancer; stroke; accidents; influenza and pneumonia (primarily pneumonia); diabetes mellitus; cirrhosis of the liver; bronchitis, emphysema, and asthma (primarily emphysema); suicide; and "certain diseases of early infancy."[15] An analysis of the reasons for the changes in the rates by cause, which account for the changes in relative rank, is helpful. We shall first look at those diseases which have decreased in importance as causes of death since 1900.

Of the combined cause, "influenza and pneumonia," pneumonia has always been the most prominent. It accounted for 175 of the 202 deaths per 100,000 in the combined diagnostic category in 1900. By 1930, in the absence of any widely-utilized specific therapy, the pneumonia death rate had dropped to about 83. During the thirties, the use of specific anti-sera for certain pneumonias came into some vogue, but it is unclear how widespread this use was. Sulfa drugs and then penicillin were discovered just before World War II. But the latter was not made available for significant civilian use until after the war. The death rate for pneumonia in 1938, the year sulfa drugs began to come into general use, was 67.7. Ten years later it was 35.2, an apparent triumph for antibacterial drugs. However, the rate was still 28.2 in 1976. Nevertheless, the largest part of the reduction in the pneumonia death rate since 1900 occurred in the absence of specific therapy.

For influenza, being a viral disease, there is of course, no known therapy. Immunization against influenza is a difficult task, as was proven during 1976–77 in the United States, at least in part because there are so many variants of the virus and authorities cannot be sure which one will be responsible for the next outbreak. In any case, the bulk of the reduction in the influenza death rate was achieved by the end of World War II, well before any vaccines were generally available. Thus for both influenza and pneumonia one must give major credit to general improvements in the standard of living for reductions in their death rates.

The story for tuberculosis is similar. The death rate for tuberculosis was already down to 30 per 100,000 population in 1948, the year streptomycin was discovered. It is likely that the additional drop since then is due to antibiotics, but even that is unclear since the decline before 1948 had been so precipitious.

Gastroenteritis has been virtually eliminated as a cause of death in this country principally by improved sanitation, although the mortality data by year show that the last sharp reduction took place coincident with the introduction of sulfa drugs. In 1937, the rate was already down to 14.7; by 1938, it was 4.0.

Continuing to refer to table 2.6., there were slightly fewer deaths due to cerebrovascular disease in 1976 as compared with 1900, although because of other changes, it had moved up in rank. The reduction in the rate has occurred in the last fifteen years, and may be associated with improved measures for controlling hypertension. Chronic nephritis has dropped off the list entirely principally because of a change in disease classification.

The reduction in the accidental death rate has been accomplished by a drop in deaths due to accidents on the railroads, in the home, and at the workplace. These drops have been accompanied, of course, by an increase in automobile accidental deaths. The reasons for the drop in the death rate from "certain diseases of early infancy" relate to improved standard of living and improved hygiene, as well as to improved obstetrical techniques and other treatment modalities.

The elimination of diphtheria as a cause of death is a clear triumph for the science of immunology and the public health programs which make sure that the vaccine is used. The sharp break in bronchitis deaths occurred just after World War I and may have been related to a change in the definitions of causes of death. It is not possible to show a relationship between changes in deaths due to bronchitis and the introduction of antibacterial therapy. On the other hand, emphysema has been increasing in importance as a cause of death since the 1950s. Suicide has changed position, but the rate has not changed significantly.

To summarize this material, an editorial in the *American Journal of Public Health* written in 1944 by the great public health leader, C.-E.A. Winslow is very helpful. Winslow analyzed the factors in the reduction of the major causes of death between 1900 and 1940, the year which marked the beginning of the antibacterial drug era. Winslow commented in particular on a matter which I have not previously stressed, the relative roles of the public health and private physician sectors of the health care delivery system in achieving this reduction. (Readers may note some slight descrepancies between Winslow's figures shown in table 2.7., and mine, apparently due to the use of different data sources and definitions. However, the orders of magnitude of the figures are similar.)

Table 2.7. Changes in Mortality 1900–1940.

	Death Rate per 100,000		Percent Reduction	Actual Deaths 1940	Deaths Which Would Have Occurred in 1940 at 1900 Rates	Number of Lives Saved per Year
	1900	1940				
Typhoid and parathphoid fevers	35.9	1.1	97	1,443	47,173	45,736
Diphtheria	43.3	1.1	97	1,457	56,896	55,439
Diarrhea and enteritis	133.2	10.3	92	13,573	175,025	161,452
Measles, scarlet fever, & whooping cough	34.8	3.2	91	4,300	45,727	41,427
Tuberculosis	201.2	45.9	77	60,428	264,377	203,949
Pneumonia and influenza	180.5	70.3	61	92,525	237,177	144,652
All other causes	1,126.1	944.5	16	1,243,543	1,479,695	236,152

Source: Winslow, C.-E.A. "Who Killed Cock Robin?" *American Journal of Public Health, 34,* 658, 1944.

In this table are shown the actual results accomplished between 1900 and 1940 in the reduction of mortality from the five causes of death with which the organized health forces of the community have been concerned, and also the corresponding reduction in pneumonia and influenza, where responsibility has been shared between the public health officer and the private physician. The last line of the table includes the changes in mortality from all other causes taken together. Many of these have also come within the scope of the public health program.

It will be noted that typhoid fever and diphtheria mortality rates have been reduced by 97 percent. The results accomplished in the case of typhoid fever have been due to the work of the engineer, to purification of the public water supplies, improvement in sanitary conditions, and to epidemiological control and immunization programs, conducted by health officers. In the case of diphtheria, administrative control, and the use of antitoxin and later toxoid, are responsible for the accomplishment. The basic discoveries in these fields were made by men like W. H. Park working in public health laboratories, and introduced by health officers like Hermann M. Biggs, often in face of vigorous opposition from the practitioner.

Diarrhea and enteritis of infants has been reduced by 92 percent through the pasteurization of milk supplies, under the leadership of public health authorities and through the establishment by boards of health and visiting nurse associations of well baby clinics for the instruction of mothers. Here again the initiative came primarily from the organized health forces representing the public interest.

The group of infectious diseases of childhood, measles, scarlet fever, and whooping cough, have shown a 91 percent reduction in mortality, due in large part to vigorous and energetic epidemiological control on the part of public health authorities. Tuberculosis, which has been cut down by 77 percent, represents the result of a program carried on in nearly all its phases through the leadership of public health departments, public health clinics, and publicly maintained sanatoria. Here, again, it should be recalled that the introduction of the first program for the reporting of tuberculosis was strenuously opposed by the medical profession.

In the case of pneumonia and influenza the practising physician deserves a lion's share of the credit.* Even here, however, it should be pointed out that the basic discoveries in regard to serum treatment and the use of sulfa drugs were made by salaried physicians in the employ of

*Actually, my analysis of pneumonia death rates above shows that the practicing physician probably played a relatively minor role in the reduction of this disease as well.

public health laboratories and foundations and universities, rather than by private practitioners.

It seems certain that the organized public health profession rather than the private medical practitioner is responsible for a major part of the gains which have been made during the past forty years.

It is no doubt true that the "Other Causes" of death listed in the last line of the table are much more difficult to control than those which the public health administrator has so successfully attacked; but it may he hoped that a sound system of prepayment which will make good medical care available to the lower economic half of the population, now woefully lacking in such services, would produce notable results in the reduction of many other causes of death than those which have so far been successfully attacked.[16]

Based on the evidence of the past thirty-five years, it appears that even so great a supporter of public health practice as C. E.A. Winslow overestimated the possible effects of treatment medicine on population health levels. Furthermore, he seems to have underestimated the potential of public health/preventive practice in dealing with the modern killer diseases, as we shall see below.

Referring once again to table 2.6., we can see that the death rate for diseases of the heart has more than tripled since 1900. Some of this is due to changing diagnostic styles. Some is due to the fact that the population is aging due to the falling infant mortality rate. More people are surviving into old age and since they are not dying of those diseases which used to kill infants, they must die of something. But a number of elements of modern living have been shown to be related to cardiovascular disease: cigarette smoking, stress, diet, and lack of exercise. These are likely the principal factors accounting for the sharp increase in the death rate.

The cancer death rate has almost tripled since 1900. The annual lung cancer rate has risen from a negligible level to over 40 per 100,000, the second most frequent cancer cause of death. The obvious relationship here is to cigarette smoking. Indeed, authorities such as Dr. John Higginson, Director of the International Agency for Research on Cancer now consider that environmental factors are responsible for about 75 percent of all cancers.[17] In addition to cigarettes, we are exposed to other air pollutants; to chemical and other industrial pollutants at the workplace, in our food, and in our water; to the residua of herbicides, fungicides, and pesticides; to food additives; and to significant changes in our diets such as a decrease in fibre and an increase in beef; as well as to other environmental hazards.

The death rate from diabetes mellitus has risen moderately. This may be due to changes in both diagnostic acumen and diagnostic style, or it may be real. The causes of diabetes are unknown, although there is a familial relationship. Its increased incidence may be related to the aging of the population as are heart disease and cancer to a certain extent. Diabetes mellitus can be neither prevented nor cured, but it can be readily detected, and its complications can be controlled by treatment. Although diabetes can kill directly, it is its complications, heart and kidney disease, blindness, and nervous system disease in the extremities which are both the most disabling factors and the principal killers. Early control, by diet, pills, or insulin, can prevent the occurrence of complications in most patients. It is thought that about 4 percent of the population has diabetes, but only half of those persons are known and under care.

Cirrhosis of the liver, related primarily to alcohol consumption (another environmental hazard) has increased both absolutely and in rank as a cause of death, as has suicide. Having reviewed what has happened to those causes of death which were the "top ten" in 1900, compared with the current members of the same category, we are in a position to make some summary comments concerning the relative importance of various health measures in dealing with the principal causes of death in our country over the last three-quarters of a century.

Factors in Changing Death Rates Since 1900 in the United States: Summary

First of all, the overall death rate has dropped by almost half. The biggest drops have occurred in influenza and pneumonia, tuberculosis, and gastroenteritis. Specific therapy has had some effect on pneumonia, none on influenza, moderate on tuberculosis and slight on gastroenteritis. The important factors are general improvement in living standards, and in the latter case, improved sanitation.

The stroke death rate has gone down slightly, just in the last fifteen years. This may well be related to specific therapy for hypertension. However, since many persons with hypertension do not know they have it, public health programs for the detection of the disease are extremely important in its control.

The overall accidental death rate has dropped, perhaps due in part to improved trauma treatment services. Part of the drop is certainly due to the demise of the railroads, improved industrial safety, and safer homes. However, automobile deaths rose steadily until the gasoline crisis forced a speed limit reduction and many of them are preventable by other means. Diphtheria has been eliminated by a public health measure. The rise in emphysema deaths is directly related to cigarette smoking, an environmental hazard. Emphysema is neither treatable nor reversible. Treatment has had some influence on "certain diseases of early infancy," but general environmental and preventive measures are important there as well.

Finally, numbers one and two, heart disease and cancer, have not been shown to be very amenable to treatment on the one hand, and are caused at least in part by controllable or potentially controllable environmental factors on the other hand.

In summary, treatment is related in part to changes in death rates for pneumonia, tuberculosis, accidents, stroke, and diabetes. Improving standards of living and/or specific preventive measures have played the sole or major role in reducing or eliminating influenza, pneumonia, tuberculosis, gastroenteritis, certain categories of accident, certain diseases of early infancy, and diphtheria. Treatment measures have not affected heart disease, cancer, the results of automobile accidents, cirrhosis of the liver, or emphysema. Furthermore, preventive measures are available, as we shall see below, which can positively affect the death rates from all of those conditions. Our record in both diabetes and hypertension-related stroke, as well as other hypertension-related conditions such as certain kinds of heart disease, could be vastly improved by better detection and organized treatment programs. It should be obvious that, at least insofar as the leading causes of death are concerned, improvements in living standards and specific preventive measures are of primary importance in their reduction, with treatment playing a secondary role. In understanding this picture more clearly, it is also helpful to look at what has happened to the cause-specific death rates for certain conditions of low fatality.

Changes of the Death Rates of Important Conditions Which Cause Relatively Few Deaths

Three of the most common surgical operations in the United States are for gall bladder disease, inguinal hernia, and peptic ulcer. These conditions cause relatively few deaths; their death rates have changed little since 1900. Bacterial Meningitis is a relatively rare, but frightening disease. Its death rate fell from 9.7 to 3.0 during World War I, in the absence of any specific therapy. It has fallen gradually to its present level below 1.0 since that time, but there is no sharp drop associated with the introduction of antibiotics. Typhoid fever, not common, but an ever-present epidemic threat in this country in the nineteenth century, has given way to sanitary sewage disposal, while whooping cough and smallpox succumbed to immunization early in the century.

More recently, immunization has controlled the rare but dangerous disease paralytic poliomyelitis, and measles and mumps, two infectious diseases which though not often fatal, can have serious side effects or complications. The death rate for scarlet fever, caused by the streptococcus bacillus, sensitive to sulfa drugs and penicillin, did drop with the introduction of those agents, but it already had fallen significantly during World War I from its early twentieth-century level, again without the introduction of specific therapy.

Finally, we may consider the most serious venereal disease in the United States, syphilis. Syphilis has never been a major killer in modern times (apparently, however, a major killer in sixteenth-century Europe) but interestingly enough, the syphilis death rate increased steadily from 1900 through the 1930s, even while specific arsenical therapy was being introduced. The syphilis death rate then declined steadily as penicillin therapy was introduced. Penicillin is specifically effective against the bacterium causing syphilis. Furthermore, in most cases syphilis must be in the body for a very long time before it kills, usually several decades. However, while the syphilis death rate has declined steadily since the introduction of penicillin, the incidence of the disease, that is the number of new cases appearing in a given time period, has not. Rather it has gone up and down, a consequence of both characteristics of the disease and the proper method for its control.

Syphilis has several stages. The first sign of infection is usually just a small pimple-like lesion on the skin or mucous membrane, called a chancre, where the person has been infected. Often this chancre cannot be recognized or is ignored. The second stage, generalized infection which can have many different manifestations, does not appear until some weeks later. Many people do not seek treatment until this time, but during the interim they can infect others, who themselves may have inapparent infections and in turn infect still others. Syphilis no longer kills many people because it virtually never gets beyond the second stage, where it is readily recognized and treated, into the again inapparent third stage, when it can kill after many years. But it is still very present in our country in the first and second stages: about 25,000 reported cases per year, likely many more than that unreported cases.

There is presently no vaccine for syphilis. Since penicillin is specific for syphilis, some medical authorities, such as Dr. Lewis Thomas, head of New York's Memorial Sloan-Kettering Cancer Center, would have us believe that controlling the disease presents few difficulties.

> With syphilis, of course, the problem now turns out to be simple. All you have to do, armed with the sure knowledge that the spirochete [bacterium causing syphilis] is the intervener, is to reach in carefully and eliminate that microorganism. If you do it quickly enough, before the whole system has been shaken to pieces, it will put itself right, and the problem solves itself.[18]

However, Dr. Thomas is focussing on syphilis in individuals. The solution is not really that simple at all, when one faces the appearance and propagation of the disease in the *population.* Since syphilis has a stage of *inapparent infection* during which a person can have the disease without realizing it and can unknowingly pass it on to others, effective control of syphilis in the population requires not just treatment of sick individuals who come in for treatment. In addition, the tracing of their sexual contacts, the testing of them for syphilis, their treatment if necessary, and secondary contact-tracing, must be carried out as well. This is the public health procedure called case-finding and contact investigation.

Case-finding and contact investigation is part treatment—for those individuals who are already infected—and part prevention—for potential future sex partners of infected persons who, if the infected persons were not treated, might get the disease as well. It is the only way in which the spread of the disease in the population can be achieved. Contrary to Dr. Thomas's position, penicillin is necessary, but *not* sufficient, to effectively deal with the disease syphilis. When it is realized that diseases manifest themselves in populations, not just in individuals, and that they have *population* characteristics, not just *individual* characteristics, this point is easier to understand.

Case-finding and contact investigation must be used to control any infectious disease having a stage in inapparent infection, for which there is no vaccine available. Two other important such diseases in our country are gonorrhea and tuberculosis. (A gonorrhea vaccine is under development. There is a vaccine for tuberculosis, but its effectiveness has not been established beyond doubt, and it is used only to a limited extent in the United States.) Case-finding and contact investigation programs require money. Since World War II in fact, the incidence of syphilis has varied almost directly with the amount of Federal government money available to support case-finding and contact investigation programs nationally. Once again, the importance of public health programs is shown, even for treatable infectious diseases. In fact, syphilis, gonorrhea, and tuberculosis are all virtually eradicable diseases, using this method, since every infected person could eventually be found and treated.

Common Problems in Office Medical Practice

Finally, we may examine the relative roles of prevention and treatment in dealing with the patient problems most commonly seen by office-based physicians in the United States, table 2.2.

After general examination and follow-up visits, the most frequent diagnosis is pre-natal care. This is primarily a personal preventive service, checking progress, advising the mother on nutrition, screening for potential complications. Next is hypertension, a treatable disease. However, a major problem in the United States is finding all those persons who have hypertension and do not know it. Doctors in their offices will not see such people. To find them, public health detection programs must be instituted. Detection or screening programs do not prevent hypertension. But they can find people who have it, bring them under treatment and thus, by and large, prevent its potentially most serious complications.

Acute respiratory infections and pharyngitis are not treatable, unless they are of bacterial origin (relatively rare). However, they are almost always self-limited. Many neuroses can be treated, but many doctors have not been taught how to deal with them. Chronic ischemic heart disease is generally not treatable, except in certain relatively rare instances where surgery is indicated. However, it is a condition which is at least partially preventable. Hay fever is treatable in some patients and preventable with appropriate desensitization techniques in others. Otitis media, middle ear infection, is treatable with antibiotics and its treatment, with the prevention of subsequent hearing loss, represents one of the most important triumphs of the antibiotic age. Obesity is both preventable and treatable. Refractive errors are correctable, some eczemas and certain other skin problems are treatable. Diabetes, like hypertension, can neither be prevented nor cured but can be detected and treated, controlling the development of complications. However, like hypertension, since many persons who have it do not know, and do not seek medical help, public health detection programs are necessary for its control.

Types of Health Services and the Nature of Prevention

Health services can be divided into three categories: personal, community, and combined. Personal health services are those provided directly to individuals for the detection or treatment of disease or the maintenance of health. These are the health services familiar to most of us provided by doctors and other direct care-givers. Community health services are provided to groups of people, often without their direct knowledge, such as sanitary sewage disposal. A combined health service is one given to an individual which also has a community health service component. For example, immunization against measles protects a child against the disease, but also prevents him from becoming a potential source of infection to others.

Prevention thus has a number of aspects. We have shown that historically it is community health services which have had the most influence on population health levels, *as we can measure them.* Community health services are always preventive in nature. Second most important have been combined services, especially immunization. However, personal health services have their preventive aspects as well. Individual health education may cause some people not to smoke cigarettes, or give them up, to control their weight, to exercise regularly, all measures which prevent or inhibit the development of several different diseases. *Early detection* obviously does not prevent the disease, but in hypertension, diabetes, and glaucoma, early detection followed by prompt and effective treatment can prevent serious complications in most cases, as we have previously pointed out. Early detection may improve the chances of survival from certain cancers, although the evidence is unclear. Early detection is sometimes called secondary prevention, a term also used to refer to treatment of diseases with potential complications.

The Primacy of Prevention

I believe that I have now demonstrated that prevention has been the most important factor in the observed improvement in health levels which has occurred in the past three centuries in Western countries.[19] This observation is hardly new. At a time when the process had barely started, Benjamin Franklin said: "An ounce of prevention is worth a pound of cure." If prevention is the principal factor in improvement of health levels and in health maintenance, logic then dictates that it should be the most important function of any *health* care delivery system. But, alas, logic does not pervade our health care delivery system, nor that of most countries with socioeconomic systems similar to ours.

Treatment services dominate our system, as Chapters 4 and 5

will show. Since the doctor dominates the health care system, as I pointed out in the previous chapter, a great deal of the responsibility for this state of affairs can be laid at his door. Doctors tend to concentrate on treatment and tend to ignore preventive services, whether of the personal, community, or combined sort. There are two principal reasons for this. First, doctors are not trained for prevention. Second, the primary reimbursement mechanism, payment of a fee for taking care of an ill person, does not reward preventive work and obviously emphasizes treatment services. We will return to these two points on a number of occasions throughout the book.

At this point, I would like to make it very clear that I am not against treatment services, nor am I underestimating their importance to sick individuals. The person with an inflamed appendix should have it surgically removed, or in some cases be treated with a combination of intravenous fluids and antibiotics, or he stands in danger of dying from generalized abdominal infection if the appendix bursts. The person with a fractured leg must have it set, or he will almost surely have a deformed limb and may become permanently disabled. The person with a bacterial middle-ear infection must have it treated with antibiotics, or he stands a good chance of having a hearing impairment resulting from scarring of the sound transmission mechanism. For the person who has a condition amenable to treatment, it must be of the best quality available. For that individual, the fact that treatment services mean little to the population's health is irrelevant. But that last fact is itself irrelevant to the population and its continued striving for improved health levels. Our health care delivery system is now precariously imbalanced towards treatment services as opposed to preventive services. This is both expensive, as we shall see, and reckless of the future development of the species. The modern world holds many health hazards. The health care delivery system must deal with them, in concert with other divisions of the political economy, if the survival of the species is to be assured and the three-century trend line of rising health levels is not to be reversed. If we are concerned about health, prevention must become primary.

A Word about "Life Style"

These days we hear a great deal about "life style" and its importance to health. Lester Breslow, Dean of the School of Public Health of the University of California at Los Angeles, and his colleagues have shown that "living a good life," that is, not smoking, drinking only moderate amounts of alcohol, controlling one's weight, eating a nutritionally balanced diet, exercising regularly, getting a reasonable amount of sleep, driving safely and wearing automobile seat belts, and the like, can lead to increased life expectancy in adults.[20] Considering the current major killers (refer back to table 2.6.), this is logical. Cigarette smoking is related to heart disease, to lung and several other cancers, possibly to stroke, and to emphysema. Lack of exercise, obesity, possibly an excess of saturated fat, and a stressful life are related to coronary artery disease. Diet may well be related to cancer of the large intestine and sexual practices to cancer of the several female organs. Unsafe highways and automobiles, and the lack of compulsory or passive passenger restraint systems contribute to the automobile accident fatality rate. Heavy drinking and alcoholism are directly related to cirrhosis of the liver. Hypertension, not itself a leading cause of death, is an important associated factor in coronary heart disease and stroke and may be related in part to stressful living. Stressful living is certainly related to suicide. Thus "life style" directly influences the four leading killers as well as numbers seven, eight, and nine.

Using only death rates as a measurement of health, then, life style is an important factor in determining today's health level in the United States. In the absence of specific therapies for most of the leading killers, and understanding the historical importance of prevention as opposed to treatment in improving health in any case, it is obvious that positively influencing life style is a route which holds a great deal of promise for the future of improving health. The question is, how is this to be done?

Dealing with Problems of Life Style

A great deal of weighty contemporary opinion puts the primary responsibility for changing life style on the shoulders of each individual. Professor Victor Fuchs, a leading health economist, said:

> The greatest current potential for improving the health of the American people is to be found in what they do and don't do to and for themselves. Individual decisions about diet, exercise, and smoking are of critical importance, and collective decisions affecting pollution and other aspects of the environment are also relevant.[21]

Professor Herman Somers observed:

> It now seems that the greatest potential for improving the health of the American people is probably not to be found in increasing the number of physicians or hospital beds, but rather in what people can be taught and motivated to do for themselves, in influencing personal behavior and attitudes.[22]

Aaron Wildavsky, the Dean of the Graduate School of Public Policy at the University of California (Berkeley), put it succinctly:

> The lesson should be that doctors should do less and that we-the-people should do more about our own health.[23]

A recent comment of the Medical Society of the State of New York is along the same lines but unfortunately rather flip:

> We've been hearing reports lately about how we could prevent much cancer if only we lived more sensibly. One of the latest is from Frank J. Rauscher, M.D., director, National Cancer Institute, who says Americans could prevent about 60 percent of all cancer cases if they stopped smoking, improved their diets, and took other precautions.
>
> This leads us to believe it's time to update the famous plaint of writer Alexander Woollcott: Everything I like to do is either illegal, immoral, or fattening. We might add: or carcinogenic.[24]

Life Style and "Freedom of Choice"

The position represented by these views is that, individual choice in the matter of life style is entirely free, that individual choices are entirely inner-determined, that individuals are or can become fully informed on the health consequences of the various choices they make, and that the primary current responsibility of the health care delivery system is to educate individuals to make the "right" choices. In his statement, Fuchs does make a slight nod in the direction of recognizing the importance of environmental influences on health, but his major emphasis is on personal responsibility. He concludes his book by saying:

> By changing institutions and creating new programs we can make medical care more accessible and deliver it more efficiently, but the greatest potential for improving health lies in what we do and don't do for and to ourselves. The choice is ours.[25]

I disagree with this position. My argument is not with its basic premise that further major improvements in health levels will come from preventive measures applied to the major killer diseases, but with how it proposes to achieve that end: principally by health education of individuals, essentially leaving the whole living environment alone, by implication at least.

Are the Choices Really Free?

Are choices in the matter of life style entirely free? Let us say a middle-aged corporate executive is under severe stress because he is suddenly unemployed. He chooses to work but cannot find a job anywhere in the country. Is that a matter of free choice? Let us say that a Puerto Rican child in the South Bronx is chronically afflicted with asthma related to cockroach leavings in the food she eats. Her parents would like to move, but (1) they are restricted in their movements by racial discrimination, (2) they cannot afford much higher rent in any case, and (3) no public housing is available. Is that free-choice?

Are choices entirely inner-directed? In 1973 the tobacco industry had the fourth highest advertising budget in the United States, exceeded only by the automotive, transportation, and food industries. The alcoholic beverage industry was fifth.[26] If these industries did not feel that they had to advertise in order to sell their products, they obviously wouldn't do it. Yet cigarettes probably constitute the single most potent health hazard today. One-half of auto accident fatalities are alcohol-related, and cirrhosis of the liver, in this country a disease related almost entirely to alcohol, is the seventh-leading cause of death.

Eating is an activity which is heavily pushed by the food industry in this country, generally without concern for total caloric intake, nutritional balance (some companies, such as a few of the margarine and bread companies, are an exception to this rule), or regular eating habits (eating between meals was shown to be detrimental to health by Breslow and his colleagues).

The drug industry plays an interesting role in influencing life style choice-making. The message of the drug companies to the lay public is generally: "Do you have a problem? Well, then, take a pill [or an elixir, or use a spray, etc.] Headache?—aspirin; indigestion? —antacid; body odor?—deodorant; insomnia?—sleeping pill; somnolence?—waking pill; athlete's foot?—powder; want to feel good?—vitamins." The message to the health professions is along the same lines, only more sophisticated: specific therapies are offered for specific diseases. This message gets through to the general public. Doctors have often told me that they feel under pressure from some patients to give antibiotics for upper-respiratory infections (against which antibiotics are generally useless), because patients "expect something" when they come to the doctor's office —and pay the fee.

In my view, it is no accident that drug abuse and addiction are major health problems in this country. Without malevolent intent, certainly, the drug industry is continually telling both the public and the health professions that in drugs lie the solutions to many problems. There are few messages which say: headache?—look for causes of stress and try to deal with them; indigestion?—watch your eating habits; body odor?—wash yourself with care, (except for the deodorant soap ads); insomnia?—try to figure out what is troubling you and deal with it; and so on. Choices in many areas of life style are not entirely inner-directed at all, but are heavily influenced by the actions of commerce and industry.

Full Information and Freedom of Choice

Are individuals fully informed concerning the health choices they make, and if not, can they be? In any case, if they can be, is that the complete answer? Individuals can be fully informed about the consequences of cigarette-smoking, alcohol abuse, and overeating, certainly. But if the economy continually subjects them to propaganda that encourages them to smoke, drink, and eat improperly, is full information really the only answer?

Turning to an area which is not generally included in "life style," but is an important external influence on health, consider the case of cancer-causing agents (carcinogens) in the environment. Suppose a worker is fully informed that substance exposures at his plant may well lead to cancer in himself, and maybe even in his family, but he could not possibly find a job in another industry. What is he supposed to do? Suppose a family finds that their community water supply is contaminated by a carcinogen? Are they supposed to stop drinking water, truck it in, or buy bottled water? How important is full information in matters of pesticides, herbicides, and fungicides in food, in the matter of food additives emplaced during the manufacturing process, or such things as sugar-added cereals promoted heavily by sponsors of childrens' television programs.

Personal and Community Preventive Measures

Taking all of these factors into account, what then is the primary responsibility of the health care delivery system in dealing with modern diseases, and the influence of life style and other environmental influences on them? The authorities quoted above certainly agree that prevention is the key. However, we have seen that there are two general classes of preventive measures: community and personal. Health education, advocated by most current supporters of the "change-life-style-and-health-will-improve" school, is a personal preventive measure. People are taught, either individually or in groups, what behaviors will produce health benefits, and then they are expected to perform in a certain way. A decision to adopt a community health measure is generally taken collectively, but the measure, once implemented, does not require individual actions for its success.

Turning to history once again, we learn that of the various preventive measures available, it has been the community-wide ones which have been the most effective. In fact, of the personal preventive measures, only immunization and case-finding and contact investigation both combined, not solely personal health services, have been significant. Consider the case of eliminating cholera in central London in the mid-1850s. A particularly perceptive epidemiologist, John Snow, figured out that cholera was related to a contaminated water supply. (By using the epidemiological approach of relating cases to particular water sources, by the way, he was able to make this deduction long before the specific bacterium causing cholera was discovered.) No treatment was available for cholera, so the solution was preventive. The personal preventive approach would have been either to educate people to go elsewhere for their water (water was not available in the home, but was obtained from street pumps), or to teach them to boil and strain their water before drinking it. The community preventive approach was to clean up the water supply at the source. The latter approach, the only possible effective one, was taken—and it worked. In fact, the whole of sanitary reform, the second most important health measure historically after improved nutrition, was based on community, not personal preventive measures.

Community Prevention and Cigarette Smoking

We can consider what a modern parallel would be in the control of cigarette smoking. Personal preventive measures consist principally in having individual health care providers tell individual patients not to smoke, in having anti-smoking advertisements, and in having programs of various kinds to help smokers quit. (The last is treatment of the smoking habit, not in itself considered a disease.) However, if smoking is stopped, its complications will be prevented. This sort of campaign has been generally underway in the United States since the release of the Surgeon General's Report on Smoking and Health in 1964. It has met with modest success in that the percentage of cigarette smokers in the population has decreased. However, quite alarming, the proportion of teenagers who smoke has increased, as have the proportion of women smoking in the twenty-one to twenty-four and over-fifty-five age groups.[27]

A community prevention program for cigarette smoking would have quite a different character. Prohibition would not be employed. That has been tried, with only limited success in alcohol consumption, marijuana smoking, and heroin addiction, and with fearful social consequences of other sorts. However, advertising would be banned completely, a proposal supported by over half the adult population in the United States. (If advertising were not so important in recruiting new smokers and keeping old smokers in the fold, the tobacco industry would not spend so much money on it. The tobacco industry spends a higher proportion of its income on advertising than does any other industry.) To help the advertising industry and the print media absorb this shock, government expenditures on anti-smoking advertising could be vastly increased. Availability of cigarettes could be restricted by banning cigarette machines, or perhaps by having cigarettes sold only in special stores, as are alcoholic beverages in certain states. Federal government subsidies to tobacco farmers would be ended. At the same time, subsidies could be offered to farmers shifting to other crops. Government subsidy could help tobacco companies diversify, while retraining their workers. Taxation policy could encourage the use of low-tar and nicotine cigarettes, and cigarette taxes could be made nationally uniform and collected at the point of production, with distribution of fair shares to states and localities, to make "boot legging" of cheaper cigarettes from low tax to high tax states unprofitable. Finally, subsidies could be offered to those companies developing and converting to an acceptable non-tobacco cigarette.

Community Preventive Measures in Other Conditions

These are all community preventive measures. Similar measures could be applied to alcohol. The epidemiologist Milton Terris, M.D., has shown that in Great Britain taxation policy and moderate limitations on alcohol availability have gradually but steadily reduced cirrhosis of the liver mortality in Great Britain since the measures were introduced during World War I, originally to combat industrial absenteeism.[28] Community prevention programs, different in detail but similar in philosophy, can also be developed to deal with traffic accident fatalities as well as home and industrial hazards, air and water pollution, industrial carcinogenesis, food additives, and pesticide, herbicide, and fungicide pollution. In fact, community prevention programs to deal with many of these hazards are already in place as we know, some working better than others. Overeating and lack of exercise are more difficult to deal with without becoming punitive (higher health insurance premiums for overweight people have been suggested, for example), but with some creative thought it might be possible to deal with these problems through community prevention programs as well. Certainly, if childhood obesity is related to adult obesity, as some authorities think it is, perhaps the addition at the factory of sugar to breakfast food should be banned.

The Importance of Health Education

All of what I have said above should not be taken as a denigration of consumer health education. It is an important, indeed, vital function. One of the sad facts of life in the United States is that people generally know so little about how their bodies work—and don't work. Neither do they know much about how their health care delivery system works: what it is supposed to do and how its quality can be judged. The "medical mystique" is too readily accepted. There must be much better health and health care consumer education. People should be able to participate in decisions concerning their own bodies. They should be able to make rational choices in dealing with the environment and its varied hazards, especially in the absence of comprehensive community preventive programs. Consumers must be educated to intelligently influence the political processes which lead to the development of effective community prevention programs. (I will deal with consumer action in medical education reform in the last chapter of this book.) Nevertheless, it must be recognized that historically, in the improvement of health levels, community preventive measures have been primary and personal preventive measures have been secondary. We thus must not expect too much from consumer health education. We certainly must not rely on it as our principal weapon in the battle against the major modern diseases.

Interference with Freedom of Choice: Real Concern or Straw Man?

Some critics of community prevention programs for modern diseases, for example R.F. Meenan, and certainly Dr. Jack Harnes, quoted at the beginning of this chapter, claim that they infringe on personal freedoms.[29] Statements are made such as "it's *their* lungs" in reference to cigarette-smoking control, "it's *their* skulls" in reference to compulsory helmet laws for motorcyclists, and "it's *their* lives" in reference to alcoholism-control programs. However, few personal habits affecting health can now be considered entirely personal matters. The public cigarette smoker is polluting the air of others. The drunken driver may kill the innocent. And anyone, such as the helmetless motorcyclist, who increases his risk of a morbid event requiring health care services, which would be less likely to occur in the presence of preventive measures, is increasing the total cost of the health care delivery system, which must be borne by the population as a whole.

Prevention and Modern Health Problems

Modern health problems can be solved. In the middle of the nineteenth century, the biological causes of the group of diseases we now recognize as primarily infectious were no less of a mystery to the scientific community of the day than are the biological causes of heart disease, cancer, stroke, hypertension, diabetes, and cirrhosis of the liver to the scientific community now. Yet the diseases were tackled, came to be understood, and were dealt with. The science of epidemiology, the study of the distribution of disease and health in populations, permitted the control of certain diseases such as cholera before the specific biological causal factor was known. Similarly, epidemiology has highlighted the relationship between many environmental hazards and a variety of cancers, for example; thus control mechanisms are available, even though the specific biological mechanisms in cancer are not known.

I have attempted to illustrate the connection between prevention and the improvement in health levels over time, and to show that the most important preventive measures are those applied to communities as a whole rather than to individuals. Of the personal preventive measures available, only immunization and case-finding and contact investigation have had significant effects on improving health levels, historically. Screening and early detection, measures not preventive of disease but preventive of complications, are important in, for example, diabetes, hypertension, and certain vision and hearing defects, and may be important in the control of certain cancers.

The Functions of the Health Care Delivery System

If prevention is primary for health, and the principal purpose of a health care delivery system is the maintenance of health, then the most important activity of any health care delivery system should be prevention. Presumably, then, the most important concern of the leaders of the health care delivery system should be prevention. However, prevention is neither the most important activity of the health care delivery system in the United States, nor is it the most important concern of its leadership.

The U.S. health care delivery system has multiple functions. One is, in fact, the maintenance of health. Prevention is practiced, just not nearly as much as it should be. The health care delivery system's most prominent biomedical function is the treatment of disease. It also conducts research, educates its personnel, and constructs its facilities, all of which are necessary for the maintenance of health as well as the prevention and treatment of disease. However, the health care delivery system has other functions as well.

All of its human component parts, like the human members of any system, are interested in self-perpetuation. It seems to be a human characteristic, which I really do not understand, that many people see self-perpetuation as being related to lack of change. A system becomes irrelevant, or never has been relevant, to social needs, but its personnel think that by saying "we are doing a great job" repeatedly, and loudly, that the problems will just go away, or will not be recognized by others as problems. The personnel then think that they will be allowed just to go on as they always have done, perpetuating themselves and their system. Life is comfortable and please, they should be just left alone, or, if anything, allowed to return to "the good old days." This attitude is prominent in many sectors of the health care delivery system.

Next, a function of the health care delivery system is to provide rewards, monetary, social, and intellectual, to its personnel. In Western countries, doctors do particularly well. Over 80 percent of practicing physicians in the United States are in private office practice, being reimbursed on a fee-for-service basis. Fee-for-service can provide an income level which is determined primarily not by level of skill or social relevance, but by hours worked, personality, and social contacts within the profession. Depending upon the geographic location, potential income is very high indeed. By the same token, academic medicine can provide important intellectual rewards and a great deal of ego-satisfaction, as well as high incomes on occasion, in the absence of social relevance. It is very easy for either the private practitioner or the academic physician to get trapped into a work pattern which brings him these kinds of rewards but benefits the population little either in terms of health maintenance or disease alleviation. Not every physician gets trapped in this wise, by any means, but certainly some do.

Finally, a function of the health care delivery system for certain of its components is the making of financial profits. The principal purpose of the commercial drug industry in this country, and there is no non-commercial drug industry, is to make a profit. The commercial health insurance industry, which sells about one-half of all hospital and other health-service insurance sold in this country, is also in business to make a profit. Neither industry routinely reveals its profits. Elsewhere, I have estimated the annual profits of the commercial health insurance industry to be over $1 billion.[30] This is made principally by investing premium payments while they have them, rather than by having an excess of premium income over benefit expenditures. Company propaganda to the contrary notwithstanding, the drug industry seems to be a profitable field as well.

The majority of institutions in the scandal-ridden nursing home industry in this country are privately owned, and operated for a profit. About 10 percent of general hospital beds are in private, profit-making hands as well. Then there are other, relatively smaller profit-making segments like some home health services, many clinical laboratories, the hospital supply industry, and the medical equipment and devices industry.

Contradictions and Functions

There are contradictions between making profits and providing the best of health services, preventive or therapeutic. For example, if a drug company has an item that sells well and provides a profit, protected by patents, why should it reduce profits by investing in research for new drugs which may come to naught. In fact, many new drugs are discovered not by drug companies, but in university laboratories. In nursing homes, why should services be improved, when all that will do, aside from providing better patient care, is reduce profits?

The contradiction between private medical practice and preventive services is particularly sharp. Physicians in our country are paid for treating sickness, not preventing it. I think that few, if any, doctors consciously fail to provide preventive services because they might reduce trade. But they often don't actively provide them either. (The reimbursement method is only one aspect of this. The other is the medical education system. But more, much more, of that later.) Further, preventive services are generally offered by government agencies. These government agencies may also be in, or want to be in, direct treatment services. Private physicians view *this,* rightly or not, as competition, sometimes labelled "unfair competition."

Since 1920 or so, organized private medicine has fought tooth and nail to contain government health services to the preventive sector, except for treatment services for certain sharply delimited categories of persons (see Chapter 4). In continually hammering away at preventing the expansion of government treatment services, the private sector has invariably hampered the expansion of preventive services, even of the community type. Organized medicine often takes the view, explicitly or implicity, that treatment services are the principal reason for the improvement of population health levels, in spite of all of the evidence cited above to the contrary. Thus, for several reasons, there is a contradiction between the private medical sector and the expansion of preventive services.

Then there is the contradiction which is one of the basic concerns of this book: the contradiction between what is taught in the medical schools, treatment medicine, and what is of most value to the people as a whole, preventive health services. If the health of the people is to prosper in the next century, this contradiction, as well as others I have and have not outlined, must be resolved. Prevention is the key to health. It must become the keystone of the health care delivery system.

3

Problems of the U.S. Health Care Delivery System

It has been popular among observers of the U. S. health care system in the 1960s and 1970s to describe it as being "in crisis." In 1960, *Harper's* Magazine devoted a special supplement to "The Crisis in American Medicine." The supplement began:

> Contradictory as they may sound, these two statements probably would be accepted by most Americans:
>
> 1. American medicine is the best in the world.
> 2. Millions of people are bitterly dissatisfied with the medical care they are getting.

The first proposition is hardly open to argument. Reports on new wonder drugs, new methods of life-saving surgery, Nobel Prize awards to American medical scientists are becoming almost commonplace. Eminent people from all corners of the world—including Sir Anthony Eden and Arab princes—come to America for treatment, as they once went to Berlin or Vienna.

The second proposition, however, has been stubbornly denied by a large part of the medical profession. Your own doctor, in all likelihood, will tell you that most Americans are perfectly satisfied with our traditional system of medical care, and that any suggestions for change are either hare-brained or subversive.

In recent months, this argument has begun to sound less and less convincing. Even some physicians—the more thoughtful ones—are now beginning to admit that something seems to be very wrong indeed.[1]

In 1968, Roger Battistella and R. McK. Southby published "Crisis in American Medicine" in the British medical journal, the *Lancet.* They began by saying:

In terms of gross national product the U.S.A. spends more on health than does any other country. But costs are rising at such a rate that more and more people will find it difficult to get complete health care. This particularly applies to the poor, the old, the Negroes, and other disadvantaged groups. Doctors and hospital beds are distributed most unevenly both in broad geographic regions and between States. There are indications, too, that the quality of care has been inferior, especially in terms of antenatal and infant mortality. The whole organization of medical care in the U.S.A. has failed to respond to changing disease patterns, the move from country to cities, industrialization, and the increasing proportion of old people in the population.[2]

In 1970, the Editors of *Fortune* entered the lists:

American medicine, the pride of the nation for many years, stands now on the brink of chaos. To be sure, our medical practitioners have their great moments of drama and triumph. But much of U.S. medical care, particularly the everyday business of preventing and treating routine illnesses, is inferior in quality, wastefully dispensed, and inequitably financed. Medical manpower and facilities are so maldistributed that large segments of the population, especially the urban poor and those in rural areas, get virtually no care at all—even though their illnesses are most numerous and, in a medical sense, often easy to cure.[3]

Listen also to Senator Edward Kennedy, as quoted by Spencer Klaw:

> "America," Senator Edward M. Kennedy told an audience of doctors in New York City in 1971, "is beginning to realize that we have a health care crisis on our hands, and that the magnitude of the crisis is enormous." He added, " 'I have seen that crisis first hand, and I challenge even the most reactionary pillars of organized medicine, even the most affluent physicians in the most affluent suburbs of this rich city, to deny that a crisis exists, or that it exists for all Americans—not just the poor, not just the black, but each and every one of us."[4]

There have been many other reports in recent years taking similar positions, some of which are listed in the Notes.[5] But social critics are not alone in holding negative views. Eliot Richardson, one of the Secretaries of the USDHEW in the Nixon Administration, said the following in Senate testimony under the title, "Health Care Crisis in America" (1971):

> In general our critical health problems today do not arise because the health of our people is worsening, or because expenditures on health care have been niggardly, or because we have been negligent as a Nation in developing health care resources, or because we have been unconcerned about providing financial protection against ill-health. We must look elsewhere. I should like to suggest that our present concern is a function of two broad problems. The first is the inequality in health status and care, and in access to financing. The other is the pervasive problem of rising medical costs . . . The impressive growth in the number of people covered by health insurance conceals the fact that only 29 percent of all personal health expenditures were paid by insurance in 1968. The indices of general improvement in health pale in importance when we look behind them and see that the poor and non-whites are doing far worse than whites and those with decent incomes . . .
>
> When we look beyond our borders and compare ourselves with other nations, any sense of accomplishment over our long-run gains in health status is mitigated by the fact that other advanced nations are doing better than we are. . . . These disparities point to a gap between what we have accomplished and what remains to be accomplished, between our achievements and our expectations, between what is and our impatience for what might be. . . .

Observations of this sort are not new. Professor Milton Roemer of the School of Public Health, University of California at Los

Angeles, has cited a number of critical studies going back to 1927.[6] Professor Roemer noted that:

> Each of these books has made a contribution to public understanding, pulling aside the mask of secrecy which shielded the healing arts from public scrutiny and accountability for too many decades. Generally these books have resulted from painstaking study of the problems of medical care, they have exposed the enormous inequities caused by the private entrepreneurial market in which American medicine is immersed, and they have offered constructive solutions for improving the system.

For an example of an early description of health care delivery problems still with us, one can turn to a work entitled, the *Final Report of the Committee on the Costs of Medical Care,* published in 1932. The Committee had been established in 1928 to look into problems of health care delivery in the United States. Its chairman was Ray Lyman Wilbur, M.D., a past president of the American Medical Association. The book began with the following statement:

> The problem of providing satisfactory medical service to all the people of the United States at costs which they can meet is a pressing one. At the present time, many persons do not receive service which is adequate either in quantity or quality, and the costs of service are inequably distributed. The result is a tremendous amount of preventable physical pain and mental anguish, needless deaths, economic inefficiency, and social waste. Furthermore, these conditions are, as the following pages will show, largely unnecessary. The United States has the economic resources, the organizing ability, and the technical experience to solve this problem.[7]

It is a striking fact that this statement could easily have been written forty years later and still have been entirely applicable.

On the other hand there are observers who think that the situation is really not so bad; in fact that it is really rather good. For example, the American Medical Association, as reported in its own newspaper, the *American Medical News:*

> The constantly improving American health system is the best in the world and must not be stifled by adopting a government-controlled national health insurance program, the American Medical Association told Congress.
>
> "When considering a national plan for this country, it is necessary to take cognizance of the strengths of our own method of health care deliv-

ery . . . this will assure that our excellent system will continue to improve and will not suffer the stifling effects experienced in other countries," AMA President Max H. Parrott, M.D., testified.

Dr. Parrott told the House Ways and Means subcommittee on health that "American medical service and technology have developed at an unparalled rate . . . presently there is more and better medical technology here than anywhere else in the world."[8]

In 1972, Harry Schwartz, a journalist, wrote *The Case for American Medicine.* The entire second chapter, "What Health Crisis?", was published in *American Medical News.* The AMN introduced the chapter by saying:

> AMN is proud to reprint here a chapter from *The Case for American Medicine* book, which concludes that "the American medical system—pluralistic, complex, and ever-changing—has served the American people well."[9]

In this chapter Schwartz says, in part:

> In the 20 years before 1970, medical science progressed with unprecendented rapidity and [certainly] some of those gains . . . have been translated into concrete health gains for the American people. It is [a] dark evaluation of American medicine that must be in the minds of many who agitate for radical change and who use the terms "health care crisis" and "health crisis" interchangeably. . . .
>
> [However,] all persons familiar with the facts know that there has been enormous progress in improving the health of the American people since 1950. . . . The facts reviewed in this chapter make evident that there is nothing resembling a "health crisis" in the United States. Those who speak in such terms betray their taste for fantasy and hyperbole and their ignorance of the enormous progress that has been made. Insofar as medical science can control illness and death, the United States in the 1970s has a population enjoying the best health and greatest longevity in the nation's history. To improve health and longevity further the primary need is for more knowledge to cure presently incurable diseases, for individual life styles and life patterns that will prevent the self-inflicted injuries and deaths that are now so prevalent, and for radical improvement in the material conditions of the most deprived groups of Americans.

Is There a "Crisis"?

The American Medical Association, Mr. Harry Schwartz, and other defenders of the American health care delivery system as "the best in the world" may be right on that score. On balance, we may indeed have the best health care delivery system in the world, although visitors from Canada, Great Britain, Sweden, the Soviet Union, and China might argue that point vigorously on a variety of grounds. But that is really neither here nor there when the system is examined using objective criteria. According to many observers, those we have quoted and cited above as well as others, the system has many serious problems. I shall review the major current ones below, in some detail. But first, the question of whether or not the system is in "crisis" should be examined.

"Crisis" is defined by Webster's New World Dictionary as ". . . a turning point in the course of anything; decisive or crucial time, stage, or event; a time of great danger or trouble, whose outcome decides whether possible bad consequences will follow. . . ." In my opinion, the facts of the U.S. health care delivery system, as they are determined by available statistical data, by data from quantitative research, and by descriptive analysis, show that major problems confront it: lack of attention to preventive services; concentration on acute care as compared with chronic care; rising costs; financial and other barriers to care; geographic maldistribution of manpower; overspecialization by providers; excess surgery; deficiencies in quality and quality control; poor planning; problems in provider-patient communication; a tendency, particularly in the physician sector, to stress the unusual at the expense of the commonplace; training and educational programs which are not always directly relevant to patient needs; and a biomedical research undertaking which suffers from a similar problem.

However, the historical record and the situation in the mid-1970s show that most, if not all, of these problems are not new. Over time they have undergone changes in magnitude. However, these changes for the most part have not been sudden and sharp, but gradual. Indeed, John Gordon Freymann has shown clearly that many of the major problems which were confronted by the Committee on the Costs of Medical Care in 1932 and which we confront today, have their origins in developments which took place in health care and its modes of delivery in our country and those of our European forebears in the seventeenth, eighteenth, and nineteenth centuries.[10] Thus, in terms of the definition of the word, we do not face a "crisis" in health care. Rather, we must deal with a health care delivery system which has some very serious problems of long standing, having deep historical roots embedded in the whole fabric of American society. This fact should not be a cause for complacency, however. It is often easier to deal with a crisis, even one of great magnitude, than it is to deal with long-standing, unchanging chronic problems. Modern medical practice itself attests to the truth of this statement.

Major Problems Faced in the Mid-Seventies

Prevention Given Short Shrift

In the last chapter, I showed that preventive measures have been primarily responsible for the improvements in health levels experienced in the Western World during the last three centuries. I also showed that a great deal is known about how the major diseases of our time are distributed in the population, and about the various environmental and social factors which increase the risk of people getting the major diseases. Thus, most of them could be ameliorated, or even eliminated, if known preventive measures were applied. This is true despite the fact that our knowledge of the basic biological causative mechanisms of conditions such as heart disease, cancer, hypertension, and diabetes is incomplete. To *cure* diseases, it is often necessary to know the biological *cause.* However, to *prevent* disease, the science of epidemiology, which elucidates the patterns in which diseases manifest themselves in populations, often provides us with sufficient knowledge.

The Economics of Prevention

Medical practice in the United States is, as I have pointed out before, cure-oriented, not prevention-oriented. This fact is reflected in the distribution of resources within the health care delivery system. The scientific reality, that a great deal could be done in disease control through known preventive measures, is largely ignored. In the fiscal year 1975, we spent approximately $120 billion on health services. Only about 3 percent of that total went to identifiable government public health activities, not all preventive services. Voluntary health agencies such as the American Heart Association spent another 0.6 percent of the total, a good deal of it on preventive services. Some of the funds spent on research and construction supported preventive services, and some of the work done by hospitals, physicians, and dentists is of a preventive nature. Estimating that $500 million of the $7.25 billion spent on research and construction, and $3 billion of the $75 billion paid for the services of hospitals, doctors, and dentists went for preventive services, we can conclude that no more than 5.5 percent of total national health expenditures, $6.6 billion, went for prevention,* and that estimate may be a high one.[12] Lester Breslow and Anne Somers, two leading authorities on preventive medicine, have estimated the rate of expenditure on preventive services at 2.0 to 2.5 percent.[13]

"Well," one might say, "how do we know that that level of expenditure on prevention is not after all the right one. Maybe it's even too much!" An examination of the economic costs of illness, the direct ones of caring for the sick, and the indirect ones of lost production, is illuminating in dealing with this point. Such an examination indicates that an expansion of preventive measures could save the nation a great deal of money, in both direct and indirect costs.

Barbara S. Cooper and Dorothy P. Rice of the Office of Research and Statistics, Social Security Administration, have provided some estimates of the economic costs of illness in the United States for 1972. They estimated costs in three categories: direct

*It should be noted that in 1975, the same year, federal, state and local governments spent about $6.7 billion on sanitation and sewage disposal, and there are significant private expenditures in these areas as well.[11] Much smaller amounts were spent on controlling other types of environmental pollution through such measures as the Occupational Safety and Health Act, the Clean Air Act, and the Toxic Substances Act. These measures, very important to health, are not counted as health services in the federal accounting system.

costs, morbidity (illness) costs, and mortality costs. Quoting the authors:

> The *direct* cost of illness represents expenditures for prevention, detection, treatment, rehabilitation, research, training, and capital investment in medical facilities.
>
> *Morbidity* losses are incurred when illness results in absence from employment, prevents a housewife from performing her duties, or results in disability that prevents someone from working at all. The lost earnings and the dollar value of the unperformed housekeeping services are the morbidity costs.
>
> *Mortality* costs [are] calculated [by] the "human capital" approach. This approach values one's life according to one's earnings or, in the case of housewives, according to the market value of one's duties. . . . Calculation of mortality costs considers earnings over a lifetime rather than a single year. . . . It is the present value of these future losses that is the appropriate measure.[14]

The major findings of Cooper and Rice are summarized in table 3.1. Recall that the year is 1972, when direct national health expenditures amounted to "only" $90 billion or so, as opposed to about $140 billion in 1976. The economic costs of illness are distributed among fifteen major diagnostic categories, plus "other." Ninety-three percent of all costs are accounted for by the fifteen categories, which are ranked in descending order of total economic cost. Note that with certain exceptions for diseases which are not major killers, such as mental disorders and diseases of the nervous system and sense organs (which in this classification does not include stroke, considered a disease of the circulatory system), the ranking parallels that of the major killers reviewed in the last chapter.

As I showed in the last chapter, preventive measures are already available to deal with significant proportions of illness in the following categories: diseases of the circulatory (including both heart disease and stroke); accidents, poisonings, and violence; diseases of the digestive system (which includes cirrhosis of the liver); neoplasm (cancer); diseases of the respiratory system; endocrine, nutritional, and metabolic diseases (diabetes mellitus is the most important one here); infective and parasitic disease; complications of pregnancy, childbirth, and the newborn period; and congenital anomalies (genetic screening and counselling, not previously men-

Table 3.1. Total Economic Costs: Estimated direct costs, and the costs of morbidity and mortality on potential lifetime earnings, by diagnosis, 1972.*

Diagnosis	Direct**	Indirect**		Total
		Morbidity	Mortality	
Circulatory System Disease	10,919	6,417	22,724	40,060
Accidents, Poisonings, Violence	5,121	3,883	17,674	26,678
Digestive System Disease	11,100	2,606	3,781	17,487
Neoplasm (Cancer, etc.)	3,872	862	12,633	17,367
Respiratory System Disease	5,931	7,089	3,434	16,454
Mental disorders	6,985	6,179	753	13,917
Nervous System Disease	5,947	3,944	1,060	10,951
Musculo-Skeletal System	3,636	5,103	209	8,948
Genito-urinary System	4,471	1,249	736	6,456
Endocrine, nutritional	3,436	1,137	1,357	5,930
Infective and Parasitic	1,412	1,200	831	3,443
Complications of Pregnancy	2,607	245	80	2,932
Skin Disease	1,525	460	67	2,052
Congenital anomalies	381	238	1,284	1,903
Blood Disease	491	220	210	921
Other	7,398	1,494	4,402	13,294
Total	75,231	42,323	71,235	188,789

*These figures are calculated on a "discount rate" of 4 percent on lifetime earnings. The concept of "discount rate" is explained by Mrs. Cooper and Mrs. Rice on pp. 35–36 of their paper.

**Amounts in millions.

Source: Cooper, B.S. and Rice, D.P. "The Economic Cost of Illness Revisited," *Social Security Bulletin,* February, 1976, p. 21, table 7.

tioned, can have great value here). Preventive measures are also available to deal with some of the illnesses in important, generally non-killer categories: dental disease (dental illness is included in the digestive disease category and accounts for about one-half of its direct costs); mental disorders (suicide is, of course, in "top ten" of killers); infectious diseases, such as syphilis, gonorrhea, tuberculosis, and the childhood viral diseases for which vaccines exist but are incompletely applied to the population; and the generally non-killing congenital anomalies such as cerebral palsy, and

German measles abnormalities. Preventive measures for diseases of the blood and blood-forming organs, the nervous system and sense organs, the genito-urinary system, the skin, and the musculo-skeletal system are not so readily available.

It appears that the thorough application of known preventive measures could save billions of dollars per year, in both direct and indirect costs. Of course, these measures would cost money to implement. Detailed cost/benefit analyses would have to be done to determine the net savings which could be achieved. Since existing preventive measures are generally of low relative cost, I am certain that cost/benefit analysis results would be positive, that is that significant savings would be achieved. Considering the potential which preventive services have for improving health levels and the quality of life, and for saving money, it would appear that the proportion of present health expenditures spent on prevention is pitifully low. In terms of *health,* this is our number one health care delivery system problem.

Separation of Services for Acute and Chronic Care

Continuing our problem list, U.S. health services concentrate on providing care for the acutely ill. The mentally ill, persons with other chronic diseases imposing significant limitations in activity, and the infirm aged generally receive short shrift. The "stars" of the health care delivery system are the large acute care hospitals, the physicians and surgeons who perform the "miracle cures"—on a relatively small number of persons—and the research labs which investigate the "interesting" diseases—usually rare. Rehabilitation receives about as much attention as does prevention.

John Gordon Freymann provides the factual basis for these statements, and also explains their historical origins.[15] The institutional separation of the acute and chronically ill can be traced back to the establishment of the forebears of our modern hospitals in the eighteenth century, institutions heavily influenced by the British tradition. The few hospitals of that time were built by private philanthropists. They were in the main, interested in "success." That meant having a relatively constant flow of patients in and out, the "curables." In fact, for most of these hospitals, strict rules were established to keep the "incurables" from being admitted.

The "incurables," regardless of what condition they had, if they required institutionalization were put in the only available long-term "care" institution (that is, where they existed), the poorhouse. The poorhouse, as it developed more rapidly in the nineteenth century, was the place in the cities where all persons who could not support themselves in their own homes were placed. Thus the unemployed and otherwise economically destitute, the chronically ill, the mentally ill, the mentally retarded, the aged, the orphans, and what have you were all lumped together. In many areas, the acutely ill poor for whom there was no other provision, also were placed in poor houses.

Gradually during the nineteenth century, separate categories of facilities were established for most of these groups. State mental hospitals began appearing during the 1840s and 50s in response to Dorothea Dix's crusade. Hospitals for persons afflicted with non-mental chronic illness began making their appearance later in the century. Separate institutions for the aged did not come into being in significant numbers until the Social Security Act of 1935 gave the aged poor some independent purchasing power. Acute care public hospitals for the poor began in the early nineteenth century as poorhouse infirmaries. Interestingly, they followed the pattern of their private philanthropic predecessors and tried to limit themselves to the care of "curables."

Thus acute care has been linked with "success" and chronic care with "failure" since institutions began in this country. Acute care has received a great deal of attention; chronic care not very much. Since most training of physicians, and other health care providers as well, takes place in acute care institutions, it is no wonder that this pattern continues relatively unchanged. This is a theme to which I will return in later chapters when I deal with the problems of the medical education system *per se.*

The Rising Cost of Health Care

Over the last ten years or so, health care costs have been rising at a rate in the 13–15 percent range, sometimes a bit less, sometimes a bit more. (The increase for fiscal 1976 over fiscal 1975 was around 17 percent.) The rate of increase has generally been about

20 percent higher than that observed in the Consumer Price Index, although for 1975–76 it was more than twice as high as the increase in the CPI. In 1950, health services consumed about 4.6 percent of the Gross National Product. In 1965, the figure was 5.9 percent. By 1975, it had reached 8.3 percent, and the fiscal 1976 estimate stands at 8.6 percent.[16] (At this rate compounded, some wags note that in less than fifty years we will be spending half of our GNP on health services!) There are many reasons for rising costs, but the principal responsibility lies with the doctors, and the hospitals.

Recall that the bulk of expenditures on health services is provider, not consumer, determined. The bulk of expenditures is on treatment services for the acutely ill, many of whom have at least partially preventable conditions. The most costly sector of the health care delivery system is the hospitals. (Hospitals account for about 40 percent of all health care spending; doctors for about 20 percent.) Over the last ten years, hospital expenditures having been rising at a rate about double that for all other health care expenditures. The most important element in this is the increasing technical complexity of hospitals, with general inflation and rising wages being somewhat less significant factors. Unfortunately, the efficacy and positive cost-benefit of many of these technical improvements has yet to be clearly demonstrated. I will deal in more detail with the linked problems of excess hospital bed capacity, overutilization of existing hospital beds, and unnecessary surgery in Chapter 5.

In December, 1976, the Council on Wage and Price Stability of the Executive of The President reported on a year-long study of rising health care costs in a work entitled, *The Complex Puzzle of Rising Health Care Costs.* The Council commented on the unique economic nature of the health care delivery system:

> Unlike the supplier-consumer relationship typical of other sectors of the economy, in the medical care transaction, the primary supplier of medical services, the physician, usually determines the level of services required by the consumer, the patient.
>
> Moreover, medical services are largely paid for through a system of third-party payors, insurance companies, and government health programs, on behalf of the patient. Often unaffected by the true extent of the costs, the consumer may tend to consume a higher level of services than if he or she were to pay for these services directly.

Hospitals, a primary provider of health services, have little incentive to provide cost-efficient services because of such factors as: retrospective cost reimbursement by third-party payors and inefficient planning which does little to stem excess capacity and duplication of expensive facilities and equipment.

The Council came to the conclusion that:

To begin with, there is no evidence that health care providers, left to their own devices, would do anything other than behave in a manner which will continue to fuel an inflationary bias already deeply imbedded in the structure of the system. Like a seamless web, the separate, individual decisions made by thousands of health care providers are, aggregately, too costly to society. As presently structured, there are few incentives within the provider system to control costs, to economize, or to weight the *costs* of a proposed action—whether it is the purchase of new equipment, the expansion of a hospital, or the selection of a course of treatment—against its *benefits.* Unless and until cost-control incentives are introduced which will exert discipline on the providers and consumers of health care, we can expect only a continuation of the present cost spiral.

The problem of rising costs is becoming more urgent, the Council noted, in terms of what people are willing to spend on health care:

. . . we have heard consumer groups and labor organizations say that their members, and the American people generally, are becoming increasingly unwilling to devote an ever larger portion of their personal income to health care. Although the full extent of the cost escalation has been somewhat hidden through the mechanism of third-party payments, taxes, payroll deductions and direct employer and union payments to insurers, the day is coming, and coming fast we were told, when the people are going to discover how much they must increasingly sacrifice simply in order to maintain the *status quo* in health care services.[17]

The most important step in cost containment which can be commenced quickly is to control hospital utilization and reduce the number of hospital beds, a problem I will discuss in more detail in Chapter 5. There are other approaches to health care cost control considered by the Council as well:

1. Increasing the emphasis on prevention;
2. Changing the organizational pattern for physicians so as to encourage the utilization of less costly alternatives to hospitalization, as in

prepaid group practice and the Health Maintenance Organization approach;

3. Controlling doctors' fees;
4. When it can be done safely, substituting less expensive personnel with less training for costly personnel where the latter are overtrained for the work they do;
5. Broadening insurance coverage to include ambulatory services;
6. Substituting other payment systems for the present cost-plus mechanism under which most hospitals are reimbursed;
7. Simplifying regulatory mechanisms on institutions, i.e., designing one reporting form to do the work of twelve;
8. Increasing competition by inhibiting professional society resistance to new modes of medical practice;
9. Improving health care system planning and controlling capital expenditure;
10. Developing less costly institutional care for persons who need to be in a bed but don't need the full range of hospital services;
11. Providing for generic drug prescribing;
12. Controlling overutilization and provider fraud under Medicare and Medicaid; and
13. Effecting significant reforms in the medical malpractice system.

It is obvious that there are many available approaches to cost control. It is also obvious that central to the implementation of many of them is the necessity for significant change in individual and institutional provider behavior.

Financial Barriers to Care

Despite the proliferation of insurance plans, and the Medicare and Medicaid programs, more than one of every three dollars spent on health care services comes directly out of the pocket of the person receiving the service. This is a significant health care delivery system problem. Over 75 percent of the United States population has some kind of insurance coverage, but it pays for only 25 percent of the total cost. Relatively few people have insurance coverage for doctors' office visits not related to hospitalization, for nursing home or dental care, or drugs. This means that some people in some areas are not getting care simply because they cannot afford to pay for it. This problem has lessened in recent years with the advent of Medicare and Medicaid, but it is still significant for many poor people in many parts of the country. Furthermore, with the continually increasing costs, many persons with insurance coverage find it insufficient; cases of serious disease can destroy a family financially. The doctor's fee itself, even when it can be afforded, can form a psychological barrier to care for some patients. Universal financial entitlement, in the form of some sort of equitable national health insurance plan, is necessary to remove the financial barriers to care, real in many cases, psychological in others, which exist. However, it should be remembered that national health insurance, in the absence of a thoroughgoing program for prevention, will do little for the population's *health.* NHI is necessary, but not sufficient for that purpose.

Geographic Maldistribution of Physicians

In 1973 there were about 170 physicians (M.D.'s and D.O.'s) per 100,000 population nationally, approximately 1 for every 600 persons. That is considered by most observers to be a fairly good ratio. However, doctors are not at all evenly distributed. By county population size, the ratio varied from 40 per 100,000 in counties with fewer than 10,000 persons to 196 per 100,000 in metropolitan counties with between one and five million people.[18] (Counties with over five million people had a lower physician population ratio, 130 per 100,000, reflecting the deteriorating health manpower situation in densely populated central cities.) A 1973 study of physician migration since World War II showed that physicians tended to follow changes in the per capita income pattern, following the movement of the higher per capita income groups.[19] I shall discuss the meaning of physician-population ratios in relationship to health care services in Chapter 5, but suffice it to say here that the distribution is quite uneven.[20]

Specialty Maldistribution of Physicians

Three categories of physician are available to provide front-line, office-based, primary care: general practitioners, internal medicine specialists, and pediatricians.* In 1931, 75 percent of all physicians were in these three categories, with 72 percent in "general practice and part-time specialty." ("Part-time specialty" for general practitioners in those days usually meant some routine general surgery and some deliveries of babies, in addition to primary care practice.) The "family physician potential" was thus 94 per 100,000 population, with a total of about 125 physicians per 100,000 population. By 1957, only 45 percent of all physicians were in the primary care specialties, with a population ratio of 60 per 100,000. The total physician-population ratio was by then over 130 per 100,000. By 1972, the office-based primary care physician ratio had fallen to the area of 40 per 100,000, while the overall physician-population ratio was about 165 per 100,000. Thus in forty years, the percentage of physicians available for office-based, front-line, primary care had fallen from 75 percent to less than 25 percent. The percentage is rising slightly now as more recent medical school graduates are choosing to go into family practice and primary

*Elsewhere I have defined primary care as "medical attention to the great majority of ills." I stated that such services *should* be "provided continuously over a significant period of time by the same appropriately trained individual (or team) who is sympathetic, understanding, knowledgeable, and equipped, who is as capable of keeping people well as he is of returning them to health when they fall ill." Also included in primary care is episodic care for acute and emergency conditions not necessarily handled by a person's ongoing source of primary care. This can be contrasted with definitions of secondary and tertiary care, the set in which the term "primary care" usually appears. According to Milton Roemer:

> Secondary care consists only of curative services . . . ordinarily obtained on referral from the primary care level . . . [It] includes the services of specialists [beyond the primary-type internist or prediatrician], whether the patient is ambulatory, or hospitalized . . . in a peripheral or district general hospital . . . Likewise, long-term care of chronic illness . . . is a part of secondary care. . . . Tertiary care includes the services of the "superspecialists" for rare disorders or the care of serious long-term conditions of relatively low frequency . . . [usually] at a regional medical center. . . ."[21]

care internal medicine and pediatrics.

In relation to the medical conditions manifested by the population (see the data in Chapter 2), we have too many specialists. This leads to a number of different problems. There is a deficiency in the volume of physician primary care services available. This deficiency is difficult to quantify, but at least if one looks at the disease profile in this country one can conclude that there are not enough physicians delivering primary care who are trained to deliver primary care. Overspecialization increases unit costs. The specialist managing a patient with an uncomplicated case of diabetes, which could easily be taken care of by a primary care physician, will usually charge more on a private fee basis, and will be reimbursed at a higher rate by Medicare/Medicaid.

Overspecialization is a likely cause of unnecessary surgery. Almost one-third of all American doctors are surgeons and anethesiologists. John Bunker compared the frequency of surgery in England and Wales with that in the United States. He said: "There are twice as many surgeons in proportion to population in the United States as in England and Wales and they perform twice as many operations. . . . Indications for surgery are not sufficiently precise to allow determination of whether American surgeons operate too often or the British too infrequently."[22] However, health levels are roughly the same in the two countries. One might frame one of those weighty "laws" of personnel functioning: "When surgeons are present they will operate." Nevertheless, it happens that there are so many surgeons in the United States that not only is there excess surgery, but even with it the average surgeon is underemployed. Studies by Dr. Walter W. Hauck and his associates have shown that surgeons perform an average of 3.7 operations per week, based on a forty-six-week working year. About 50 percent of all surgeons perform one operation per week or less. This is relatively little work indeed for a doctor who has spent at least five years in training after medical school and who could easily and safely do at least two operations per day. Nevertheless only 1 percent of all surgeons do ten operations per week or more.[23]

The training of specialist physicians is not subject to any rational planning process. The results are apparent.

Deficiencies in Quality and Quality Control

In Chapter 6, I will deal with this problem in some detail.[24] It is sufficient to say here that study after study over a twenty year period has shown that there are serious deficiencies in the quality of medical care practiced by a significant minority of American physicians. Related to this finding, and perhaps a significant cause of it, is the fact that control mechanisms dealing with one-on-one doctor-patient interactions, the overwhelming majority of patient contacts with the system, are woefully weak.

Lack of Planning

We have many health services planning agencies and have had a series of (mostly failed) national and state legislative efforts in planning.[25] (See also the next chapter.) The basic reason for this is that the principal sector determining the commitment and expenditure of health care resources, the physician, is at present virtually uncontrolled and uncontrollable. The main decision-makers are over 200,000 independent, private entrepreneurs, accountable to virtually no one for decisions they make in their use of resources. Furthermore, few doctors are trained to have any consciousness of the economic power which they exert collectively. Therefore, there is really no reason to expect them to have such a consciousness. Nor do most physicians receive even the most elementary training in methods of rational planning and use of the health care resources over which they exert so much control.

Strong efforts have been made in recent years to control the actions of the other prime economic decision-maker in the health care field, the hospitals. Of course, hospital corporations cannot admit patients to hospital beds, make diagnoses, or give treatment; only doctors can do that. But hospitals do make many important decisions on expenditure of resources. They also seem to have been remarkably successful in many parts of the country in resisting efforts to impose some mechanisms of rational planning on them.

The principles of health care planning are really quite simple (although the practice is not nearly so simple). First, one determines the levels of medical need in a community using the tools of epidemiology. Then one evaluates the existing health care resources available to meet those needs. Third, one determines what the unmet needs are. Fourth, one determines the content and dimensions of the new resources necessary to adequately meet the unmet needs. Fifth, if adequate resources cannot be made available to deal with all of the unmet needs, one must set priorities among them, to use the available resources wisely. Finally, one establishes a system for evaluating one's work.

A variety of health care planning systems have been created by legislation in the last fifteen years to attempt to deal rationally with our nation's unmet health care needs. However, until the private physicians who make the majority of health care resource utilization decisions are properly trained and brought into the planning system on the one hand, and until a sensible series of controls over their work is created on the other hand, planning efforts are, by and large, doomed to failure. It is simply impossible to redesign an arch without doing something about the keystone.

Provider-Patient Communication

My impression is that the communication gap between doctors and patients is one of the most serious problems in the health care delivery system, as those problems are perceived by patients. (The other most serious problem perceived by patients is cost.) Communication problems are difficult to document scientifically. However, there is some evidence. Jay Lebow reviewed a series of studies of patient evaluations of medical care in a variety of settings.[26] In many of them, it is clear that effective doctor-patient communication is one of the most important criteria used by patients to evaluate care received. For example, in one study "satisfaction was found to be related to improvement in condition, personal interest of the staff in the patient, and explanation received about their conditions." A second study found that "most dissatisfaction involved the patients' feeling that, although the physicians did understand their physical problems, they did not adequately disclose the nature of the illness to the patient."

In a study of hospital nursing care "satisfaction levels were found to be directly related to the *amount* [my italics] of care given." A study of a group practice found that "technical accuracy, personal interest of staff, and accessibility" were the most important criteria used by patients. Another group practice study found that the rating factors were "personal interest of the physician, accessibility of the service, and convenience for the patients." In a study of an outpatient clinic the most frequent patient complaint was that the explanations offered were poor. In yet another clinic study, "patients expected that physicians would be friendly and communicative and when the physicians did not meet their expectations, satisfaction was decreased."

There is evidence from the arena of medical malpractice litigation as well to support the view that doctor-patient communication, and the lack of it, is a serious problem. In 1973, the Commission on Medical Malpractice of the Secretary of the Department of Health, Education, and Welfare noted that:

> A malpractice suit reflects not only a patient's dissatisfaction with the result of treatment, but frequently it is an expression of anger by the patient directed towards the doctor who treated him, the hospital in which the treatment was provided, or both. What prompts such anger? What factors in the treatment process seem to give rise to the greatest frustration and disappointment, and how can they be prevented?
>
> The importance of human relations in the malpractice problem has been recognized by nearly everyone who has attempted to analyze the cause of malpractice litigation. In fact, there are those who believe the malpractice problem is essentially a human relations problem, and that greater attention to the human component is the only sure solution.

The Commission went on to say:

> The quality of the relationship between the patient on the one hand and the doctor or hospital on the other may stimulate the patient either toward or away from filing a malpractice suit. In plain truth, the suit itself is often merely tangible proof of the final breakdown of that relationship.
>
> "If understanding between physician and patient is not commensurate with the necessary diagnostic and therapeutic activities, there is a strong possibility of a failure of treatment, the collapse of the relationship, or both. If both occur at about the same time, chances for a lawsuit are strong."*

*The Commission quoted here from Louisell and Williams, *Medical Malpractice,* Matthew Bender and Co., New York, Sec. 5.02, p. 137.

The Commission then pointed out that:

> Doctors themselves are acutely aware of this problem. Indeed, of physicians who responded to a questionnaire sent out by a professional magazine [*Medical Opinion,* December, 1971], 37 percent of 420 who had been sued or threatened with suit and 44 percent of 448 who had been sued or threatened named "poor communication between physician and patient" as the single most common cause of malpractice suits.[27]

This view has been confirmed to me in private conversations with a number of practicing physicians. Since patients are not in a position to judge the technical quality of care in many cases, except in instances where the outcome is grossly poor, this phenomenon is really to be expected. A large scale study of patient attitudes by Janet Birch and Samuel Wolfe showed that most people never seem to question the technical competence of their physicians.[28] Patient complaints about health services are more likely to focus on provider attitudes, waiting time, the physical environment of care, availability and accessibility of services, and costs. Studies currently underway by the American Bar Association are likely to show that there is little relationship between malpractice suits and the technical quality of care. The two key factors seem to be on the one hand the relative risks of a bad result from the treatment procedure involved, no matter how good the technical quality of the care (orthopedic surgeons and anesthesiologists are much more likely to be sued than are pediatricians), and on the other, the quality of the famed (ill-famed?) doctor-patient relationship.

Marvin Belsky is an internist in New York City who has done pioneering work in teaching patients how to evaluate medical care in the private fee-for-service sector. He is the first physician I know who has set up regular "feedback" sessions with groups of his patients so that they can discuss with him the manner in which he practices medicine and relates to them. In his book *Beyond the Medical Mystique: How to Choose and Use Your Doctor,* Dr. Belsky says:

> Faulty communication between physician and patient wastes the time and effort of both, leads to treatment on the basis of inadequate information, causes needless patient dissatisfaction. The communication gap and

educational vacuum between physician and patient is the most serious and significant impediment to their therapeutic relationship.[29]

In certain cases, the fault for poor communication does lie with patients who simply will not listen or ask questions, and who seem just not to care. However, it seems to me that we doctors have a professional responsibility to make sure that explanations are made in language and in such a manner that patients can understand. We must be interested in people, not just diseases or organs. We must not assume that most people are stupid. They may be ignorant of medical matters, but many can learn if messages are given clearly. Further, a friendly word, an unrushed, relaxed feeling, a nice smile, a couple of minutes of explanation are not really difficult for doctors to manage, if they give it a little thought. A fourth-year student of mine, then on the surgical service in the hospital at which we were working, once made an interesting remark on this point during a discussion about doctor-patient communication. "Why," she said, referring to the house staff and attendants with whom she worked "can't they at least face the patient when they are talking at the foot of the bed?"

My sample is certainly not a random one, but so many times when patients I know talk to me about their personal physicians, they begin with words to the effect of: "My doctor won't talk to me." I find myself explaining diagnoses, or disease processes, or treatment plans to these patients when they really should already have that information. In most cases, reasonable explanations can be made in a few minutes. Most patients seem to catch on quickly and are often reassured.

Of course I am not at all surprised that many doctors are unable to construct simple explanations in English, not Greek or Latin, that doctors are at times lacking in simple good manners and exhibit behavior bordering on the grossly impolite, that doctors don't seem to mind keeping people waiting, or that many doctors appear to their patients to place themselves on pedestals from which they on occasion speak to their patients. In fact, I am surprised that so many doctors do manage to communicate reasonably well with their patients, and do manage to treat them as people, not simply diseases.

I am not surprised in the first instance and am surprised in the second because in so few medical schools is any significant amount of time given to the problem area of doctor-patient communications. (In fact, little time is even given to doctor-doctor communication, so that it is little wonder that peer review of quality of care is a process with many problems.) There are techniques for establishing rapport. One can be trained to listen, and listen sympathetically. Politeness is easily taught, by example. So is thoughtfulness. The techniques for making explanations simple, or making them at all can be taught as well. But in most schools, as far as I can tell, these things are not done. In fact, the opposite is often done, either consciously or unconsciously. The Medical Mystique, that quintessential barrier to communication is carefully nurtured, consciously and unconsciously, and each medical student is imbued with its aura.

In describing the Medical Mystique, Dr. Belsky cites Eliot Freidson, the medical sociologist. Belsky lists, and comments on, Freidson's six components of the Medical Mystique:

> The first is that the doctor is always saving the life of every patient he sees. That is simply not so. Most illness does not involve life and death, which means that many elements of judgment and training are not all that arcane.
>
> A second element of the modern medical mystique is that medicine is a precise, effective science. The truth is that it's neither precise nor effective on many occasions; to the contrary, it may be imprecise and ineffective.
>
> A third rationalization of the mystique is that judgment is so complex in medicine that the physician exercising it can't, himself, be judged. Not so—the diagnosing physician is often comparing symptoms to criteria that may be as basic and fixed as multiplication tables. To be a good diagnostician, he has to know his fundamentals.
>
> The fourth is that doctors are perpetually rational. This assumes that doctors are immune to human frailties, that they don't get tired or lose their edge. Doctors are human. They do get tired. Their interest does flag.
>
> A fifth aspect of the mystique is that the quality of medical work is "assured by a long, arduous course of professional training." Actually, much of what was learned may be forgotten. Doctors' knowledge becomes stale. It requires constant replenishment through continuing education.
>
> Finally, the medical mystique assumes that doctors comprise a re-

sponsible, organized profession dedicated to the public good. The truth is that dedication is variable, and doctors are no more or less dedicated than members of other professions.[30]

The most important failing of the health care delivery system in relationship to the population as a whole is that the system is failing to prevent preventable disease. It appears as if the most important failing of the individual doctor in dealing with the individual patient is the inability to adequately communicate with and personally relate to their patients. Both of these problems begin —and could be easily resolved—in medical school. They are both products of the Medical Mystique.

Professional Irrelevance

The final serious problem I see is that of professional irrelevance. This is produced by the "we know best" and "we will do what we want to do when we want to do it" philosophy of the Medical Mystique. One can look at the population disease and illness profile which I presented in the last chapter. Most patients have relatively common problems. The common diseases in the population are—well—just that: common.

Most patient-care contacts, about 80 percent of them in fact, take place in doctors' offices. On the average, each American sees a doctor in his office between five and six times per year. On the average, only one in seven Americans is hospitalized during the course of a year. Kerr White, formerly Professor of Health Care Organization at the Johns Hopkins University School of Public Health, now Director of the Institute for Health Care Studies of the United Hospital Fund in New York City, has pointed out that during 1970, of every 1000 persons in the population, 720 consulted a physician (become a "patient") in an ambulatory setting at least once during the year, 100 were admitted to a hospital at least once, and only 10 were admitted to a university hospital at least once.[31] Since university hospitals by choice focus both their research and patient-care work on the relatively uncommon, persons with relatively rare conditions are likely to be admitted to university hospitals in numbers out of proportion to their frequency in the general population. Since medical education is carried out primarily in university hospitals it is little wonder that it tends to focus on the relatively uncommon. Let me give you a few examples, some anecdotal, some with a broader factual basis.

I remember clearly the introduction to the first lecture on glucosuria (sugar in the urine) given to my second year class in medical school. One of the bright young men from my school's world-renowned endocrine system research lab had come bounding across the street to give this lecture. "Nine hundred ninety-nine out of 1000 cases of glucosuria are due to diabetes mellitus," he began, introducing an epidemiological reference (a rare event in itself). "Therefore, I am going to talk to you about idiopathic glucosuria" (sugar in the urine due to an unknown cause). I remember little of the rest of the lecture, have never seen a patient with idiopathic glucosuria, and have never even heard of one, except in the literature. On the other hand, it is estimated that 4 percent of the United States population has diabetes mellitus, with only half of those people knowing that they have the disease.

One is generally taught in medical school to equate rare with "interesting" and common with "uninteresting." Pity the poor majority. Although the bulk of care is given to ambulatory (literally, walking under their own power) patients, the vast majority of medical education, both in medical school and in the postgraduate years, takes place in hospitals—in medical school hospitals.

I recall sitting in a curriculum committee meeting at my school discussing the organization of so-called "clinical correlative" sessions for second-year medical students so that they could see some of the clinical applications of the basic medical science they are learning at the time. I suggested that it might be useful to run the clinical correlation sessions in ambulatory care settings so that the students could see the elucidation of basic medical science principles in ordinary patients with ordinary problems. One of my colleagues, who happens to be both a physician and a basic scientist objected, saying, "What can students learn in the clinic?" In other words, only the hospitalized patient has anything worth learning about.

It is instructive to look at the tables of contents of our leading medical journals. A great deal of the research reported in them just bears no relationship to the disease profile of the population. I am not saying that the rare and unusual should not be investigated. Of course it should. For patients with rare diseases, it is important that someone, somewhere understands them, and if possible knows how to treat them. Nor am I condemning basic biological research which may someday lead to a better understanding of common—or rare—diseases. What I do strongly criticize is the imbalance which now exists in our research establishment. The Medical Mystique, or perhaps better expressed, the Biomedical Mystique, is as pervasive there as it is in medical education and clinical medicine.

As a second year medical student, I was taught microbiology, the biology of bacteria and viruses, by a department in which *no one* had worked on infectious disease for seven years. And that was in 1959! The faculty were all bacterial geneticists. The one thing I remember from the final examination in that course was that we were asked a series of questions about the physiology of a bacterium which doesn't even cause a disease!

These are all examples of professional irrelevance. Our population has a particular disease profile, but our training and research establishments do not appear to be interested in it; they focus on quite a different picture. This is, of course, a theme with which I will deal again. We now turn, in the next three chapters, to a description of how our health care delivery system presently operates.

SECTION II

U.S. Health Care Delivery System: Current Status

4

Government and Financing

Let us all strive to be bigger than government, not in arrogance of power but in loftiness of spirit and demonstrated concern for the public we serve.

—*Raymond Holden, M.D.*
Chairman of the Board of Trustees
American Medical Association, 1977

In a free enterprise system, the practicing physician is, in a sense, an entrepreneur. As a businessman, he has the right to charge on a fee-for-service basis, which can be described as a "social contract." The fee-for-service arrangement protects the interests and the freedom of patient and physician alike.

—American Medical News

Government plays a variety of roles in the U.S. health care delivery system. It licenses and regulates both individual and institutional providers of care. It is a direct provider of health services —personal, community, and combined. It engages in planning. It carries out biomedical and health services research and educates many categories of health care personnel. It constructs health care facilities. Finally, through many different programs, government finances the provision of health services, planning, research, education, and construction by nongovernmental institutions and individuals. Government in the United States does not provide the single framework for the system, as it does in so many of the other advanced capitalist countries. Nonetheless, it is a very important factor in the system. Before I go on to describe government activities in some detail, I will present the briefest outline of governmental structure in our country, to aid in an understanding of the very complex involvement of government in the health care delivery system.[1]

Principles of Government in the United States

The two basic constitutional principles on which the structure of government in the United States is based are the sharing of sovereignty between the federal government and the states, and the separation of powers. Sovereignty is the basic power a government has to assert its will over its constituents. This power is ultimately backed up by the force of arms. The original founders of the United States were, in effect, thirteen independent sovereign entities which banded together and agreed, through the Constitution, to share some of their sovereignty with a new entity, the federal government.

Among the powers retained by the states is the police power, i.e., the power "to enact and enforce laws to protect and promote the health, safety, morals, order, peace, comfort, and general welfare of the people."[2] The police power is not specifically mentioned in the Constitution. Therefore, under the terms of the tenth Amendment, "The powers not delegated to the United States by the constitution, nor prohibited by it to the states, are reserved to the states respectively, or to the people," the states have the police power. It is the basis for their authority in health matters. Among the states' other inherent powers is delegation of authority. The states have used it to create the third tier of the governmental system, local government. Most states have delegated some of their powers in health matters to local government.

Because of the sharing of sovereignty, the federal government has some power in health affairs as well, although health is not specifically mentioned in the Constitution. The federal government's health authority is derived from its power to tax and spend for the general welfare, and to regulate interstate and foreign commerce, as provided for in Article I, Section 8 of the Constitution. Thus the Constitution directly created a two-tiered governmental system. The inherent delegatory powers of the states have led to a basic three-tiered system of government in this country: federal, state, and local. (In many states, there is more than one level of local government, but since all their powers are delegated by the states, for our purposes it is simpler to just subsume the several possible levels of local government under one heading. At any rate, in most areas it is only county or municipal government, rather than town or village government, which has any significant health functions.) As we shall see below, all three levels of government are active in health matters in a variety of ways.

In addition to the horizontal, federal-state-local division of government, there are the vertical divisions created by the Constitutional provisions for separation of powers at the federal level—the clear creation of three independent and interdependent branches of government: executive, legislative, and judicial. The independence/interdependence is achieved by the famed system of "checks and balances." The tripartite form, with checks and balances, is followed fairly closely by state governments. At the local level, the boundaries between branches become rather blurred: for example, in some areas the local chief executive officer presides over the local legislative body.

Basic Functions of the Three Branches of Government Legislatures

Each branch of government has an important role to play in health affairs. Legislatures enact the legal framework within which the health care delivery system functions. They may impose certain requirements for planning and development of the system and for quality measurement and control. If the government is to participate in health care financing or directly deliver service, those programs must first be established by legislative acts. Overall, it is the responsibility of legislatures to set policy and define programs.

The Judiciary

The judicial branches in the three levels of government have important health powers too, both civil and criminal. Since they cannot apprehend, prosecute, or punish transgressors, the courts must work in concert with the law enforcement arms of the executive branches. Together they form the civil and criminal justice systems. The civil and criminal justice systems, of course, enforce laws as created by the legislatures.

The civil and criminal justice systems support the work of the other components of the government in adjudicating disputes related to health care, and in protecting the rights of individuals under the due process and equal protection clauses of the Constitution. Most importantly, although a legislature creates a licensing law for physicians and an executive branch administers it, the criminal justice system enforces it, if necessary by sending to jail a person who "practices medicine without a license."

Legislatures are passing an increasing number of laws attempting to regulate one or another part of the health care delivery system. Often one or another provider group feels that its ox has been gored. As gored oxen often do in our country, the offended provider group may turn to the civil justice system for relief. Through litigation, providers avail themselves of the functions of one branch of the government to deal with what they feel are unconstitutional, illegal, or unwarranted intrusions into their work by one or both of the other branches.

Finally, malpractice litigation is one method by which dissatisfied consumers attempt to get some kind of satisfaction from providers who the consumers feel have wronged them in some fashion. The civil justice system is the arena in which malpractice litigation is carried out.

The Executive—An Overview

In speaking of "government in health care," we usually mean the executive branch that administers programs, not the legislature that creates them, or the courts that adjudicate disputes arising from them. In the remainder of the chapter, the term "government" will generally mean "the executive branch of government," but I will use the shorter term because it is common parlance, and much less cumbersome. In addition to administering specific direct service and financing programs, a large and ever-growing responsibility, executive branches regulate the work of both individual and institutional providers. They also have an important role to play in setting policy. The executive branches cannot write legislation or create new programs. However, they can and often do make proposals to the legislative branches. Also, by indicating in advance how it would respond to legislative initiatives, the executive branches can strongly influence the shape of legislation. The courts, too, have an influence on health policy, through legal decision-making and the creation of case-law.

Government Activities in Health and Health Care

Licensing

Since medical practice (the treatment of ill individuals) is the centerpiece of health care delivery systems as we know them today, the overall character of any health care delivery system is determined by the mode of medical practice within it. By mode of medical practice I mean the content of the work of the physicians and its theoretical basis, the accepted norms and standards of good medical care, the degree of control that physicians have over the utilization of health care resources and how they exert that control, their hierarchical relationships with other health care providers, the character of their relationships with their patients, and the degree to which they have exclusive authority to practice that body of work defined as medicine.

The legal basis of any mode of medical practice is determined by the licensing system, which establishes and codifies the various elements of medical practice. Thus licensing of individual providers, which determines who may and may not deliver what kinds of health services, and, in theory at least, establishes minimum standards, is the most important function of government in the health care delivery system.

The licensing system, which is discussed in detail in Chapter 6, gives physicians tight control over the central product of the system: medical services. By exercising this control, physicians largely determine the structure of the health care delivery system—how it is organized, the types and functions of the institutions, and the powers of personnel.

Certain kinds of institutions are licensed in our system. Institutional licensure sets minimum standards for their work and to some extent investigates the qualifications and characteristics of owners and providers. However, institutional licensing is fundamentally different in its basic nature from individual licensing, as I shall explain further in Chapter 6.

In the United States, licensing is carried out primarily by the states, and all three branches of government are involved: the legislatures enact the statutes, the executive branches administer them, and the courts interpret and enforce them. Related to licensing, a process occurring at discrete points in time, is regulation which is, in theory at least, an ongoing process. There is government regulation of both individual and institutional providers and I shall return to its consideration in Chapter 6 as well.

Direct Provision of Health Services

Personal Health Services

The federal government generally provides care to categories of persons, defined by present or former occupation, or, in the case of American Indians and Alaskan Eskimos, by a special historical relationship to the federal government. Merchant seamen, employees of the United States Public Health Service (USPHS) and their families, and certain other federal government beneficiaries can receive care in USPHS hospitals. Veterans with service-related disabilities, recipients of Veterans Administration pensions, veterans sixty-five years of age and older, and medically indigent veterans can receive care from Veterans Administration health care facilities. The Department of Defense is a major direct provider of health services to military and civilian employees of the armed forces and their dependents, both in this country and overseas.

The USPHS provides health services to American Indians and Alaskan Eskimos.

State governments, in comparison, offer direct services for person with categories of disease. The two main health problems for which state governments have historically taken responsibility are mental illness and tuberculosis. Local governments have traditionally provided direct health services to categories of persons defined by socioeconomic class. Care for the poor and the medically indigent* is generally the responsibility of county and municipal governments. There are some overlaps: the federal government cares for persons afflicted with leprosy and narcotics addiction, and operates St. Elizabeth's Hospital, a mental institution in the District of Columbia; governments at all levels provide care for prisoners; but the distinction holds for the most part.

Community and Combined Services

Government at all levels is a major provider of community health services such as pure water supply and sanitary sewage disposal; food and drug inspection and regulation; communicable disease control; vital statistics and public health laboratory work. However, there are certain activities which are shared with the private sector. In public health education the voluntary agencies—for example, the Cancer Society and the Heart Association—are very important. Private refuse collectors are important in solid waste disposal. Private organizations are very active in environmental protection. Private institutions of course play a vital role in health sciences education and research.

Government is an important factor in the delivery of combined health services, those which have both personal and community aspects—for example, immunization and treatment of venereal disease and tuberculosis.

Planning for Health Services

Legislated efforts in planning for health services at the federal level go back to the so-called "Hill-Burton Act" of 1946. It provided federal money, channeled through state government agen-

*Persons not able to afford medical care but otherwise self-supporting.

cies, to assist in the construction of general hospitals, usually of the voluntary type. (See Chapter 4.) Certain planning efforts were required of state governments if they were to be eligible to receive funds for distribution to hospitals. There have been several pieces of federal health care planning legislation since then, as well as individual efforts in certain states. As of 1977, the existing federal health planning legislation was the National Health Planning and Resource Development Act of 1974 (Public Law 93–641). It may be renewed, or completely revised by Congress in 1978.

This is not the place to go into detail on the planning act, but a few comments might be made.[3] This legislation combined provisions of the original Hill-Burton Act and its subsequent modifications with two pieces of legislation created by the 89th Congress: the Regional Medical Program Act of 1965 and the Comprehensive Health Planning Act of 1966, and their subsequent modifications. It provided for combined federal-state-local government efforts in health services planning, with significant input from health services consumers at the local and state levels. The principal organs for planning are the Health Systems Agencies, HSAs, which now blanket the country; there are about two hundred Health Systems Areas, designated by the Secretary of the USD HEW in cooperation with the state governors. Policy-making bodies under this legislation must have consumer majorities.

The Health Systems Agencies have a great deal of responsibility on paper, however their actual powers are limited. Although the HSAs are required by law to write forward, positive plans for the development of health services in their areas, they have no power to implement those plans. They can only react to proposals made by institutions and agencies. They do have significant authority in this regard. They must approve or disapprove proposals by any hospital receiving federal funds of any kind (including Medicare/Medicaid), to expand, significantly renovate or build new facilities, or to purchase expensive equipment. This is called the "certificate-of-need" power. The institution must be able to clearly demonstrate a need for the new beds and facilities which it wishes to add, otherwise it will not be permitted to do so. HSA decisions are reviewed and formally approved at the state level, but it is as yet unclear whether or not the state planning agencies are significantly altering HSA decisions. The HSAs have similar review powers over applications for grant funds under the Public Health Service Act.

HSAs thus operate under two severe limitations. First, they have no control over the principal resource utilization decision-makers in the health care delivery system, the doctors, at least as the law is now interpreted and implemented. Therefore, HSAs, and their parent state agencies, cannot deal with the twin problems of geographic and specialty maldistribution. They can attempt to deal with the over-supply of hospital beds through certification-of-need, but they have no powers to deal with over-hospitalization in existing beds and with excess surgery—both the responsibility of doctors.

Second, and most important, HSAs have no positive planning powers. They can only react to the proposals of others; they cannot implement, except possibly by cajolery and exhortation. I pointed out in the previous chapter that health services planning consists primarily of identifying unmet needs and then developing services to meet them. HSAs can do the former but not the latter. To use a simile of our times, planning without implementation is like sex without orgasm, while its opposite, implementation without planning, which is carried out by too many providers, is like orgasm without foreplay.

Research and Education

In later chapters, I shall return to the very significant government role in these areas in some detail. The bulk of financing for medical education and research comes from government sources. The federal government directly participates in the medical education system through the Veterans Administration hospitals. Most state governments operate medical schools, sometimes the only ones in their states. The federal government, some state governments, and an occasional local government directly engage in biomedical and health services research; they also provide a great deal of financial support through grants and contracts for research carried on in non-governmental agencies and institutions. Payments for medical services provided in medical school hospitals under Medicare and Medicaid provide an important source of both institutional and faculty support.

Financing

Government participates in financing in three ways. First, the three levels of government directly finance the operation of their own programs. Second, the federal government provides money to state and local governments, and state governments provide money to local governments (so-called "grants-in-aid") for program operations. As I have noted, various government jurisdictions finance education, research, construction, and health services program development and operation by non-governmental institutions and agencies. For example, there are federal government grants for the development of health maintenance organizations and the operation of neighborhood health centers. (See next chapter.) This can be called indirect governmental program financing, since the government provides the money but does not operate the program. Third, the federal government operates the Medicare program, and, with state and some local governments, the Medicaid program. Thus the government acts as a third-party payor (neither the provider nor the patient), running a health insurance program.

Summary

Government has a multiplicity of roles in the health care delivery system. Its involvement increases every year, particularly as costs continue to escalate. However, it operates only part of the system and shares its control with many other loci of power.

Financing for Health Services

Health services is the third largest industry in the country in terms of gross annual product; only manufacturing and retail trade are larger. There are four major categories of health care expenditures: how much money is spent, where does it come from, where does it go, and how is it paid out. In this section I will refer only occasionally to dollar amounts. They change (mostly upwards) every year. I will primarily report percentage distributions, which for the most part change relatively slowly over time.

How Much is Spent?

According to the Social Security Administration in fiscal 1976 we spend around $140 billion, 8.6 percent of the Gross National Product—a large sum and in comparison with most other countries a high proportion. Even so, this is probably a low estimate for several reasons. One is that the figures on doctors and dentists incomes are obtained from the Internal Revenue Service.

Where Does the Money Come From?

Ultimately, of course, all the money to pay for services comes from the pockets of the people of the country; thus I am really discussing the routes which money takes on its way from the consumers to the providers.

PUBLIC OUTLAYS. About 42 percent of all health care expenditures are made by governments.[4] Two-thirds of this amount (28 percent of the total) is paid by the federal government, the balance by state and local governments. About 70 percent of all federal government outlays are in the form of third-party payments, while about 53 percent of state and local expenditures are in that form.

The two principal public third-party payment programs are Medicare and Medicaid. Although they were passed together as amendments to the Social Security Act in 1965, Medicare and Medicaid are in principle quite different measures (besides being designed for different population groups). Medicare is a uniform federal program, originally based in the Social Security Administration,* financed primarily by social security taxes, available to all persons sixty-five and over regardless of income. (Persons ineligible for Social Security may buy into the program.) It has copayment and deductible features (co-insurance),** offers a limited

*In 1977, a USDHEW reorganization took Medicare out of the Social Security Administration, and Medicaid out of the Social and Rehabilitation Service (abolishing the service at the same time), and placed them together in a new Health Care Financing Administration.

**A copayment is a percentage of every charge, paid by the patient. A deductible is a set amount the patient must pay for each major category of service each year, before the insurance plan begins to pay.

range of benefits and separate plans for in-hospital and out-of-hospital services (Parts A and B), uses fiscal intermediaries (insurance companies) to make payments to providers, and pays hospitals on a cost-reimbursement basis and individual providers on a "usual and customary fee" basis.

In July 1973, patients under sixty-five who were disabled and receiving social security payments and who had chronic kidney disease were made Medicare beneficiaries as well. Part A, the institutional care part, automatically covers everyone who is under Social Security. Part B is a voluntary program for which a premium must be paid. Since 1972, both parts A and B have been available to non-Social Security Beneficiaries who wished to pay premiums. Part A of Medicare is paid for from Social Security taxes while Part B is supported by general tax revenues and the premium payments. Medicare expenditures are large and growing, but they pay less than 40 percent of the health care bill for the population sixty-five and older. The remainder comes primarily from Medicaid and personal payments (around 40 percent).

Medicaid, unlike Medicare, is run jointly by the federal and state governments. It is in fact fifty different programs, because each state has its own variant developed within Federal guidelines. Medicaid is designed to serve the poor, primarily those on welfare. If they wish to do so, states may extend coverage to the medically indigent. Thus Medicaid embodies the means test principle. A "means test" is a measure of a person's net worth and income to determine if they are financially eligible (that is, poor enough) to be a beneficiary of a particular financial or service program. There is a certain basic set of services which states must offer, but they can adjust the amount of service available and they determine the eligibility levels. Medicaid is financed from general taxation, has limited provision for co-insurance, may or may not use fiscal intermediaries, pays hospitals on a cost-reimbursement basis, and individual providers on a fee basis.

PRIVATE HEALTH INSURANCE. About 24 percent of all expenditures are made through health insurance plans.* There are

*The term "insurance" in this context is actually a misnomer. "Insurance" originally meant, and usually still refers to, the contribution by individuals to a fund for the purpose of providing each contributor with protection against financial loss following the occurrence of a relatively rare but damaging event. Thus,

three kinds of health insurance plans.[5] About 300 or so private, commercial, profit-making companies of the stock or mutual variety, sell both group (primarily through employers) and individual policies. The commercial companies take in about 49 percent of the total premium income and provide about 45 percent of the benefit expenditures. Blue Cross is a group of private, nonprofit companies providing primarily hospitalization insurance. Blue Shield is a group of private, nonprofit companies often associated with the Blue Cross companies in their respective areas, which provides coverage primarily for in-hospital doctors' fees. Blue Cross/Blue Shield takes in about 44 percent of the premium income while providing about 47 percent of the benefit expenditures.

The third group consists of the so-called "independent" plans. These are private, nonprofit health insurance companies usually associated with a medical group practice plan or with a trade union. The beneficiaries of the independent plans receive health services directly from their plans, in many cases. Beneficiaries of Blue Cross/Blue Shield and commercial health insurance either have care given to them by an institution or an individual under the terms of their policy paid for by insurance (a "service benefit"), or receive a cash payment which can be used to offset fees and charges directly from the insurance company. This so-called "cash-indemnity" benefit is usually found in individual health insurance policies of the sort advertised through an insert in your Sunday newspaper.

It is very important to know that although approximately three-quarters of all Americans have some kind of health insurance coverage, less than 25 percent of the nation's health care bill is paid through insurance. Furthermore, I have estimated elsewhere that the profits of the commercial insurance companies, derived from the investment of premium income while they have it, is in the $1 billion range, annually.[6]

there is insurance against fire, theft, death at an early age. All of these events occur within a group of people at a predictable rate but are rare occurrences for any one individual in the group. However, use of health services is a relatively common event, at least over a period of years. Thus health "insurance" is really more of a prepayment mechanism which has some insurance features in case of very serious, costly illness. Nevertheless, I will use the simple term health insurance, because everyone else does.

OTHER PRIVATE SOURCES OF FUNDS. Thirty-four percent of all health care expenditures are from other non-governmental sources. About thirty percent of the total is paid by patients directly out-of-pocket. The remaining 4 percent consists of philanthropy, expenditures by private foundations to support research, private investment in construction, and expenditures by industry for in-plant services. Thus despite insurance plans, direct government expenditures for health services, and government third-party payment programs, Americans are still paying almost one-third of their total bill for health services directly out-of-pocket.

Where Does the Money Go?

Almost 40 percent of all money goes for hospital services. About 19 percent goes to physicians, 9 percent for drugs, 8 percent for nursing homes, 6 percent for dentists, 4 percent for prepayment and administrative expenses, 4 percent for construction, 3 percent for government public health activities, and 2 percent for research. (The total does not reach 100 percent; the balance is for other, smaller categories. We spend almost as much on eyeglasses and other medical appliances as we do on research.) Note that 25 percent of all expenditures go to the principal decision-makers; the physicians and the dentists.

There are different primary sources of payment for different kinds of services. Fifty-five percent of payments to hospitals are from public sources, while about 35 percent comes from private health insurance and only 8 percent is out-of-pocket. However, only 27 percent of private physicians' fees come from public sources, while almost 40 percent is from private insurance and over one-third is out-of-pocket. On the other hand, about 85 percent of payments for dental services and for drugs are out-of-pocket.

How is the Money Paid Out?

The health care delivery system is a labor-intensive industry. About 70 percent of all expenditures are for personnel. The vast majority of health care workers are paid by wages or salary. However, about 400,000 physicians, osteopaths, dentists, optometrists and opticians, chiropractors, psychologists, social workers, speech pathologists, and physical and occupational therapists, among others, are paid on a fee-for-service basis by their patients or third parties.

INDIVIDUAL PROVIDERS. The fee-for-service system has provoked a great deal of controversy.[7] Proponents of the fee-for-service system usually argue, especially in relation to fee-for-service reimbursement for physicians, that direct payment cements the necessary bond between provider and patient, a bond on which effective treatment often hinges; that it gives the provider an incentive to work that is not present under any other system; that it is justified by the special life-and-death responsibility that physicians, especially, must accept. I must say that I can see no "natural" justification for the fee-for-service system: it is simply a product of the special status of physicians, established and protected by the licensing system (see Chapter 6). Remember, the majority of health care providers are paid by salary.

The fee-for-service approach is responsible for several serious problems in the United States health care delivery system. (For a further development of this argument, see Chapter 12.) Foremost, it creates the two-class system of medical care in the United States about which there is so much complaint. If fees, which some people cannot afford, were not charged at the time of service, then there would be no need to have one set of health care facilities for those who can afford to pay the doctor and a second for those who cannot. Further, it is certainly an important factor in the problems of specialty and geographic maldistribution, over-hospitalization, and unnecessary surgery.

In fee-for-service, the cash exchange is a barrier to utilization and in some cases interferes with rather than helps the provider-patient relationship. As for the argument based on the life-and-death relationship, providers are only rarely in a life-and-death relationship with their patients. But even if this were the case more often, the argument is weak. The airplane pilot does not collect a fee for service, and he certainly has a life-and-death relationship to his passengers. The fireman does not request personal payment before he turns on the water or even after he has put out the fire. Indeed, when a fireman undertakes a life-and-death responsibility for a person in a burning building, he does not ask for a fee, even though he is also putting his own life on the line in carrying out his responsibilities, which doctors rarely, if ever, do.

Nor can I understand why a fee system should be necessary as incentive for doctors to work. It seems to me that to hold that position demeans the medical professions. Airline pilots, teachers, and many other professionals, including many health professionals, are paid on a salaried basis and work hard, doing a good job. Part of the original definition of professionalism is the existence of both an inner drive and peer group pressure to do one's job to the best of one's ability, regardless of external rewards. Furthermore, if the fee-for-service system really motivated all doctors to do quality work, we should expect much higher quality ratings for the profession as a whole than we customarily see.

The alternatives to fee-for-service are salary and capitation. Salary is self-explanatory. Under the capitation arrangement—used primarily for doctors providing continuing care—the physician receives a flat annual fee for each person who agrees to be under his care, regardless of the degree of frequency of service utilization. Both salary and capitation have significant advantages over fee-for-service, principally because the doctor's income is no longer simply related to the number of units of work that he does. Financial incentives for doing more and/or better work can remain in the form of raises. However, under this system, the profession is given the opportunity to implement and stress non-financial incentives to more and better work.

The medical profession is now organized principally in the private, entrepreneurial mode, which means fee-for-service private practice. It seems to me that the major organizations representing the mass of physicians view the protection of that organizational mode, and the high incomes that go with it, as their major task. I think that this holds back the development of the medical profession. Less occupation with money and more with the quality of our work would be healthy both for ourselves and the people we serve.

PAYMENTS TO HOSPITALS. There are four major modes of hospital reimbursement. The first, oldest, and most rapidly disappearing, is that based on charges. This method is used by private, profit, and nonprofit hospitals. A price (which may or may not bear some relationship to the cost of that service) is put on each item of service—a day in bed, use of the operating room, a lab test—and the patient, and/or his insurer under cash-indemnity plans, is billed for that price, usually called a charge.

A more sophisticated reimbursement mode is based on cost. The determination of cost never involves individual patients. It is a matter for negotiation between hospitals and the major insurance companies in their areas. In certain states, the Insurance Department and/or Department of Health may be a party to the negotiations in either an advisory or approval capacity. Cost reimbursement is used when insured patients receive their benefits as services rather than as dollar indemnities. (Almost all group health insurance policies in the United States now provide service benefits rather than dollar indemnities.) In the usual approach, one of several accounting techniques determine the cost of various services per unit of service; the hospital is reimbursed for those costs as it provides the services. Thus, if the agreed bed-day cost figure is $150 for each day of care provided to a patient with Blue Cross insurance, the hospital will receive $150 from Blue Cross. This method is sometimes called "retrospective cost reimbursement."

A still more sophisticated approach, "prospective reimbursement," is used in certain parts of the country. The hospitals and major area insurer get together and attempt to predict, on the basis of previous experience and current rates of cost-increase what costs will be for the coming year. The hospital then receives that rate per service (or in some instances, per hospital stay or even per time-period without relation to number of units of service actually provided), regardless of its actual cost. There is an obvious stimulus for hospitals to attempt to control costs because under prospective reimbursement they receive a given amount of money for providing a given service without regard to the cost of the service at the time it is rendered. This method, particularly when applied to the total hospital budget, obviously approaches annual budgeting for hospitals as related to total program, rather than to individual units of service. However, in most cases reimbursement to the hospitals is still based on the number of items of service delivered.

Finally, government hospitals at all levels operate on total annual budgets, and have always done so. The costs of various inputs, salaries, and expenses are determined; and then a budget is prepared, which is not related to units of service in any way. Although some third-party payments, primarily Medicaid/Medicare, are available to them with reimbursement rates calculated on a cost basis, for most government hospitals the proportion is small. The bulk of government hospital monies come from tax revenues. Thus, government hospital budgets are subject to other considerations besides costs and programs. As health care expenditures, particularly for hospitals, continue to rise at a high rate, and as we move toward national insurance, it is likely that prospective reimbursement or annual budgeting will be applied to increasing numbers of hospitals outside of the public sector in an attempt to control costs, if nothing else.

We have now had a quick run-through of the role of government in and the financing system for health care services. In the next chapter, I turn to a description of the institutional and personnel resources of the system, as well as some measures of utilization.

5

Institutions and Personnel

Hospitals

The hospital is the institutional center of the United States health care delivery system. Although the antecedents of the modern hospital can be traced back to the church-operated *hospices* of the middle ages, the prototypes of the institutions with which we are familiar did not make their appearance until the latter part of the eighteenth century. It is said that not until the end of the nineteenth century did a person entering a hospital have better than a 50 percent chance of emerging alive. Since that time the hospital has evolved from a place where one went to spare his family the anguish of watching him die to a multiservice institution providing interdisciplinary medical care to ambulatory as well as bed patients. In addition, the present-day hospital has functions other than delivering health and medical services. It is the center of most clinical medical training, both graduate and undergraduate; it is the principal locus of continuing education, formal and informal, for most physicians. It also trains other categories of health provider and conducts health and medical research. It is the principal institutional workplace for most United States physicians (in addition to their office practices) and the only place at the present time where they are likely to encounter peer review. And the hospital has symbolic importance: being the most visible component of the health care delivery system, the hospital becomes that system in the minds of many laymen; its increasingly complex and sometimes bewildering structures and methods have come to represent the growing complexity of the delivery system as a whole.[1]

Types of Hospitals

The American Hospital Association principally classifies hospitals by size, type, mode of ownership, and length of patient-stay. There are also cross-tabulations by geographic location, medical school affiliation, and an all-inclusive descriptor combining several of the principal characteristics: the "community hospital" is defined as "all nonfederal, short-term general or other special hospitals, excluding hospital units of institutions [such as prisons and universities], whose facilities and services are available to the public." Hospital size is determined by number of beds, excluding bassinets for newborns. There are four types of hospitals: mental, tuberculosis, other special, and general. The "other special" category includes all remaining specialty hospitals. A general hospital is the category that includes the majority of hospitals in the United States.

There are two principal modes of ownership: private and public. Private hospitals are categorized by the use to which they put their surplus income. They may be investor-owned for-profit (proprietary) or not-for-profit (voluntary). Public hospitals are categorized by the level of government jurisdiction that owns and operates them: federal, state, or local. Length-of-stay categories are long and short, as one might imagine, thirty days being the dividing point.

Some Data on Hospitals

In 1976, there were about 7100 hospitals in the United States, with over 1.4 million beds.[2] They provided almost thirty-seven million admissions, representing fewer than 36 million individuals because some persons had two or more admissions during the year. On any given day, almost 1.1 million people, about 0.5 percent of the population, were in hospital—an occupancy rate (proportion of total available beds that are filled) of just under 76 percent. Among the short-term hospitals, the principal groups are the voluntary, proprietary, local government, and federal government general hospitals. Local government general hospitals are primarily for the poor while federal government general hospitals serve principally veterans on the one hand and Department of Defense employees and dependents on the other. The state mental hospitals comprise the principal group of long-term hospital. For selected data on these hospital categories, see table 5.1.

In 1975, the average community hospital had 158 beds while the average state long-term mental hospital had 1055 beds. From 1965 to 1975 the number of community hospitals has increased by only about 4 percent. However, the number of beds has increased by about 28 percent, quite a bit faster than the population, which went up by only about 11 percent. Obviously, community hospitals are getting larger and the bed-population ratio is rising.

In 1976, the average number of days a patient stayed in a community hospital was 7.4. The average length of stay (ALOS) has remained virtually unchanged for three years. There is wide variation by age, as one might expect. Patients sixty-five and over stayed an average of about 11.8 days while those under sixty-five stayed about 6.3 days. There is also variation in ALOS by region and hospital bed-size. For example, for persons sixty-five and over, in January 1976 the ALOS in community hospitals ranged from 8.7 days in the Pacific states to 14.3 days in the mid-Atlantic states, and from 8.7 days in hospitals of 25–49 beds to 13.2 days in hospitals

Table 5.1. Selected Characteristics, Major Categories of Hospital, United States, 1976.

Type of Hospital	No.	Beds (×1000)	Admissions (×1000)	Occupancy Rate
Short-term				
Voluntary general	3291	664	23,855	77.2
Local government general	1672	182	6,348	69.2
Proprietary general	715	75	2,667	65.0
Federal government general	331	86	1,827	76.5
Long-term				
State government mental	268	261	351	79.4
All hospitals	7,082	1,434	36,776	76.0

Source: American Hospital Association, *Hospital Statistics,* 1977 edition, tables 1 and 2.

with 500 or more beds. Variation in ALOS by hospital size may be explained in part by variation in severity of disease, but regional differences are difficult to explain on medical bases alone. Measured by type of short-term hospital, the ALOS in 1975 was shortest in the proprietaries (6.7 days), longest in the voluntaries (7.9 days), with local government hospitals falling in between (7.5 days). Doctors make the decisions both on patient admission and discharge. The figures for geographic differences in ALOS are an indication of the degree of control doctors have over the utilization of health services, although time of discharge of patients with chronic disease obviously is also related to the availability of alternative forms of institutional care.

Of the admissions to all hospitals, in 1975 92 percent were to community hospitals (although only 63 percent of the patient-days of care were in community hospitals). Seventy percent of these admissions were to voluntary hospitals, 19 percent to local government hospitals. Although only 1.0 percent of admissions were to state long-term psychiatric hospitals, these accounted for 22 percent of the patient-days of care. In terms of volume of care, the dominant group is obviously the community hospital, the type of institution people usually think of when the word "hospital" is mentioned.[3]

Teaching Hospitals

In medical education, we are particularly concerned with those institutions called "teaching hospitals." The term generally refers to hospitals in which undergraduate and/or graduate (interns, residents, and specialty fellows) education takes place. The term is not applied to hospitals with teaching programs for nurses, technicians, therapists, and other allied health workers who are not physicians. The AHA publishes information on hospitals affiliated with medical schools, which account for most teaching hospitals. In 1975, there were 687 of them (10 percent of all hospitals), with over 300 thousand beds (22 percent of all beds). Their average size, excluding mental hospitals, was around 450 beds, while the average size for all hospitals, excluding mental hospitals, was around 160 beds. They provided 10.7 million admissions (29 percent of the total), and on the average day, cared for 26 percent of all hospitalized patients. They provided one-third of all out-patient visits. Their occupancy rate was 80.1 percent and the average length of patient stay was 8.5 days.[4] Both because of these figures and their obvious influence on both the quality and quantity of personnel available to the system, teaching hospitals have an importance in the health care delivery system quite out of proportion to their number in the hospital system.

Conditions Requiring Hospitalization

In terms of pathology, the ten most common diagnoses listed at time of patient discharge from short-stay hospitals in 1975 were: childbirth and its complications; ischemic heart disease;* cancer and other malignancies; diseases of the urinary system; fractures; non-cancerous tumors; pneumonia; enlarged tonsils and adenoids; cerebrovascular diseases; and disorders of menstruation.

*"Ischemia" means decrease in blood supply. "Ischemic heart disease" is due to problems with the so-called "coronary arteries" (blood vessels which supply the heart muscle itself)—the heart does not get energy from the blood which it pumps through its major chambers.

The most common surgical procedures, not counting either normal delivery of babies nor circumcision of newborns as surgical procedures, in 1975 were: biopsy (taking a small piece of tissue for microscopic examination, often done in cases of suspected cancer); dilation and scraping of the uterus; hysterectomy (removal of the uterus); tonsillectomy; repair of hernia in the groin; removal of the ovaries; removal of the gall bladder; dental surgery; female sterilization; and operation on muscles and tendons. It is striking that the second, third, sixth, and ninth most common operations are female-only procedures. It also happens that eleventh in frequency is removal of a breast.[5]

Too Many Hospital Beds?

I discussed the problems of overbedding, overutilization of existing hospital beds, and unnecessary surgery briefly in Chapter 3. I will review that material in more detail here. In 1948 there were approximately 3.4 nonfederal general medical and surgical hospital beds per 1,000 civilian resident population, with a geographical range from a low of 2 beds per 1,000 population in the south to a high of 6 beds per 1,000 population in the industrial north and far west. By 1973, the community hospital bed-population ratio was approximately 4.3 per 1,000. There was some variation around the mean, ranging from 3.1 per 1,000 in New Mexico to 6.5 per 1,000 in North Dakota among the contiguous states and overall from 2.1 per 1,000 in Alaska to 7.2 in the District of Columbia. The ratio in a majority of states lay within $\pm$ 0.5 beds per 1,000 of the mean.[6] Nevertheless, there are no known variations in health status, positive or negative, which can explain the variations that do exist.

Although improvements in bed distribution and increase in bed supply since World War II have been regarded as an achievement in providing access to hospitals for people in rural areas, the overall number of hospital beds in America has come to be regarded as excessive. This is difficult to quantify because a generally accepted definition of an excess bed cannot be found. The number of beds required for a given geographic region is a function of the number of patient-days of hospital care needed by the population (expressed as average daily census) and the occupancy level deemed appropriate for the hospitals of a given area. However, beds have not always been built in accordance with such a rational formulation, but rather because of doctors' wishes, local wealth, civic pride, and competition.[7]

Once built, the availability of hospital beds promotes their use. The popular formulation of this relationship is known as Roemer's Law, abbreviated as "a built bed is a filled bed."[8] Thus, adding beds can cost the system money unnecessarily even if the beds are all used, because they may be filled with unnecessary admissions.

A relatively high proportion of hospital costs are either fixed, or varied with difficulty in the face of short-term changes in utilization. Personnel costs accounted for about 53 percent of community hospital costs in 1975.[9] Of the balance, capital costs for a plant already purchased do not vary and utility costs can be reduced only slightly. Only expenditures for food and consumable supplies do not have to be made when a bed is empty. For these reasons, it can be estimated that on a short-term basis an empty bed costs about 70 percent as much to maintain as does a filled one.[10] High occupancy provides a stimulus to shorten length of stay, and pressure for maximum use of diagnostic and therapeutic facilities. However, increased occupancy raises hospital costs only modestly, while raising hospital income dramatically, assuming that the patient has a payment source. Thus, the incentive for hospitals is to admit paying patients. The only way to really save money in the hospital sector is to close beds and eliminate those high fixed costs. Simply holding down admissions will not solve the problem: it saves third-party insurers money in the short-run, but does not reduce to any great extent total health expenditures in the long run.

Overbedding

A great deal of controversy has been generated in recent years over the related, but different, questions of overbedding and overutilization of beds. Overbedding means an excessive bed supply, resulting in unused beds. Researchers at the University of Michigan's Program and Bureau of Hospital Administration have determined that a general hospital of 300 beds or more can easily operate in the 85–95 percent occupancy range. In 1975, the community hospital adult bed occupancy rate for hospitals of all sizes was around 75 percent nationally.[11] Although in 1974, John Alexander McMahon, the President of the AHA said, "We've already got more beds than we need,"[12] in 1975 the AHA officially took the position that the 75 percent occupancy figure does not necessarily mean that there are too many beds: the ideal bed-population ratio has not been determined, flexibility is needed to meet emergency situations, there are variations in occupancy rate by region and medical service which are not reflected in national figures.

Nevertheless, in 1975, as part of an effort to control hospital costs, the American Hospital Association took an official position against building new hospitals or expanding existing ones, but did not argue against replacing dilapidated ones or recommend closing existing ones.[13] In the 1975 AHA Annual Report the president of the AHA warned the membership against allowing costs to continue to increase and provided an eleven-point anti-inflation package.* However, a simple end-to-expansion policy may not be sufficient. Legally acceptable means of closing beds down must be devised. Financial resources to provide support for geographically necessary but underutilized hospitals must be generated so that these hospitals will be able to survive.

In the study cited above, Sattler and Bennett concluded that for 1975 the estimated national community hospital bed excess was about 70,000.[14] They assumed that although larger hospitals could safely operate with a 90 percent occupancy rate, smaller ones could not: enough beds to allow for emergencies must be provided. They suggested that a weighted national average occupancy rate of 81 percent for hospitals of all sizes would be optimal. Estimating the average cost of carrying an excess bed to be $18,-250, the authors found that the 81 percent rule would produce an annual saving of over $1 billion.

In 1975, the Health Research Group (HRG) of Public Citizen, the Ralph Nader organization, issued a report called *The $8 Billion Hospital Bed Overrun: A Consumer's Guide to Stopping Wasteful Construction.*[15] The author, Barry Ensminger, used 85 percent as his optimum community hospital occupancy rate, rather than 81 percent,

*This "voluntary" approach, which didn't work well in 1976, was endorsed again by the AHA, this time joined by the American Medical Association, in late 1977, as President Carter's hospital cost-containment program was stalled in Congress.

and thus arrived at a figure of 100,000 excess beds. Using a conservative construction-cost-figure of $50,000 per bed, he estimated the cost of building these beds at $5 billion; the annual maintenance cost he estimated to be $2 billion. The "$8 Billion Overrun" refers only to annual operating costs: the $2 billion for maintaining excess beds, plus $6 billion for claimed unnecessary admissions, a subject to which we shall turn shortly.[16] In 1976, a special committee of the prestigious Institute of Medicine, came to conclusions on overbedding similar to those of the HRG, although the IOM group estimated the oversupply at not quite so high a level as did the HRG, about 7 percent versus the HRG's 10 percent. The IOM committee concluded that:

> . . . significant surpluses of short-term general hospital beds exist or are developing in many areas of the United States and that these are contributing significantly to rising hospital care costs. [See note 7.]

Overutilization

Overutilization means that a significant proportion of hospital admissions are unnecessary. If they were not made, the occupancy rates would be even lower than they already are, and the excess bed figure would be even higher. There is significant evidence to support the position that there is over-hospitalization in the United States. A lengthy review of the performance of Health Maintenance Organizations by Milton Roemer and William Shonick cited a series of studies over many years showing that prepaid group practice subscribers have hospitalization rates that average 40 percent below those of beneficiaries of Blue Cross/Blue Shield and other item-of-service reimbursement plans.[17] Ensminger cited a short series of studies making the same point.[18] A 1976-study published in the *Social Security Bulletin* reported on the utilization experience of persons covered by Medicaid in ten Health Maintenance Organizations with a combined enrollment of almost 1.3 million people, of whom about 225,000 were on Medicaid.[19] The Medicaid group-practice subscribers were compared with matched controls. The experimental group used less than one-half of the hospital services used by the control group, measured both by admissions and days of care. In none of these studies is there any evidence that the health status of one group is different from that of another. The logic behind these findings is straightforward. Group practices tend to stress personal preventive services. Some feature early detection programs. All of them, by providing financial coverage for doctors office visits as well as hospitalization, make the former readily accessible so that patients tend to seek care earlier in the course of an illness. Furthermore, group practice doctor reimbursement mechanisms do not offer the incentive to hospitalize patients that fee-for-service does. Finally, most present health insurance packages encourage hospitalization because they provide payment for that kind of service, and not much else.

Assuming that this evidence is correct, we may have not just 10 percent too many general hospital beds, but perhaps up to twice as many hospital beds as we would really need under a balanced insurance program and a group practice mode of physician organization. The occupancy figures cited are for the country as a whole, of course. There are many regional and even local variations producing bed shortages by any objective measure in certain areas.

Unnecessary Surgery

A corollary of overhospitalization is unnecessary surgery, a subject which has received a great deal of publicity in the past few years. As I mentioned in Chapter 3, several different studies, examining both recommendations for surgery and surgical outcomes, have come up with unnecessary surgery rates in the 10–20 percent range.

Barry Ensminger, citing studies by Eugene W. McCarthy and Geraldine Widmer, Charles Lewis, and a book by a pseudonomymous Dr. L. Williams, estimated that the national excess surgery rate is 20 percent.[20] He estimated the dollar cost of that surgery at $3 billion. (Added to the $2 billion for excess beds and an estimated $3 billion for overlong hospital stays, Ensminger arrived at his $8 billion overrun total.) Ensminger also raised the issue of unnecessary death as the ultimate side effect of unnecessary surgery. He estimated that if there are three million unnecessary surgical operations each year, there must be about fifteen thousand unnecessary deaths (assuming normal surgical and anesthetic mortality) resulting from the unnecessary operations.[21] This dispute really blossomed when in early 1976 the *New York Times* projected McCarthy and Widmer's figures nationally.[22] Their estimates were somewhat lower than Ensminger's, but still substantial: 2.4 million unnecessary operations and almost 12,000 needless deaths.

The response of organized medicine to these charges was as sharp as the AHA's response to the overbedding instigations. Dr. Francis D. Moore, chief of surgery at the Peter Bent Brigham Hospital in Boston said: "Fraudulent operations are extremely rare and it's irresponsible to suggest otherwise. . . . The person who wrote that story in the *New York Times* ought to be horsewhipped."[23] The *American Medical News,* the AMA newspaper, criticized the *Times* "for exaggeration, for distortion of admittedly true facts, for extrapolating sound data beyond reasonable limits."[24] A former AMA president Malcolm Todd, quoted by AMN, said: "These figures are outrageously exaggerated."

Few surgical voices called for vigorous investigation of problems in surgery, George Zuidema of Johns Hopkins being one exception.[25] However, it is an issue with a long history. *Medical World News* compiled a lengthy bibliography with citations going back to 1946.[26] As with overbedding, the question is not whether unnecessary surgery and overutilization occur, but to what extent they prevail. It is up to the hospital industry and the medical profession to determine the true state of affairs and then to take action to save dollars and lives.

Controlling Hospital Costs

Since hospital fixed costs are so high, significant amounts of money cannot be saved by "capping" hospital reimbursement rates and controlling hospital length of stay, although measures of this sort do have some utility and should be carried out. As I noted above, the only approach having any hope of real success is the further reduction of hospitalization rates and the closing of hospital beds. It must be realized that the amounts of money paid to hospitals by insurance companies, Medicare, and Medicaid, for a day of patient care is related to the cost of operating the whole institution, whether all the beds are occupied or not, not just the cost of operating the filled bed. So all of those empty beds are costing you, and me, and everyone else who pays taxes and/or an insurance premium for himself or his employees a great deal of money.

Closing a significant number of hospital beds will require major changes in several powerful sectors of the economy. First, no institution or set of institutions likes to be reduced in size, even if it makes economic sense. Thus, the hospitals themselves will likely fight significant shrinkage tooth and nail. Second, insurance coverage will have to be broadened to become comprehensive. Third, a reduction in the hospital bed stock and a major reduction in renovation, addition, and new construction will hurt the building industry, the hospital supply industry, and the banking industry which now provides so much of the capital to the hospital sector. Fourth, a significant number of hospital workers would be put out of work, and provision for retraining and reemployment would have to be made for them. Fifth, and perhaps most important, the working habits of most physicians, those people who decide who is hospitalized when, for what, and for how long, would have to be changed. This might be the most difficult change to accomplish.

Modes of Ownership and Control

There are three principal modes of ownership of hospitals: private not-for-profit (voluntary), private for-profit (proprietary), and government (federal, state, and local). As we have seen, the dominant mode in the United States is voluntary. In this case, a not-for-profit corporation is chartered by a state government to operate the institution and be responsible for all phases of its activity. The ownership, ultimate responsibility, and ultimate control (in theory), reside in a board of trustees. The key to the voluntary principle is that any accumulated financial surpluses do not go to the owners but are put back into the institution in the form of capital investment, additional staff, or salary increases.

Proprietary hospitals are owned like any other businesses, by individuals and partnerships (often physicians) or stock holder corporations (often publicly held). Financial surpluses may be reinvested in the institution, but they may, and often do, accrue to the owners as profits. The private owners (or board of directors in the case of a corporately owned institution) have the ultimate responsibility and authority for the hospital.

Government hospitals are owned by their respective government agencies. They may have the equivalent of a board of trustees, usually appointed by the chief executive and/or the legislature for the owning jurisdiction, or they may be operated directly by the government agency. The former is the case with many county hospitals, and the federal government's hospitals.

Hospital Staff Organization

Despite the differences in mode of ownership and control, United States hospitals tend to have rather similar patterns of staff organization. A marked feature of it is the relative independence from the hospital's administration of the two principal professional groups, the doctors and the nurses, especially the former. There is somewhat less independence in government institutions for the doctors, since they are paid by salary rather than as independent contractors, but their professional status continues to set them apart.

Most hospitals in the United States do not have a unitary organizational structure.* The principal hospital operating divisions are medical, nursing, other diagnostic and therapeutic support, financial, personnel, hotel, and community relations. Most hospitals provide services both to inpatients (who are admitted to the hospital and assigned a bed) and to outpatients (who come to an emergency department, an outpatient clinic, or to a diagnostic or therapeutic service for a procedure not requiring admission). The first two named divisions, medical and nursing, are the domains of self-defining and, to a great extent, self-governing professional groups. In most hospitals, most physicians (except for house staff and certain other full-time doctors who may be employed by the hospital to chair depart ments or staff such hospital services as the emergency room)

*We are here considering primarily community hospitals, as defined above. Although some of the broad generalizations and principles apply to other kinds of hospitals, many of the details do not. However, community hospitals comprise the majority of hospitals, as we saw above.

are paid directly by the patients or third-parties. They do not have an employer/employee relationship with the hospital, but are independent contractors, using hospital facilities to carry out their work. The hospital thus becomes "the doctors' workshop."

The Medical Staff

The medical division is generally organized along the lines of the medical specialities. The larger the hospital and the more specialized the medical services, the more medical departments are found, particularly in teaching hospitals. There is no universal logic to the way in which medical departments are categorized. Some are separated from the others by type of skill involved (surgery, non-surgery), some by the age or sex of their main patient group (pediatrics, obstetrics-gynecology), and some by the organ or organ system (cardiology, neurosurgery) which is their primary purview.

Hospital medical staffs have their own organizational structures and are considered to be self-governing. The Joint Commission on the Accreditation of Hospitals, the voluntary agency which accredits hospitals (see Chapter 6), has specific requirements for medical staff governance. There are numerous medical staff committees. The more important ones deal, in theory at least, with policy issues and the control of the quality of care. In 1976, a court in South Dakota ruled that despite the fact that a voluntary hospital's lay Board of Trustees, the theoretical owners of the hospital, originally authorized the establishment of the hospital's medical staff and its bylaws, that the bylaws of the staff had become the staff's own property as it were, and that the Board of Trustees could not interfere with them.[27]

There is a hierarchical structure for medical staffs, with several grades of appointment, leading up to Chief of Service. Although the hierarchy has considerable meaning in teaching hospitals, in most non-teaching hospitals, once a physician gets admitting privileges, he is a co-equal independent contractor, along with everyone else.

Nursing

Nurses are employed and paid by the hospital, but consider themselves to be a self-governing profession and have, or strive for, a great deal of independence in controlling their work, both from the physicians and the hospital administration. Nurses have a hierarchical structure too, like the physicians. If anything, it is more rigid. In some hospitals a semi-military command structure is retained, stemming from the days when Florence Nightingale originated the modern hospital nursing service to meet the needs of the British armed forces in the Crimean War.

At the top sits the General, the Director of Nursing (formerly called superintendent of nursing or matron). Below her are the Assistant Directors (the Colonels and Majors), then the Supervisors (the Captains and Lieutenants), the Charge or Head Nurses (the Sergeants), and then the privates, the floor and clinic Registered Nurses. These are all considered "professional" nurses. Beneath them still are the people who do a great deal of the direct patient care in many hospitals today, the Licensed Practical Nurses and the nurses' aides (the laborers and field hands). Before the recent explosion in the numbers of L.P.N.s and aides, a great deal of the direct patient care work was done by nursing students.

Other Health Services

In the modern hospital, there is a whole set of diagnostic and therapeutic services some of which are directly in the domain of neither the medical nor nursing service. These include: laboratory (usually under the direction of the department of pathology), electrocardiography (usually a part of internal medicine), electroencepahlography (part of neurology), radiography (part of radiology), pharmacy, social service, inhalation therapy (often part of anesthesiology or pulmonary medicine), therapeutic nutrition, physical, occupational, and speech therapy (often attached to the department of rehabilitation medicine, if there is one), and medical records. However, even where one of these services is attached to a medical department, its personnel usually have their own director and report to him or her. For example, radiography, the actual taking of x-ray pictures, is done by radiographic technologists (more training) and technicians (less training), not by the physician radiologists who read the x-ray films. In most institutions, the radiographers are supervised by a radiographer, not the Chief of Radiology.

Administration

Health administration encompasses planning, organizing, directing, controlling, and coordinating the resources and procedures by which needs and demands for health and medical care and a healthful environment are fulfilled, by provision of specific services to individual clients, organizations, and communities.[28] The hospital's chief administrator is the direct representative of the Board of Trustees or other governing authority in the management of the hospital, and is responsible to the governing authority alone for the performance of his or her duties. The administrator is responsible for seeing that all policies approved by the board, including medical staff bylaws, are implemented.

The major operating functions of the hospital administration are finance, personnel, and hotel service. The hotel services include maintenance of plant and equipment, housekeeping, laundry, and dietary (cooking and delivery of meals). Other primarily administrative functions include community/public relations, organizing volunteer services, operating the medical library, and long-range planning.

What Really Happens

In theory, the Board of Trustees and their chosen hospital director (also called the administrator, executive vice-president, and what have you), run the hospital. In practice, in many institutions it really doesn't work that way. Because of the professional status of the doctors and the nurses, a product of both history and the law, there are really three vertical lines of authority, rather than the one observed in most enterprises. These three lines, for the doctors, the nurses, and the supporting staff, sometimes meet in the office of the director. Sometimes they never meet. This kind of separation can make it very difficult to provide integrated programs of patient care in which unitary direction is required at the functional level in order to best meet patient needs. For example, in outpatient services, it is very difficult to provide a program of comprehensive patient-centered care when there is no coordinated leadership at the functional level of service for the medical, nursing, social work, and clerical personnel who are all essential to providing that care. On the in-patient side, there is no one person who can really "run the ward," when the doctors, the nurses, and the clerical personnel all have different administrative reporting lines.

For the most part, doctors will not take orders from administrators, and nurses often find it difficult to do so, both citing their special (mystical?) patient care responsibilities and biomedical knowledge. At the same time, ward clerks find it difficult to respond to orders from nurses or doctors, when it is an administrator who controls personnel matters (vacation, sick time, grievances) for them. But it is the independence of the doctors which causes the hospitals their most serious problems. Although in community hospitals most physicians are independent contractors, they have tremendous influence over hospital operations. The physician makes most of the decisions regarding the commitment and use of hospital resources, yet he has no direct financial relationship to the hospital, nor any responsibility for its financial status. It is as if modern school boards provided everything necessary for education except payment of the teachers, who would proceed to collect fees directly from the students, as indeed they did before the educational reforms of the mid-nineteenth century. To better understand these relationships, it is useful to examine the nature of private medical practice in the United States.

Private Medical Practice

The primary mode of organization of physicians in the United States (and, indeed, of most other health care providers who are licensed to practice independently, such as dentists, chiropractors, podiatrists, and optometrists) is in private practice.[29] The physician in private practice may provide a range of health care services limited only by the licensing laws of the state in which he or she may be operating as an independent entrepreneur by requirements of malpractice insurance companies, and by hospital medical-staff bylaws. The physician, in effect, contracts directly with patients (although almost never in writing) to provide a set of services in return for payment of a fee, that is, fee-for-service. Physicians in private practice provide care on a fee-for-service basis in settings that include premises owned or leased by the physician, the patient's home (on rare occasions), or in an institution. Under this arrangement, a patient hospitalized under the care of his or her private physician pays the hospital for all services other than physician care. The physician's fee is paid directly. Thus, even when working in a hospital setting, the private practitioner's relationship to the patient remains that of an independent contractor.

About 62 percent of all active United States physicians are in office practice. About 28 percent of all active United States physicians are house staff (interns and residents in training), 11 percent are full-time hospital-based practitioners (including those in federal service), and the balance are in non–patient-care positions. Of those in office practice outside hospitals, 90 percent are in private practice, the balance working in prepaid group practices, federal service, public health centers, neighborhood health centers, and other organized settings.[30] Thus, taking into account all physicians who are in active practice, including hospital-based physicians but excluding house staff, about 80 percent are in private practice. As one might expect, about 80 percent of all visits to a physician are made to private offices.[31] Clearly, the dominant mode of physician organization in American medicine is private practice.

Although there are reasonably good measures of the number of private practitioners and of the volume of their practices, we are much less certain about exactly what physicians do. Private practice is at once the most important and the least studied sector of the United States health care delivery system. Since private practitioners of any profession are loath to have outside researchers looking into their work, this is not surprising. Other than by anecdote and personal experience, it is thus difficult to describe the typical workday of a private practitioner. Little is known about how a doctor distributes his or her time among history-taking and examination, diagnosing, giving or explaining therapy, talking with patients, supervising staff, doing paperwork, traveling, teaching, attending meetings, reading, and what have you. There is little idea of what the vaunted "doctor-patient relationship" really consists, although we have anecdotal material of the negative sort, discussed in Chapter 3 and appearing in some of the vignettes distributed throughout this book. It is not known what doctors really talk about with their patients. Although there have been some studies of intradoctor referral mechanisms,[32] we do not know very much about how private physicians interact. The decision-making methods in private practice are not clearly under stood and the ability to measure the quality of care in that setting is limited (see Chapter 6). Also, little information is available about the business aspects of private practice.

We do know, of course, that American medical practice is highly specialized, causing deficits in primary care, among other problems (see Chapter 3). One of these is in patient mode-of-entry to the system. Patients, especially those using the private sector, who can thus can pick their own points of entry, face a bewildering array of physicians from which to choose. Although the question has not been studied on a national scale, many patients using the private sector seem to have what might be called a "group-practice-in-the-head," having, perhaps, "my" internist, "my" psychiatrist, "my" neurologist, "my" allergist, "my" surgeon, "my" obstetrician-gynecologist, and so on. (Fortunately only a few patients have "my" pathologist, choosing to go to him or her at the appropriate moment, but you never can tell.) This means that when a new symptom (something a patient feels or experiences) or a new sign (something a patient or other observer notices objectively) appears, it is the patient, usually an untrained observer, who evaluates its meaning and picks an entry-point in the spectrum of specialists. Unfortunately for many patients, few if any members of the patient's particular "group-practice-in-the-head" know each other. Thus communications between them are poor.

An important feature of the private practice sector in the United States is that the majority of physicians see patients both on an ambulatory basis in their own offices and as hospital inpatients. (A minority of doctors do not have hospital appointments, but the number is unknown. Most of them are probably in urban areas.) In most other countries, physicians either see only ambulatory patients or work full-time in hospitals. The unusual American arrangement offers some significant advantages. For conditions for which one physician is technically competent to provide both ambulatory and inpatient care, as in many medical specialties, there is continuity of physician care for the hospitalized patient. For surgical conditions, in many cases the nonsurgical physician who referred the patient for surgery will participate in the pre- and postoperative phases of care in the hospitals, or at least will follow his or her hospitalized patient.

The average American physician spends about fifty hours per week working, the rural physician working slightly longer hours than his or her urban counterpart, for about forty-eight weeks per year. About 90 percent of this time is spent in direct patient care. During this time, the average American physician provides about 100 visits per week. The range is rather broad, from about 35 for psychiatrists through approximately 80 for surgeons to 135 for pediatricians and 145 for general practitioners. For all specialties, rural physicians see about 30 percent more visits than do urban physicians. At the same time, the average American physician made about 40 hospital visits per week, ranging from 50 for rural physicians to 30 for urban physicians, again confirming the primacy of ambulatory care in the system. As might be surmised, surgeons made the highest average number of hospital visits per week (about 50), and psychiatrists the fewest (about 15). These figures, all for 1973, but still probably valid, confirm that the American physician does both hospital and nonhospital work. They also portray him or her as being rather busy. For this level of work, the average physician's income, as reported by themselves in 1973, was around $50,000 per annum.[33]

Ambulatory Services in Organized Settings

Hospital Ambulatory Services

An organized setting for an ambulatory service is one which has an administrative structure and an existence of its own separate from the existence of the physicians working in it. The most common forms of organized ambulatory service are found in hospitals. Hospital "outpatient" services, as they are called, are those given to patients not immediately requiring admission to a bed. The two major outpatient divisons are the emergency unit and the clinics. Hospital staffs and administrations are becoming increasingly more confused as to the differences in role and function of the two divisions; they and the patients themselves have trouble deciding who should go where for what.

Historically, it apparently has been easier for hospitals to determine that emergency services should be provided than that clinic services should be. About 85 percent have emergency units. Their original intended function was to take care of people acutely ill or injured—particularly with life-threatening or potentially life-threatening problems that require immediate attention, personnel and/or equipment not found in private practitioners' offices, and, potentially, prompt hospitalization. Most hospitals have found it desirable or necessary to provide such services.

Historically, two kinds of hospitals have offered clinic services: those located in areas where patients could not or would not attend private practitioners' offices for more routine care, usually for economic reasons and/or those that have teaching programs. Only about one-quarter of community hospitals have clinics. Regarding this fact, it is probably not coincidental that while emergency outpatient services are not among those services that private physicians can easily provide in their own offices, the type of service provided in clinics can usually be given by the private physician, economic considerations aside.

Clinic service was part of the functions of most hospitals serving the poor in urban areas in the nineteenth century. Hospitals were relatively uncommon in the United States until the late nineteenth century. In 1875, there were fewer than 200 of them. A building boom then took place and, by 1909, there were 4,359 hospitals with a bed capacity of 421,000.[34] As I pointed out above, local government hospitals were established for the sole purpose of taking care of the poor, both inpatients and outpatients. Care of the sick poor was separated from the general custodial functions provided by the poorhouse/workhouse system for persons not self-sufficient for all reasons. At least in part, voluntary hospitals were also established to fulfill charitable purposes. One way they did so was by providing free clinic care to the poor. However, the 'voluntaries,' which were much more important in setting the style for the organization of medical practice than were the local government hospitals, established clinics on their premises only grudgingly.

Hospital Clinics

Clinic services started growing in the voluntary hospitals in the latter part of the nineteenth century. By 1916, 495 hospitals had clinics, in many cases serving an educational as well as a charitable function. However, the clinics were accorded secondclass status. When, for example, a clinic was built onto the archetypal nineteenth-century voluntary hospital, the Johns Hopkins in Baltimore, it was added at the back. This typified the approach. As John Gordon Freymann says: "It was and still is an appendix tacked on the periphery of the bed-filled tower that soaks up the pride and wealth of the community. The ambulatory services huddle at the neither end of the pecking order. . . ."[35]

In 1965, John Knowles, then Director of the Massachusetts General Hospital and now president of the Rockefeller Foundation, described the scene cogently, in terms that still largely apply, particularly to teaching hospitals:

> Turning to the outpatient department of the urban hospital, we find the stepchild of the institution. Traditionally, this has been the least popular area in which to work and, as a result, few advances in medical care and teaching have been harvested here for the benefit of the community. Ever since the day of the Flexner report, university hospitals have treated outpatients and outpatient departments as if they all had the plague. Heads of departments and professors have never toiled in these vineyards, preferring the prostrate inpatient with florid disease and the convenience of multiple test results for obvious reasons: the situation was easier to grasp, diagnosis and treatment were simpler, and all the not-so-easy to settle social and mental diseases were screened out or not admitted. Similarly, the practicing, part-time, and courtesy staff were given the outpatient labor assignment while the full-time department men (academicians) were given two rewards. They were, (1) excused from going to the outpatient department and (2) given choice of times for visiting the wards filled with inpatients. Those on the 'inside' saw inpatients; the "outs" worked with the "outs."[36]

Although little "free" care remains, clinics today still play their historical role of caring for the poor. At best, patients have some third-party coverage; at worst, they are faced with a means-test–related sliding fee scale. Second, despite their second class status, clinics do have a teaching function for medical students and house staff. Finally, many clinical researchers have found the outpatient clinics to be a useful place to work. However, the last function, and, to a considerable extent, the second one, have led to organizational problems resulting in confusion and conflict.

The best way of organizing outpatient clinics to provide opportunities for teaching and research—especially in view of the way contemporary medical education is structured—is to have a large number of disease-, organ-, or organ-system-specific clinics. The typical contemporary teaching hospital has three groups of clinics: medical, surgical, and other. The medical clinic group, which may or may not have a "general medical clinic" approximating the function of the general internist, includes cardiology, neurology, dermatology, allergy, gastroenterology, and so on. Patients may stay in one or more specialty clinics for long periods of time, particularly in the typical situation in which the general medical clinic is small or nonexistent and specialty clinics admit patients directly without referral from a general clinic. The surgical clinic group includes general surgery, orthopedics, urology, plastic surgery, and the like. Since surgical care is usually more episodic than is medical care, patients are not as likely to remain in these clinics for long periods of time. The third group includes pediatrics and the pediatric subspecialties, obstetric gynecology and its subspecialties, and other specialties such as rehabilitation medicine.

Teaching hospital clinics are staffed by four categories of physician. Voluntary attending staff may draw clinic duty as part of their obligation to the hospital for admitting privileges. Full-time, inpatient physicians, usually more junior ones, may be assigned—generally to carry out teaching, supervisory, and research functions. House staff, usually residents but occasionally interns, are assigned to clinics on a rotating basis to provide direct patient care. In most hospitals the stress is on teaching and research rather than patient care. Since house staff are usually rotated frequently between various subspecialty clinics for learning purposes, patients with stable conditions coming to a subspecialty clinic, say, once every three months, may see a different physician each time. Finally, for very busy clinics, hospitals may hire outside physicians on a sessional or salaried basis, exclusively to work in the clinics. They are usually not part of the regular hospital staff, do not participate in the educational program, and are truly what Knowles called the "outs."

Most hospital outpatient departments are open all day every day, but many individual clinics, particularly when they are highly subspecialized, meet once or twice a week. Some teaching hospitals have over 100 different specialty and subspecialty clinics. Thus, a hospital-based physician working in the usual hospital clinic organization can concentrate on diabetes, peripheral vascular disease, or stroke in his or her teaching and/or research. This is advantageous to the provider who has a focus confined to a particular disease or condition. It may also be advantageous to the patient who has a single disease problem of a rather complex or unusual nature.

Three kinds of patients face difficulties in using such clinics. First is the patient with the ordinary problem for which no specialty clinic exists; few hospitals, for example, have "sore throat" clinics. Second is the patient with a categorical disease, like diabetes, which, however, is uncomplicated. Going to a diabetes clinic, such a patient is likely to have to take a back seat to a diabetic patient who has complications. Third is the patient with multiple problems. These patients, often elderly, may end up attending diabetes clinic on Tuesday, stroke clinic on Wednesday, peripheral vascular clinic on Thursday, and cardiology clinic on Friday. (Fortunately, Monday is a free day.) This is distinctly disadvantageous for two major reasons: it necessitates multiple trips to the clinic and precludes looking at the patient as a whole person rather than as a collection of diseased organs and organ systems.

Thus the basic conflict in hospital ambulatory services is established, between the needs of specialty-oriented providers on the one hand and patients with either ordinary problems or several different problems on the other. This situation is not new; neither is professional recognition of it. In 1964, at a conference on "The Expanding Role of Ambulatory Services in Hospitals and Health Departments" held at the New York Academy of Medicine, Cecil Sheps, M.D. said:

As I saw through the sessions yesterday and today I had a persistent feeling of deja vu. I possess a book written by Michael M. Davis [*Clinics, Hospitals and Health Centers,* New York: Harper, 1927] and published in 1927. In it there is quoted a statement prepared in 1914 that describes the purpose of an outpatient department just as clearly as anything said at this conference: that the focus must be on the patient, that care must be organized around the patient, and that the hospital must take the community as its venue and not simply the patients who come to it.[37]

Hospital Emergency Services

The hospital emergency unit serves a variety of functions. It does, of course, take care of critically ill and injured patients. In many hospitals, it serves as a secondary, well-equipped private doctor's office, in which staff physicians can see their own patients for whom more sophisticated care than that available in the doctor's own office is required. A third role, particularly for emergency departments in local government hospitals, is that of primary admitter of patients to the hospital. In the Morrisania City Hospital, Bronx, New York, where I once worked, a busy emergency department was responsible for about 75 percent of hospital admissions. A fourth, increasingly important, role is the provision of care to persons who are not injured or critically ill, who do not have or cannot reach a private physician, and/or who do not use the hospital clinic, if one exists, or another organized ambulatory service, or find that it is not open when needed.

The late Dr. E. Richard Weinerman and a colleague correctly analyzed this situation:

> The ultimate solution must be found outside the walls of the hospital. It must encompass an integrated system of medical care for the entire community assuring availability of appropriate medical care at all hours and to all classes of the population. When this dream is realized, the emergency service will again be appropriately named, and triage* will no longer be necessary.[38]

*Triage, a term taken from French military medicine, describes the sorting of patients presenting to hospital emergency departments into three groups for purposes of determining appropriate treatment: "emergent" (those with life-threatening conditions); "urgent" (those with serious, but not life-threatening conditions); "non-urgent" (all other patients).

Organizational Structure of Hospital Ambulatory Services

The tripartite organizational structure seen in many hospitals is reflected in their ambulatory services. Generally each medical department is responsible for physician services in its own clinics. The pattern may extend to the emergency unit as well, or it may be the primary responsibility of one department, say surgery. Alternatively, physician staffing in the emergency unit may be entirely the responsibility of a separate entity, an Emergency Department, which may stand on its own, may be part of a Department of Ambulatory Services or Community Medicine, or may be attached to the office of the hospital's director. In teaching hospitals, Departments of Ambulatory Services, when they exist, may exert some control over emergency unit physicians but only rarely have any true control over clinic physician staffing.

The Nursing Department generally controls the nursing services for both clinics and emergency units, sometimes designating an Associate or Assistant Director of Nursing for Ambulatory Care. Likewise, the hospital's administration runs the clerical and other support services, often through an associate or assistant administrator or director.

This tripartite approach works well as long as one is not particularly interested in establishing one coordinated program in ambulatory care. When there is not one person, or office, in charge of all the resources required to provide ambulatory services, it is very difficult indeed to mount such a unified program. If one wishes to provide ambulatory services of a comprehensive nature in which the patient, rather than the disease or injury, is the focus (as discussed above), coordination of physician, nursing, and support under unified leadership is essnetial.

Group Medical Practice

There are a number of forms of organized ambulatory care besides hospital outpatient services. There are emergency medical service systems, which are concerned with bringing the victims of accidents and sudden, serious illnesses to medical care as quickly as possible and preserving life or resuscitating the patient during transport; local health department personal health services, like well-baby and venereal disease clinics; industrial, school, and university health services; neighborhood health centers, comprehensive services based on multidisciplinary team health care practice, usually funded under special government programs and located in poverty areas; and organized home care, usually hospital-based, in which the full range of hospital, diagnostic, therapeutic, and rehabilitative services are made available on a coordinated basis to patients largely confined to be din their own homes. The most prominent type of non-hospital organized ambulatory service is group practice.

The AMA defines group practice as "the application of medical services by three or more fulltime physicians, formally organized to provide medical care consultation, diagnosis, and/or treatment through joint use of equipment and personnel, and with the income from medical practice distributed in accordance with methods previously determined by the members of the group."[39] This definition excludes any combination of physicians who simply share space. There are a number of different types of group practice defined by different characteristics—the types of providers included, types of specialties included, mode of physician reimbursement, and mode of patient payment.

In terms of types of providers included, some groups can be defined as multidisciplinary, i.e., other health care providers besides physicians are included, in a health care team. Multidisciplinary groups, the most inclusive type, are also the newest in the United States. They are usually found in neighborhood health centers although this pattern is now to be seen in some independent prepaid group practices, and also in some hospital ambulatory services.

Physician-only groups may be single-specialty or multispecialty. Single-specialty groups are particularly popular in fields in which out-of-regular-hours calls tend to be fairly frequent. Multispecialty groups usually divide the physicians into two ranks, primary and referral. The primary care rank may consist of internists and pediatricians doing frontline medical practice, or general practitioners, or both. In the referral rank are the medical subspecialists and the surgeons.

The mode of physician association in group practice varies

widely. In some groups, physicians may simply share space and perhaps a common billing procedure, but not share patients. This sort of arrangement becomes a bit more sophisticated with the addition of a partnership arrangement among the participating physicians. Beyond that some groups are based on a corporation. The pattern of medical practice may be true group or essentially solo. In the latter, physicians have complete responsibility for their own patients with no other physician ever involved, except on formal referral for consultation, or for night or weekend coverage, which is usually shared by group members on a regular rotation basis. In true group practice, physicians share patient-care responsibility.

The mode of physician reimbursement may be fee-for-service (paid either directly by the patient or by the group even if the patient does not pay the group on a fee-for-service basis), capitation, or salary. The mode of payment to the group by the patient may be fee-for-service or what is called prepayment, in which the patient or, more usually, the patient's employer or union health fund, pays a premium to cover a set of agreed-to services for a particular time period. Almost every possible combination of the three methods of physician reimbursement and the two methods of patient payment is used somewhere, but the three most common combinations are fee-for-service patient payment with fee-for-service physician reimbursement, patient prepayment with physician reimbursement by capitation, and patient prepayment with physician reimbursement by salary. Although group practice has been growing ever since the first one was established by the brothers Mayo in Rochester, Minnesota, in 1887, only about 20 percent of all physicians are engaged in group practice. The five most popular specialties for single-specialty grouping are radiology, anesthesiology, orthopedics, internal medicine, and pediatrics.

Prepaid Group Practice

Although it receives a great deal of attention, particularly from persons who believe that the United States health care delivery system needs significant improvement, prepaid group practice (PPGP) is a relatively small phenomenon. The first PPGP was created by Dr. Michael A. Shadid in Elk City, Oklahoma, in 1929. A good working definition of PPGP is provided by the *Harvard Law Review:*

> Prepaid group practice may be broadly defined as a medical care delivery system which accepts responsibility for the organization, financing, and delivery of health care services for a defined population. Essentially, it combines a financing mechanism—prepayment—with a particular mode of delivery—group practice by means of a managerial-administrative organization responsible for ensuring the availability of health services for a subscriber population.[40]

There are relatively few PPGPs, although the number is increasing, stimulated by the federal government's Health Maintenance Organization program (see below). The AMA listed only 142 prepaid groups nationally in 1975, in which at least 50 percent of patients were covered by prepayment. About 7000 physicians worked in these groups, about 3.5 percent of all physicians in office-based practice. Since 1969, the number of prepaid group practices has increased by two-thirds, and the number of physicians employed in them has risen by almost 80 percent. It can be estimated that about 5 percent of all physician office visits are made to prepaid group practices.[41]

I have noted above the positive effects of PPGP on hospitalization. In 1963, George Silver summarized the advantages and disadvantages for physicians of group practice, including PPGP, in comparison to solo practice.[42] The advantages include a regular work schedule, reasonable competitive income, provision of malpractice insurance, the opportunity for collegial medical practice, better access to ancillary personnel and services, and freedom from concern with the business aspects of medical practice. Disadvantages include possible deterioration of the "doctor-patient relationship," limited professional contacts and choice of consultants, and a possible rigidity in practice modes and conduct. Advantages for patients include no or low charges at time of service, one-stop shopping for 24-hour, 7-day service, continuity of care, and protection against unnecessary hospitalization and surgery. Disadvantages for patients center around the possibility of the development of a clinic atmosphere impersonality, long waits for service, and, particularly in profit-making group practices (a recent development, not analyzed by Dr. Silver), abuse of patients through overenrollment and understaffing, the result of overselling in relation to service capabilities.

However, the most serious problems of prepaid group practice may be ideological rather than practical. Dr. Weinerman, an early, strong advocate of prepaid group practice, reviewed the experience and was disappointed. His observations, although made some time ago, are still pertinent. In essence, he said that PPGP looks great on paper, but the practical results are inconclusive; moreover, the idea really has not caught on to a great extent. He concluded that the mechanical-financial elements of the list of advantages cited above have been implemented, particularly for the physicians, but that the ideological aspects of true group practice have not. Most groups maintain physician elitism. "Group conferences," he said, "medical audits, and informal office consultations are, in my experience, more common in the descriptive literature than in daily practice." He went further:

> Perhaps most disappointing has been the hesitation on the part of most medical groups to effect changes in the "way of life" of the medical team itself. This would involve acceptance by the group as a whole of collective responsibility for the health of its patients or members . . . would mean actively reaching out into the community for . . . early detection . . . [and] identification and special protection for those at specific risk of disease . . . [and] would imply particular concern for those patients who do not use the service . . . It implies as much concern with rapport as with diagnostic labels, as much with education as with prescription.[43]

Weinerman concluded that only if such ideological changes take place, along with the organizational and financial ones, will prepaid group practice be successful. His thoughts have important implications for medical education, to which I shall return in later chapters.

Health Maintenance Organizations

In 1971, the term "Health Maintenance Organization" (HMO) was introduced in the American health care scene. Although many persons thought, and some still think, that HMO is the same as

PPGP, this is not the case. The 1971-statement of the USDHEW based on the work of Paul Ellwood and his colleagues, clearly defines HMO:

> An HMO can be organized and sponsored by either a medical foundation (usually organized by physicians), by community groups who bring together various interested leaders or organizations, by labor unions, by a governmental unit, by a profit or non-profit group allied with an insurance company or some other financing institution, or by some other arrangement. The HMO may be hospital based, medical school based, or be a free standing outpatient facility or group of such facilities.[44]

The statement went on to say that an HMO is (1) an organized system of health care that accepts the responsibility to provide or otherwise assure the delivery of (2) an agreed-upon set of comprehensive health maintenance and treatment services for (3) a voluntary enrolled group of persons in a geographic area and (4) is reimbursed through a prenegotiated and fixed periodic payment made by or on behalf of each person or family unit enrolled in the plan. This is all basic to "the health maintenance strategy [which] envisions a series of government and private actions designed to promote a highly diversified, pluralistic, and competitive health industry." Thus an HMO can be a PPGP, but it can also be a pre-payment mechanism combined with other practice forms. For example, in a Foundation for Medical Care, the prepayment system is combined with private, fee-for-service office practice.

Health Care Personnel

The Hierarchy of Health Workers

Health care providers may be divided into three major groups, in terms of their mode of functioning: independent practitioners, dependent practitioners, and supporting staff.[45] The lines separating the three groups are rather unclear at times.

Health care providers are allowed by law to deliver a delimited range of services to any persons who want them, without supervision or authorization of the practitioner's work by third parties form the *independent practitioner group.* Among them are physicians (osteopathic and allopathic), dentists, chiropractors, optometrists, and podiatrists.

Health providers allowed by law to deliver a delimited range of services to persons, under the supervision and/or the authorization of independent practitioners, often of a particular type specified by law, from the *dependent practitioner group.* It includes nurses, psychologists, social workers, pharmacists, physicians' assistants, dental hygienists, and the various therapists: speech, physical, and occupational. In certain situations, however, in relation to certain patients, many of the workers in those occupations may and can assume the role of independent practitioner. The source of many conflicts at present is the definition of the line between the independent and dependent groups.

Rather than providing a range of services to patients, supporting staff carry out specific work tasks authorized by and under the supervision of independent and/or dependent practitioners. The work of supporting staffs may or may not be regulated by laws directly pertaining to them; but if there are not special laws, they work under the legal sanctions provided for their supervisors. Included in this group are clerical, maintenance, housekeeping, and food-processing workers, research workers, administrators, recordkeepers, nurses' aides, dental assistants, and technicians, primarily laboratory and radiological. Some of these persons may assume the role of dependent practitioner in certain situations. The struggles over status and responsibility between certain categories of supporting staff and dependent practitioners sometimes mirror those between independent and dependent practitioners.

These three groups are reflected in, or reflect the three vertical lines of authority in hospitals which I discussed above. The separation of the groups is determined in part by law, in part by custom and history. A great deal of the authority of one group over another which exists in the real world of health care delivery is related to the intangibles of rank and status, in which there is a strong psychological component. Also, the majority of health workers are female, while the majority of physicians, dentists, other independent health care practitioners, administrators and other persons in policy-making positions are male. A good deal of authority has accrued to the males because of traditional concepts of male-female relationships. These, of course, are now breaking down as a result of the Womens' Liberation Movement.

There is only a certain amount of logic in the authority relationships found in the health care delivery system, since it is based only in part on a clear division of labor, resulting from rational task analysis. Although the authority structure is old and drenched in tradition, it is really rather fragile because it does not rest on a clear foundation related to the work of the health care delivery system. Thus, when a strong movement like Womens' Liberation comes along, cracks begin to appear in the structure rather quickly and easily. The doctors, having sat atop the heap for so long, with so little awareness of its fragility, are really ill-equipped to deal with the changes they are now beginning to face. Of this, more, presently.

The Size of the Health Manpower Pool

Over four million people are officially counted as health workers in the United States. Actually, several hundred thousand more people work in the health care industry, but are not denoted in labor statistics as "health workers": hospital and other institutional maintenance, clerical, housekeeping, and kitchen help. Thus the total number of health care workers is probably over five million, the largest categories being: nursing and related services (over 2,000,000), physicians (approximately 350,000), dentists and allied services (about 275,000), secretarial services (about 300,000), clinical laboratory services (about 165,000), pharmacists (about 135,000), and radiological technologists (100,000).[46]

The United States, compared with other nations, is amply supplied with health workers. The United States has one of the highest physician-population ratios in the world, about 170 per 100,000. This ratio is expected to exceed 250 per 100,000 population by 1990. The types of health manpower in the United States are also more varied than elsewhere—in the independent category, osteopaths, podiatrists, and optometrists are virtually unknown in most other countries for example. Also unique tc the United States is the number and variety of allied health manpower categories. In contrast, other nations have experimented more widely with substitutes for physicians of a scope and nature not found in the United States—for example, the feldsher in the Soviet Union, the barefoot doctor in China, and other types of auxiliaries in Africa. However, the United States is beginning to catch up in this regard too, with the development of physicians' assistants and clinical nurse practitioners.

The Question of the "Doctor Shortage"

In 1932, a Commission on Medical Education which had been organized by the Association of American Medical Colleges in 1925 issued its Final Report. Concerning doctor supply, the Report said:

> There are more physicians in the United States than are needed to provide an adequate medical service for the country.
>
> The United States has more physicians per unit of population than any other country of the world; twice as many as the leading countries of Europe . . .
>
> The present medical schools in the United States are producing more physicians than the country needs.
>
> The oversupply is being increased by additions to the profession from unapproved medical schools in this country, from physicians from foreign countries, and from an increasing number of American students who are studying medicine in Europe, a very large proportion of whom were unable to secure admission to a medical school in this country.[47]

Its conclusions were based principally on doctor-population ratios.

In 1959, a Surgeon General's Consultant Group on Medical Education concluded that:

> A growing America will need more physicians. Over the next decade the population is expected to increase by more than 3.5 million a year, with growth proportionately greater among old people and children who require more medical care. Utilization of services is increasing as incomes and educational levels rise, more people have health insurance, more hospital beds are available, and there is wider understanding of the value of medical care. Aside from the need of our people for personal medical services, a continuing and increasing supply of physicians must also be assured for research, teaching, industry, public health, and other essential functions.[48]

Again, its conclusions were based largely on the use of physician-population ratios, for which use the Group even felt constrained to apologize. In 1970, a Carnegie commission report said:

> The United States today faces only one serious manpower shortage, and that is in health care personnel. This shortage can become even more acute as health insurance expands, leading to even more unmet needs and greater cost inflation, unless corrective action is taken now. It takes a long lead time to get more doctors and dentists.[49]

Once more, this conclusion is based on physician-population ratios. On this basis, the Commission estimated that we were short 50,000 physicians, and that a raft of new medical schools were needed along with expansion of existing ones.

However, a 1976-Report of the Carnegie Council on Policy Studies in Higher Education, the successor to the Carnegie Commission, said:

> We are in serious danger of developing too many new medical schools, and decisive steps need to be taken by both federal and state governments to stop this trend.[50]

Again, with many apologies for so doing, the Council based its recommendations on physician-population ratios.

These reports all recognized that national physician-population ratios mask regional differences. They all agreed that without specific planning, with virtually any physician-population ratio one could imagine, there would be problems of supplying physicians to rural areas, and to underserved areas of our large cities (a prominent feature of our present era). However, they all ignored the central point that to rationally determine whether there are too many or too few physicians, one has to take into account what doctors *do,* and *how* their volume and content of work is determined.

Dr. Rashi Fein, in one of the first studies that attempted to go beyond simple use of doctor-population ratios, said:

> Medical manpower policy, therefore, should move beyond the maintenance of specified historically derived manpower-population ratios. It must ask whether goals can be reached in alternative less costly ways with fewer resources (or, putting it differently, whether even higher goals can be reached). It must consider the usefulness of various kinds of person-

nel. The quest is for policies that promote efficiency, if efficiency is lacking; that conserve scarce resources, if they are being wasted; that permit us to deliver more medical care to the population even at today's costs and that will enable us to meet tomorrow's demands more fully.

He added, in his conclusions:

> . . . the question that must be asked is whether at this time the greatest contributions to health would be made by increasing the number of physicians' services, whether alternative ways of spending and using limited resources would contribute more to health levels, or what combinations of both are appropriate. This question cannot be easily answered, yet it is answered all the time—whenever resources are allocated to some, but not to other programs, or when the percentage of dollars and resources going to the various programs is determined.[51]

Actually, with the present physician-population ratio, one can conclude that we have too many physicians, that we have too few, or that we have just the right number. It all depends what doctors are doing with their time. Is their work related to their training? Are they over-trained for what they are doing? Under-trained? Inappropriately trained? Does their work relate to the health and illness-determined needs of the people? What do measures of population pathology indicate about medical care needs? Are doctors doing things that other persons with less training could do? One approach to answering these questions is *rational task analysis.*[52]

In rational task analysis, the set of tasks which need to be carried out in order to achieve certain ends are analyzed. Then the tasks are divided into groups, such that each group of tasks could be carried out by one category of personnel. Then training programs, provisions for licensing, and quality controls, are devised to create people who can carry out the several task groups as defined. The aim is for a high degree of discreteness between the several task groups, for some logical ranking of degree of difficulty, for congruence between training and tasks, and for some logical hierarchy of personnel related to their real levels of responsibility in carrying out the tasks.

The organization of health care providers meets none of these criteria, because rational task analysis has never been carried out.

Table 5.2. shows a series of health care tasks, and the various health care workers who presently can and do carry them out, in different settings. This situation makes no sense. It is a waste of time and money, and most likely harms quality. I do not pretend that rational task analysis is an easy job, and will not pretend to attempt it in its entirety in this book. Towards the end of the book, I will attempt to lay out in general terms what I think is a sensible job content for physicians, as a necessary prelude to discussing a rational approach to medical education.

It must be recognized that as difficult as rational task analysis is, putting into practice a program based upon it would be infinitely more difficult, because of the legal and historical barriers to professional change. Nevertheless, if we do not make a beginning in this endeavour, we will be forever hopelessly mired in the mud of irrationality and waste.

Finally, when considering the problem of doctor supply, one cannot forget the fee-for-service system in which 80 percent of

Table 5.2. Health Care Tasks and Persons Carrying Them Out.

Task	Personnel
Suturing a laceration	Physician, medical corpsman, physician's assistant
Delivery of a baby	Obstetrician, general practitioner, nurse midwife
Giving anesthesia	Anesthesiologist, nurse anesthetist
Bedside nursing	Registered Nurse, Licensed Practical Nurse, nurses' aide
Taking a medical history	Physician, physician's assistant, clinical nurse practitioner
Cleaning teeth	Dentist, dental hygienist
Assisting at surgery	Surgeon, general practitioner, nurse, operating room technician
Directing a hospital	Physician, nurse, hospital administrator
Perform psychotherapy	Psychiatrist, mental health nurse, psychologist, psychiatric social worker

non-house staff clinical practitioners work, and the fact the doctors are so influential in determining the level of use of their services. Fee-for-service is something with which physician manpower studies seem not to deal. However, it is critical. Doctors make the majority of utilization decisions, as I have pointed out several times. The existence of the fee-for-service system (considered in some more detail in Chapter 12) means that some doctors in some cases make decisions on patient care not related solely to patient needs. To have any validity, statements on doctor supply must take these facts into account or risk being utterly irrelevant and meaningless. Unfortunately, the bulk of health manpower studies ignore both rational task analysis and the existence of the fee-for-service system.

On this sour note concerning the quality of most work in health manpower supply, I will now turn to a description of quality control mechanisms in the United States health care delivery system.

6

Quality Control and Medical Licensure

> *. . . physicians are the only people truly qualified to render high quality general medical care.*
>
> *Unfortunately, what we see today is an attempt on the part of government and persons untrained in medicine to completely dominate and take over our practices. The legislators, by law and edict, are not only unwisely interfering with our profession; but they are also opening the road to those who have not had the proper and adequate background to engage in medical practice. There is no doubt that people are entering our calling through the "back door."*
>
> *The physician is maligned, castigated, and taken to task, for the most part unjustifiably. Actually, we have become the whipping boys of the "do-gooders" of our society.*
>
> *Once my qualifications as a doctor of medicine have been established, I should be permitted to practice within the area of my capabilities, without the sword of Damocles hanging over my head. I should be given my earned privilege of pursuing the art and science of medicine unfettered.*
>
> *As a physician, I am willing to be judged solely by my peers (according to the standard dictionaries, the definition of peer is clear—"One of equal standing"). However, I will fight the mechinations of legislators and other totally unqualified individuals, as far as medical education is concerned, to judge what is right and wrong in medicine. I resent deeply being told by those who know little or nothing how I am to conduct my*

profession. I resent being told how to write a prescription, when to write it, and what to put into it. I am tired of being told when to admit a patient to a hospital and when to discharge him. I am tired of being forced by law to seek consultation whether or not there are indications for this course. I resent being told exactly what my fees should be no matter in what area and how I practice. In other words, I detest the fact that those without any expertise are trying to regiment a noble and honored discipline. They are taking over what rightfully belongs to the doctor of medicine—by education, experience, and training.

—Henry I. Fineberg, M.D.
Executive Vice-President
Medical Society of the State of New York

My Faith in Doctors

My faith in doctors
is immense.
Just one thing spoils it:
their pretense
of authorized
omniscience.

—Piet Hein

On Reputation

Nurse: "Doctor, you've given this hospital a bad name."
Doctor: "I know. Fred is a terrible name for a hospital."

—Anonymous

Several years ago, to a class of third-year medical students at an institution other than my own, I posed the question, "Why should we be concerned with the quality of medical care, and why should we want to deliver good care?" The first answer was "to protect our incomes," and the second was, "to fend off malpractice suits." A bit later on in the discussion, a student did say that there was something to good care in and of itself. Another brought up the issue of professionalism. The class eventually did agree, influenced I suppose just a bit by the discussion leader, that good work for its own sake, and the positive aspects of professionalism, were the basic motivations for concern with quality of care. This was not to say that pecuniary and selfdefensive motivations are entirely wrong, and it was not to say that they do not exist in the real world, but at least we agreed that they are, from society's point of view, at least, secondary.

Few if any of the papers on quality which I have come across deal with the question "why control quality," but I think that it is the basic one. If the various groups concerned with quality, providers, payors, politicians, and the people could agree on the "why," and *mean it,* the "how to control quality" would become much easier. I think that the basic motivation is what seems to be a natural human striving, intangible as that concept may be, to do a good job of whatever one is doing. Surrounding that basic motivation are cultural influences, which strengthen the striving feelings with ethical and moral imperatives: "Be the best;" "Just being good isn't good enough;" "Winning is everything." "Everybody loves a winner." Competition is a basic element of American life and culture, indeed of the life and culture of all countries which follow the Judeo-Christian tradition. Being "the best," however that is measured, gets rewarded in business, the professions, the academic world, in athletics. (Parenthetically, one should note that manual labor is one area where being "the best" often doesn't mean too much.)

But basically, doesn't such striving to do a good job have real survival value and thus is it not thus very explicable in terms of evolutionary theory? The bird which builds a good, safe nest, apparently by instinct, out of which eggs will not fall, is certainly improving the chances of survival of his or her immediate family, and ultimately his or her species, vis-a-vis the bird which builds an unsafe nest. Early men who somehow knew how to find or construct safe habitations, "good" ones that is, were more likely to survive than those who did not. When in modern times one adds the culturally determined ethical, moral, and indeed aesthetic imperatives, which themselves are probably at point of origin related to species survival, to the survival value of "doing a good job," the seemingly intangible "good for the thing in itself" becomes a very strong force indeed. And of course, in health care, there are many measures and procedures which do have direct individual or species survival value, if done well. Thus one major motivation for the provision of medical care of good quality is the natural human striving to do things well, which is most likely at its origin related to survival, but which has been strongly reinforced by the culture. Indeed, the fact that few if any papers on quality of medical care even bother to discuss the "why" is a strong indication of just how deeply entrenched the feeling is: most writers don't feel the necessity of discussing it, it seems to be so taken for granted.

The other major motivation to do good work in medicine is, in my view, professionalism. Like all things, professionalism is a concept which has many internal contradictions, both productive and counter-productive ones. I have not fixed in my own mind what I regard as an entirely satisfactory definition of "profession," but it does have some aspects which relate to the matter of quality. A profession is in part a field of human endeavour to which the practitioners themselves control entry and exit, that is, the members of a profession have a high degree of independent control of their own work. There is, or at least there is supposed to be, loyalty to the defined tasks and a set of professional ethics, rather than to the goals of a particular company or institution. In a profession, there is a common body of knowledge, and a continuing attempt to expand and develop that body of knowledge, so as to improve the quality of human life and extend our understanding of the nature of our existence. This last aspect of professionalism, aside from personal pecuniary and self-protective interests, adds a strong impetus to the thrust of at least part of the medical profession to regulate and improve the quality of medical care. One might say that this motivation is a particular subset of the first one which I identified.

A third reason that the quality of medical care is a matter of concern is that, in fact, the medical care delivered in this country is not of uniformly good quality, as we shall see below. While a great deal of it is good, a significant portion of it is not. Care that is not good should be identified as such, and something should be done to improve it. Related to this is the principle, *primum non nocere*, "primarily do no harm." This precept is at least as old as the Hippocratic Oath, of which it is a part. Some medical care may not be helpful; it is vital that at least an absolute minimum should be hurtful.

Finally, as I have pointed out in previous chapters, we are spending vast and increasing amounts of money on health services in this country. We should be certain that we are getting our money's worth, that we are buying the highest quality of medical care possible. Furthermore, we are concerned that the money spent is actually going to help those persons who need health and medical care, and is not being spent to meet other needs or satisfy other purposes.

Techniques for Measuring Quality of Care

If you are in the market to buy a new car, and you engage in the process of shopping around for one, you can choose from among several techniques to evaluate the various available choices. You can evaluate the company that builds the car, and the dealer that sells it. You might (although you probably wouldn't) look at the quality of the materials used by the manufacturer, the number of workers involved in building each car, the quality of the factory in which the car is built, and the table of organization of the company. You might evaluate the dealer's service department in terms of the number of mechanics working there, their qualifications in terms of training and experience, and the kind of equipment they have. This evaluative technique could be called *structural.* You make a judgement about the car based on the qualifications of the people building and servicing the car, and the quality of materials used.

Alternatively, you could look at production procedures: is the car built in one place, how much of the construction is sub-contracted out, how many cars are being built per hour, what tests are performed on the car when it comes off the assembly line to be certain that it is in working order? In terms of the dealership, you might find out how long a wait there is to get an appointment for service, how long it takes to have a car serviced, how well testing routines are adhered to during service checks. This kind of evaluative technique could be called *process* evaluation. You make a judgement based on the quality of procedures used in building and servicing the car. If they are good, you assume the car will be good too.

Finally, you can evaluate the car itself: is it comfortable, does it drive well, is it attractive to look at, does it have a good frequency-of-repair record, does it suit your needs? You can evaluate the dealer the same way: has the sales department delivered you the car you ordered, in the time promised; is the service satisfactory? You can make these kinds of judgments in two ways: from personal experience and from what others tell you. These are what can be called *outcome* measures. You are directly evaluating the product itself.

In essence, we use the same kinds of techniques in measuring the quality of medical care that we use, or could use, in evaluating the quality of an automobile: structure, process, and outcome measures. In health care systems we apply them to both individuals and institutions.

Structure

In a structural evaluation of an institution, one actually begins with its physical structure: is it safe, is it well-constructed, does it have enough space to carry out its intended program, and so forth. Then one looks at personnel: how many, what job function, what are their qualifications, how are they organized, do they examine the quality of their own work, and if so, how often and by what standards? Various criteria have to be established in advance in order to make these judgments. The assumption is then made that if an institution meets the specified structural criteria, it will provide care of good quality. This is sort of like saying that an automobile company that has a clean assembly line and an efficient table of management organization builds good cars.

The structural evaluation of individual health service providers looks at their education, work experience, and knowledge (usually measured by examination), at a particular time. Then, applying predetermined criteria, a prediction is made concerning the ability of the individual to provide care of good quality in the future. In this technique, the specific work of the individual is rarely evaluated. It is like assuming that an automobile mechanic who was graduated from a good vocational high school, has worked in a garage for a couple of years, and has passed a written exam, is (and always will be) a good mechanic. This assumption is made without actually looking at some of the work the mechanic does.

In the health care delivery system the structural technique is widely used in the *licensing* of individuals and institutions, the *accreditation* of institutions, and the *certification* of individuals. I will describe these functions in more detail below. The process and outcome techniques are also used in the health care delivery system, usually in the evaluation of individuals, rarely in evaluating institutions.

Process

Process evaluation looks at what goes on between the provider(s) and the patient, again based on predetermined criteria.* Take a medical history. Experience has taught us what goes into a good history. Were the correct questions asked, and in the correct order? If certain patient responses occurred, were the correct follow-up questions asked? Turning to the physical examination, was it done properly? If the history turned up certain information, did the physical examination follow the established lead? If the history and physical exam indicated thus and so, were the correct presumptive diagnoses (estimations of what is wrong with the patient) made, and were the correct laboratory examinations or-

*Criteria can be *explicit* or *implicit.* Explicit criteria are written down. Implicit criteria are in the head of the evaluator, e.g., what he or she thinks is "good" care. For the application of implicit criteria, evaluators are chosen on the basis of reputation and demonstrated ability. Because it is inherently impossible to reproduce and is dependent on intangibles, the implicit method is being increasingly abandoned for the explicit.

dered? The emotional and psychological quality of the doctor-patient relationship and their level of communication can be evaluated as well.[1]

As an example of this method of evaluation, one might consider what a doctor does when a patient complains of tiredness, drinking a lot of water, and urinating frequently in large amounts. These are indicators of possible diabetes mellitus. There are certain questions that should be asked in the history concerning such things as appetite, weight gain or loss, urinary tract symptoms, itchy skin, family background, and so forth. Certain signs should be looked for on the physical examination, for example, changes in the retinae of the eyes, and certain laboratory examinations should be ordered, for example, urine and blood sugar tests. If a positive diagnosis is made, certain therapy should be instituted depending upon how bad the disease is.

The degree to which the doctor follows accepted practice can be measured and evaluated. In the process technique, the assumption is made that if the correct procedures are followed, the doctor is practicing medicine of good quality. The technique can be applied to surgical practice as well. The analogy for the automobile mechanic is obvious: if the mechanic asks the right questions of the owner, and uses the right testing instruments in the right way, one will make the assumption that he is doing a good job.

Outcome

The outcome technique evaluates the results of the encounter, or lack thereof, between the patient and the health care delivery system. Outcomes can be measured in a variety of ways. Did the patient die or survive? Was the disease cured? Was functioning, of the whole patient, or say, an injured limb, restored after a serious illness or an injury, and to what degree? Was a diseased organ completely removed at surgery, without complications? Was the procedure worth the cost, financial and otherwise? Was the patient satisfied? The analogy for the automobile is again obvious. Does the new car run well? Is it trouble free? Is it worth to the owner the money it cost? Is the owner happy with it? In reference to a mechanic, did he fix the car, did he take care of what was wrong with it, does it run well, was what he did worth the money?

Positive outcomes are what we are really after in medicine: the maintenance of health, the prevention of disease, the curing of illness, the restoration of normal functioning. On the face of it, then, it appears as if we should just go ahead and use the outcome technique. Why beat around the bush? Why not get directly to the heart of the matter?

Choosing a Technique

In one of the earliest known references to quality evaluation, it was the outcome technique which was recommended as the evaluative tool. Dr. John Lister, an English physician who is a regular contributor to the *New England Journal of Medicine,* has noted that:

> . . . the need for evaluating the quality of care by outcome is not a new concept and was a matter of concern to a certain Dr. Francis Clifton as long ago as 1732. In that year Dr. Clifton suggested that "three or four persons should be employed in the hospitals to set down the cases of the patients from day to day candidly and judiciously without any regard to private opinions and public systems, and at the year's end publish these facts just as they are—leaving everyone to make the best use he could for himself."[2]

Dr. E. A. Codman, a surgeon at the Massachusetts General Hospital practicing in the early part of this century, is recognized as the grand-daddy of efforts in quality of care evaluation in this country. He advocated the use of outcome, or as he called them, "end-result" studies. He asked:

> Has the time come when hospital organization can be based on the idea of giving the patients successful and effective treatment as well as care and kindness? Is it possible to compare therapeutic results in medicine and surgery, or must we admit that no matter how much we read, study, practice, and take pains, when it comes to a showdown of the results of our treatment, no one could tell the difference between what we have accomplished and results of some genial charlatan or some less painstaking and energetic colleague? Comparisons are odious, but comparison is necessary in science. Until we freely make therapeutic comparisons, we cannot claim that a given hospital is efficient, for efficiency implies that the results have been looked into. Hospital efficiency is mainly therapeutic efficiency.

Dr. Codman proposed a system designed:

> . . . simply to follow the natural series of questions which any one asks in an individual case: What was the matter? Did they find it out beforehand? Did the patient get entirely well? If not—why not? Was it the fault of the surgeon, the disease, or the patient? What can we do to prevent similar failures in the future?
>
> We believe that the general acceptance of a system of hospital organization based on the truthful record of the answers to these questions means the beginning of True Clinical Science.[3]

However, there are a variety of problems in implementing outcome measures, the end-result system. First of all, the results can be very embarrassing. Codman had developed his technique for use by the American College of Surgeons. He carried out a study of surgical outcomes in 692 United States hospitals having over 100 beds, using criteria established by the College. He had planned to present the results to an ACS meeting in 1916. His study showed that only 89 of the 692 hospitals met the criteria. The College destroyed both the survey results and the standards before they could be released to the general public.

A second, more rational reason is that for many conditions, the outcome of diagnosis and therapy, even when both are done to the best of anyone's ability, making use of the latest and best knowledge, is far from clear-cut. We know when an appendix is removed. However, if ulcer symptoms disappear after a medical regimen (diet, antacids) and if the ulcer no longer appears on X-ray, does that mean that the ulcer is really gone? We know when a broken leg has fully healed. However, how does one precisely measure the restoration of functioning after a heart attack? What is possible for one person to do may be simply beyond the reach of another, although both have been exposed to the same program of rehabilitation. We can tell, (most of the time), when a person has been cured of gonorrhea. How do you measure success, or lack thereof, in treating a person with a disorder of sexual functioning? There are therapies for which the efficacy is unknown; there are many conditions for which the definitive therapy is not understood.

Third, there are a number of procedures in medicine in which good practice is *not* doing something. For example, it is not good practice to give antibiotics for a viral upper respiratory infection, since antibiotics affect only bacteria, not viruses. It is not good practice to use amphetamines ("pep pills") in control of overeating, except in extremely severe cases where all other attempts at weight-reduction have failed. And even then, the pills must be used with great care. In evaluating weight reduction therapy, if one uses weight loss as the only measure, one could end up saying that a formerly fat person now hooked on "uppers" represents a good outcome. It is not good practice to give a depressed person who nevertheless cannot sleep well a large supply of barbiturates, even if the outcome of that procedure turns out not to be suicide.

Fourth, it is useful to be able to catch incorrect procedures, especially not doing something that should be done, before they can lead to bad outcomes. For a person giving the history indicative of diabetes outlined above, it is imperative to test for sugar in the urine. If the urine is positive for sugar then the blood sugar level should be tested as well. Doctors have been known not to order these tests when they are indicated by history, and diabetes has been missed. If a diagnosis of bacterial infection is made in a patient with a sore throat, because white spots are seen at the back of the throat, it is imperative if at all possible to take a throat culture before starting treatment. Throat cultures must grow for a day or two before they can be read. Although one may have started treating a patient with the wrong antibiotic, one ineffective for the particular bug, if a throat culture was taken before treatment began, the correct antibiotic could then be intelligently selected without delay.

Finally, outcome studies can be very expensive and cumbersome to carry out, depending upon the condition being measured. It does seem obvious that the outcome technique is the preferred one. It deals directly with the objectives of health care delivery, outlined above. But it is also obvious that it cannot always be used, for one reason or another. Therefore, we must turn to the process technique. Even though it is indirect, it has great value in certain circumstances.

It may surprise you to learn after all this that the most commonly used technique in the United States is the structural. Dr. Avedis Donabedian of the University of Michigan School of Public Health, a leading analyst of quality assessment methodology, has said that: "It is generally conceded that the appraisal of structure is too indirect to be definitive."[4] Tom Christoffel, formerly of the Joint Commission on the Accreditation of Hospitals, has noted: "While the presence of various input measures (elements of structure) in no way assures good care, the converse—good care is unlikely where such inputs are lacking—probably makes sense."[5] Nevertheless, it has never been shown that there is any relationship between quality as measured by structural standards, and quality as measured by process and/or outcome techniques. Bad care can be, and is, given in "good" hospitals. "Well-qualified" doctors can, and do, make mistakes at a higher rate than one would ordinarily expect them to. The structural technique has fallen into such disfavor that it is no longer considered as a possible alternative in the academic literature on quality assessment methodology. The discussion continues, rages sometimes, on the relative merits of process and outcome, but structure is ignored. Why then is it so popular? To answer that question, we must turn to a consideration of the politics of quality assessment: what methods are used for what purposes and who supports their use for what reasons.

The Politics of Quality Control

Systems for Quality Assessment

In the real world, the measurement and control of the quality of medical care are not accomplished by techniques, but rather by systems for using them. For ease of analysis, I like to divide the quality control systems we have into two groups. I call them the general and the case-specific.

The general quality control systems evaluate individuals and institutions at a given point in time using structural techniques. If the results of the evaluation are positive, the conclusion is drawn that the individual or institution is providing good medical care, and the prediction is made that good care will continue to be provided in the future, for a fixed or indefinite time depending upon the particular system in question. Examination of what is going on during the care of particular patients plays little or no part in the general quality control systems. Thus in them, institutions are evaluated on the basis of physical structure, administrative and staff organization, minimum services, and personnel qualifications. Individuals are evaluated in terms of experience, education, and knowledge (usually measured by examination). Only in rare instances is measurement of what the individual or institution can *do,* what the level of competence is in actual work situations, included in the general systems. There are four general systems: licensing of individuals, licensing of institutions, accreditation of institutions, and certification of individuals.

The case-specific quality control systems, on the other hand, do look at discrete instances of patient care, using the process and/or outcome techniques. The case-specific systems are used only for individuals. We have not yet adopted the approach developed by Dr. Codman in 1915, in which an institution would be evaluated on the basis of the collective outcome of the work of its entire staff. There are three case-specific systems in use in our country: hospital medical staff review committees, professional standards review organizations, and patient satisfaction, with its subset, malpractice litigation.

The General Systems

Licensing of Individuals

A more detailed explanation of individual licensing will follow.[6] I only define it briefly here. In the United States, licensing is a function of state governments. Individual licensing represents a compact between defined professional groups and state legislatures in which the profession is granted control over individuals' entrance into, maintenance of good standing in, and exit from the profession. Most professions generally define the content of their own work and thus gain a virtual monopoly over the provision to the public of that body of work. In return, the profession, in theory at least, guarantees to the several state legislatures that the work will be of good quality. The States use the criminal justice system to enforce the agreements. The nature of medicine is such that "practicing without a license" constitutes assault and battery. Approximately twenty-five health professions and occupations are licensed by one or more states. Among the health professions and occupations licensed in all or most states are chiropractic, dental hygiene, dentistry, allopathic* and osteopathic medicine, nursing, optometry, pharmacy, physical therapy, podiatry, and psychology. Individual licensing is usually the responsibility of a professional board established by statute. The membership of professional licensing boards is usually dominated by the licensed profession itself, although physicians are at least represented on all of them.

Licensing of Institutions

Institutional licensure[7] is also a responsibility of state governments. The theoretical and legal basis of institutional licensure is different from that of individual licensure. In the former, the state is directly exerting its inherent police power to protect the public welfare. Institutional licensure is thus a regulatory function, rather than a compact between a professional group and a governmental agency. The state itself clearly defines the different kinds of institutions to be licensed and writes the regulations under which they are to operate. Regulations for institutions are usually quite detailed, in contrast to those for licensed professions, which are often quite vague and sometimes virtually nonexistent. Furthermore, institutional licensure is invariably for a limited time period, after the end of which the institution is subject to a complete reinspection.

All or most states require licensing of psychiatric, short- and long-stay general hospitals, hospitals and homes for the mentally retarded, nursing and other homes for the aged, and homes for unwed mothers and for dependent children. State health departments are the agencies most commonly responsible, with social welfare, mental health, and occasionally other departments involved as well. Licensing of major health care facilities did not become common until the 1940s. There are statutory boards involved in institutional licensing, usually including representatives from the health care field. They are much less likely to be completely dominated by providers, from the type of institution being regulated, than are statutory boards in individual licensing. Fur-

*Allopathic medicine is what is practiced by the vast majority of licensed physicians (M.D.'s) in the United States. It is based on the theory that specific diseases have specific causes, and, therefore, specific treatments.

thermore, in institutional licensing, unlike individual licensing, the state departments responsible usually have considerably more control over the actual licensing process than do the statutory boards.

Accreditation

Accreditation is another general system for quality control. It is used only for institutions. Unlike licensing, however, it is a voluntary system, rather than one based in law. Groups of like institutions or organizations with mutual interests get together, set up an organization, establish standards and an examination program, and proceed to inspect and "accredit" (or not accredit) themselves, or the institutions in which they have an interest, on a periodic basis. Certain types of institutions that deliver care, and most of those that educate health care personnel, are subject to accreditation. There is a national voluntary agency originally called the National Commission on Accrediting, now called the Council on Postsecondary Accreditation, which recognizes accrediting bodies for educational institutions. (If educational institutions are to be eligible to receive federal funds under various Acts of Congress, their accrediting bodies must also be approved by the Office of Education of the USDHEW.)

In general, accreditation involves the use of structural techniques of quality assessment. Institutions are evaluated on the basis of their physical and organizational structures and the qualifications of their personnel, who themselves are evaluated mostly by structural techniques. The basic principles of accreditation are similar to those of institutional licensure in that it is assumed that if the institution meets certain standards of physical and organizational structure at one point in time, then: (1) good quality health care, or health personnel education, is being delivered at that point in time, and (2) it can be predicted that the care will continue to be of good quality for a discrete period of time.

Accreditation is not a legal procedure, but there are strong legal and economic incentives for accrediting certain kinds of institutions. For example, the Medicare law restricts payments which may be made to unaccredited hospitals and unaccredited hospitals cannot conduct house staff training programs. State medical boards will not grant licenses to graduates of unaccredited medical schools without requiring such persons (that is, most foreign medical graduates) to meet conditions not required for graduates of accredited medical schools. Most hospitals and all medical schools in the United States have received accreditation from their respective accrediting bodies.

Certification

Certification* combines features of licensing and accreditation. Applied to individuals, it uses standards of education, experience, and achievement on examination to determine qualification. However, it is a voluntary system undertaken by health care provider professions and occupations and is neither directly sanctioned nor backed up by the force of law. Nevertheless, as in accreditation, there are incentives for individual certification. For example, speech therapy is a health profession licensed in some, but not all, states. The American Speech and Hearing Association has a national certification program, however, and many school districts in non-licensing states will hire only speech therapists who are certified by ASHA, thus providing strong impetus to ASHA's certification program. A similar situation obtains in social work.

The Case-Specific Systems

Hospital Medical Staff Review Committees

The most common case-specific system in the United States is the institution of hospital medical staff review committees. The Joint Commission on the Accreditation of Hospitals, the national hospital accrediting body to which most hospitals subscribe, requires that a hospital medical staff be organized to provide for committees to review at least the following: the quality of physician care; the products of surgical operations; deaths; the utilization of

*Confusion may arise in the terminology here. Some occupations, like medical records librarianship, use "registration" in the sense in which I use "certification," while some states use the term "registration" instead of "licensing" in dealing with certain health occupations, such as nursing. In studying a particular state, one should determine exactly how that state uses the various terms.

hospital services, in particular length of patient stay; the use of medical consultation services; and the general operations of all hospital divisions, whether direct patient care or support. The committees dealing directly with physician services all evaluate discrete instances of care delivery. They are usually concerned with physician performance in a particular case, although they may become involved with the work of other hospital staff as well. The major committees are Tissue, evaluating surgical procedures, Medical Records or Medical Audit, evaluating care in general as it is reflected in the medical records, and Mortality, reviewing all deaths in the hospital and their causes.

Before July 1, 1975, the Joint Commission on the Accreditation of Hospitals required only that hospitals demonstrate the existence of medical staff committees, and that they function to certain minimal standards. Since that time, the JCAH has gradually been implementing a program under which hospitals are required to use a particular evaluation system, the "Performance Evaluation Procedure for Auditing and Improving Patient Care," PEP for short, or its equivalent.[8] The PEP uses both process and outcome techniques, concentrating on outcomes. The JCAH does not engage in discrete-case evaluation itself, but requires that the medical staff do so, and demonstrate that they are doing so. Since the majority of physicians are hospital staff members, there is obviously a tremendous potential for quality of care measurement and control through hospital medical staff review committees. However, little is actually known about how they work and what they do; they have never been comprehensively studied. It is to be hoped that as the JCAH enforces its PEP standards, it will engage in such studies. If hospital medical staffs can be shown to be effectively using the PEP, there should be a significant upgrading of the quality of American medical care.

Professional Standards Review Organizations

Government has been very active for many years in operating general quality control systems: individual and institutional licensure. It is only recently that government, this time the federal government, has become involved in case-specific quality measurement and control. Professional Standards Review Organizations (PSROs) were established in 1972 by amendments to the Social Security Act (Public Law 92–603). According to the original PSRO Program Manual, PSRO's are:

> . . . designed to involve local practicing physicians in the ongoing review and evaluation of health care services covered under the Medicare, Medicaid, and the Maternal and Child Health programs (of the USD-HEW). The legislation is based on the concepts that health professionals are the most appropriate individuals to evaluate the quality of medical services and that effective peer review at the local level is the soundest method for assuring the appropriate use of health care resources and facilities. . . .[9]

The Secretary of the USDHEW divided the country into about two hundred geographic areas in which the physicians have or are in the process of forming themselves into PSROs, which must operate according to fairly rigorous federal regulations. The law provides that non-compliance with the terms of the law can lead to the imposition of penalties by the Secretary. Although in the beginning evaluations were to be confined to hospital care, there is nothing in the law preventing the expansion of PSRO review to office practice.

The law and the regulations make it clear that it is discrete cases of patient care which are to be evaluated. The simple application of the same old structural standards simply will not do. Case-specific process and outcome techniques must be used. Thus this legislation is a landmark: for the first time the institution of case-specific quality measurement and control systems is required by law, and one that has some fairly sharp teeth in it. PSROs thus represent a distinct departure from the American tradition of quality control.

The program was beset by under-funding problems in the beginning (now generally resolved) and is still meeting with physician resistance in some parts of the country.[10] Furthermore, not all theoretical and technological problems inherent in case-specific medical care quality review have been solved, to say the least. Thus it is still too early to determine how effective PSROs are and will be. However, their potential for positive achievement is significant.

Patient Satisfaction and Malpractice Litigation

I examined these problem areas to some extent in Chapter 3. Patient satisfaction is almost always a case-specific measure. It is poorly understood and not frequently evaluated. In most instances where it has been examined, it has been found that patients tend to evaluate care on different criteria than do professionals. Patients are more likely to consider provider attitudes, communication, surroundings, and waiting time rather than the technical content of the care, unless the outcome is very noticeably bad.

Of course, it must be understood that most patients are biased in the direction of positively evaluating the care they receive. Medicine is a mystery to most people. To deal with illness, patients place themselves and their trust in the hands of physicians. Thus patients find themselves having to believe in the professional competence of the doctor whom they have chosen to treat them. Most people want to believe that they are going to get better; therefore they want to believe that their doctor knows how to make them better. Doubt is a powerful inhibitor to successful therapy. Therefore in most cases patients are reluctant to doubt. Patient satisfaction is an important parameter of quality evaluation but cannot be used alone.

Malpractice litigation is an important subset of patient satisfaction. I do not intend to go into the medical malpractice problem in great detail here. I pointed out in Chapter 3 that malpractice litigation does not seem to be directly related to poor care per se, although in cases of certain kinds of medical disaster, unnecessary death, total paralysis from anesthesia, it certainly is. Thus malpractice litigation is neither a good measure of nor control for quality of medical care. In certain instances the existence of the malpractice litigation system and its extensive use may even lead to bad care: physicians refusing to treat certain kinds of patients with certain kinds of diseases, physicians practicing what is called "defensive medicine" and ordering tests, including X-rays, only for the purpose of protecting themselves against possible suit. One of the measures which must be taken to deal with the medical malpractice problem is improved physician quality control efforts, particularly in the identification, reeducation, and supervision of suit-prone physicians. Identification and treatment of suit-prone patients could be helpful too.

Making Choices, and the Distribution of Power

Why is one quality control system overwhelmingly accepted, indeed strongly supported by physicians, while another is condemned and resisted? Licensure, a government operated system, has always been strongly supported by physicians. Indeed, as we shall see below, physicians have played a significant role in both instituting and maintaining licensing systems. Yet PSRO has been strongly condemned by many voices of organized medicine, the American Medical Association certainly among them, as "government interference in the practice of medicine." However, this argument suffers from a certain logical fallacy when it comes from organized medicine.

Licensing certainly constitutes not only government interference in the practice of medicine, but outright suppression of the rights of the unlicensed. Government, through the force of law and the criminal justice system, gives the medical profession a monopoly over that which it defines as the practice of medicine and prevents anyone else from competing with them. In return, the profession provides a structure-based approach to quality assurance, operated independently. The highest form of governmental interference—a refusal to allow those who have not met organized medicine's requirements to practice—receives the profession's strongest support. Obviously the problem for the medical profession here is not "government interference" per se, but the ends to which that government interference is put.

In the 1880s and 90s the forerunners of the current medical licensing laws were being debated and passed in most of the states. Passage was strongly supported by the American Medical Association and the state and county medical societies of the majority group of physicians, the allopaths (see below, "Medical Licensure") who hoped to control the licensing process. Many of the other then current medical disciplines opposed passage of licensing, fearing in reality domination by the allopaths. However, that is not how they put it. They talked about "government interference," in a tone which reminds one of the tone of those representatives of modern organized medicine who so shrilly attack PSROs, (while, of course, defending licensing). An editor of the *American Homeopath* writing in 1893 said:

> . . . every man has the right to employ any other man to do anything for him, whether it be to take care of his horse . . . or his health. . . . We would not submit to legislative enactment compelling us to patronize John, the butcher, and Dick, the baker, and we see no reason why they should be compelled to have a doctor endorsed by government.[11]

When government uses or endorses a general quality control system, especially when that system guarantees the profession a monopoly, the profession is all for it. When government uses, endorses, or requires the use of a case-specific quality control system, it is described as "government interference in the practice of medicine" and is attacked. Research has shown that structure-based evaluation tells us little about the quality of medical care in terms of outcomes. Structure-based evaluation can tell us little about past performance and is at the same time a poor predictor of future performance. By definition, all licensed physicians have passed a licensing examination. Theoretically, they should then practice good medicine for the rest of their lives. Yet there is a tremendous variation in the quality of physicians' work as measured by case-specific process and outcome techniques, as we shall see below. Obviously, what physicians are objecting to when they label PSRO as "government interference in the practice of medicine" is mandated case-specific medical quality of care assessment and control.

There are several reasons for this. One certainly is that a significant minority of care is not, in fact, of good quality, as measured by physicians themselves. Another is that to recognize that some physicians almost all of the time deliver less than good care strikes a heavy blow at the Medical Mystique. To err is in fact human, and to admit it would in the minds of many doctors make them something less than the Gods they consciously or unconsciously think they are.

Third, most physicians have been taught from the beginning of medical education, consciously or unconsciously as the case may be, that while doctors do make mistakes from time to time and sometimes forget things, or even, heaven forbid, don't know something, admitting the flaw is just not done. Simply, we are not taught to say "I don't know"—as if that were an admission of weakness. On hospital rounds, as the flock of white-jacketed students and white-suited housestaff follows the white-coated attending physician from bed to bed (the category of white outer covering denoting one's status in the medical hierarchy), heaven help the person who doesn't *know* the answer. Better to mumble, answer a different question, go off on a tangent, or ask for the patient's blood porcelain level than to say simply "I don't know." What an admission of weakness, amply chastised by the disdainful glances both of one's peers and one's superiors. This type of behavior may well be related to the personalities of those people attracted to medicine too, as well as the way in which they are taught.

Fourth, in few schools are students taught how to engage in peer review and other forms of group work. Nor in many schools are students taught the techniques of quality assessment and control themselves. If this kind of approach to physicians' work is not built into medical training, it can hardly be expected that doctors will warmly embrace it once they are out in supposedly independent, private practice. An internist friend of mine, well-trained and conscientious, told me of his experience as chairman of the medical audit committee in his medium-sized, non-teaching community hospital. After five years of trying very hard, he finally gave up in disgust after being told repeatedly to "mind your own business" when raising issues of blatantly poor care with various of his colleagues.

Finally, mandated case-specific quality control measures, even when they are to be carried out by one's peers and colleagues, strike a blow at the concept of independent entrepreneurship which is the basis of the private fee-for-service practice system in which the vast majority of American physicians in clinical practice work. If one's actual work can be reviewed and criticized, if one can be subject to discipline and re-education or continuing education, does not that make one something less than a completely independent entrepreneur, so the thinking goes? (See Dr. Fineberg's statement at the beginning of this chapter.) And if one is something less than a completely independent entrepreneur might not that affect one's ability to set and collect one's own private fees? These are all important considerations in the resistance to PSROs.

But isn't American medicine "the best in the world?" Am I not really making much ado about nothing? American medicine may be the best in the world, but that question is really irrelevant. The evidence shows clearly that it is not nearly as good as it could be, as we shall see in the next section.

The Quality of Medical Care in the United States

The extent to which quality of care can be evaluated has been a subject of debate. A former president of the American Medical Association, Russell Roth, said in a presidential address that "good quality in medical care is not something which can be expressed in dollars of cost, hours of time, or for that matter, in decibels of political oratory. Quality of such medical care is not a tangible qualifiable thing."[12] He added there are "immense difficulties" inherent in properly identifying high-quality care.

On the other hand, many authorities in the field have thought it possible to measure and regulate the quality of discrete instances of care delivery. Dr. Codman's suppressed work was referred to above. Two eminent physicians, Drs. Roger I. Lee and Lewis Webster Jones did pioneering work on quality determination for the prestigious Committee on the Costs of Medical Care. Based on their studies of the content of medical practice, they wrote in 1933 that "good medical care is the kind of medicine practiced and taught by the recognized leaders of the medical profession at a given time or period of social, cultural, and professional development in a community or population group," and that the work of any physician could be measured against those standards.[13] Dr. E. Richard Weinerman, reflecting the 1949-statement by the Subcommittee on Medical Care of the American Public Health Association, *The Quality of Medical Care in a National Health Program,* said: "The quality of medical care is a composite of all the technical, organizational, and financial aspects of any program for personal health service. Good quality can be defined, consciously planned, and evaluated."[14] David Kessner and his coauthors, who in the 1970s did landmark work in advancing the technology of quality assessment, said: "The question is no longer whether there will be intervention in health services to assure quality, but who will intervene and what methods they will use."[15] Finally, another authority who has done a great deal of work in quality assessment technology, Dr. Robert Brook, said in 1973: "Even though the perfect system for assessment and assurance of quality of care may not yet exist, innumerable simple efforts can be made to improve quality of care. If applied in a systematic manner, many are likely to be successful."[16]

Measurements of Quality

Over the years, a large number of research studies have been carried out in the problem area of measuring and controlling the quality of discrete instances of medical care delivery.[17] Certain studies can be considered landmarks. In 1953–54, a study of general practice in North Carolina by Dr. Osler Peterson of the University of North Carolina used both structural and process techniques and explicit criteria, in a direct observation method. It was found that: "Many physicians were performing at a high level of professional competence. Of greater importance is the fact that other physicians were performing at a lower level . . ."[18] Of the various characteristics of the physicians evaluated, only the length of the doctors' postgraduate hospital training in internal medicine was consistently related to the quality of their clinical work. Academic performance in medical school, for example, was related to quality of clinical work only for physicians aged thirty-five and less. Dr. Paul Lembcke of Johns Hopkins was one of the pioneers in developing methods for auditing the work of physicians in hospitals, using analysis of clinical records. For example, in the midfifties he evaluated major female pelvic surgery in several hospitals and found that the introduction of auditing techniques reduced both the population hysterectomy rate and the proportion of unnecessary hysterectomies which before auditing started stood at 70 percent! After auditing, the unnecessary hysterectomy rate dropped to 20 percent.[19]

In the period 1957–1961, a study of 406 admissions of members of the Teamsters Unions and their families to hospitals in New York City used review of medical records, process and outcome techniques, and implicit criteria. The chart reviews were done by eminent physicians from leading hospitals in the city. The study was carried out by Drs. Ray Trussell and Mildred Morehead of the

Columbia School of Public Health. The results caused an uproar in the New York City medical community at the time. It was found that 88 percent of the hospital admissions were justifiable. However, only 57 percent of the patients were considered to have received "good or excellent medical care," while a fifth received fair and a fifth poor care. A second study by this group in 1962, using a slightly different evaluation technique, arrived at similar conclusions.[20]

In the early 1970s Dr. David Kessner and his colleagues at the Institute of Medicine of the National Academy of Sciences developed a quality assessment technique called the "tracer method." It combined process and outcome measures. They applied the tracer method to the study of the quality of care received by a sample of children from different sections of Washington, D.C. They concluded that "inappropriate or ineffective treatment for specific tracer conditions was documented in a large proportion of the children." For example, in the treatment of middle-ear infection, "regardless of the diagnosis, inappropriate antibiotics were given to 20 percent of the patients." In dealing with vision problems, "more than 70 percent of the children with glasses did not actually benefit from them. Moreover, 40 percent of the children who were tested with their glasses failed the [vision] test."[21]

In another important study in the early 1970s, Dr. Robert Brook and his colleagues measured the care given to 296 hospitalized patients with urinary tract infection, hypertension, or ulcer, by five different methods—some process, some outcome. Depending upon which method was used, only from 1.4 percent to 63.2 percent of patients were judged to have received adequate care. The outcome measures gave the higher percentage, indicating that perhaps the process criteria were unnecessarily strict, but even so, more than one-third of patients were judged to have received less than adequate care.[22]

In a study of care given to patients in the clinics of a university-related city hospital, Drs. Charles Kelley and Joseph Manlon found physicians were relatively frequently unaware of the existence of a variety of abnormalities as demonstrated by testing in their patients.[23] For example, 28 percent of patients with abnormalities on their chest X-rays were not known to have them by their physicians, while clear evidence of urinary tract infection was missed in 93 percent of patients.

A study of physician's knowledge of the proper usage of antibiotics was carried out by administration of an examination to over 4500 physician volunteers across the country.[24] The average score on this test was 68 percent. This means that among physicians who chose to be tested on their knowledge of antibiotic therapy, the wrong decision was made in one-third of hypothetical cases.

Finally, there is a 1976 report by two physicians from a teaching hospital in the New York City area who are involved in training medical students and housestaff in history-taking and physical diagnosis. The two, Drs. Stanley Wiener and Morton Nathanson, have developed a detailed technique for observing and recording the work of doctors-in-training in acquiring the basic information from patients necessary to begin the process of making the diagnosis and planning therapy. Wiener and Nathanson unfortunately did not quantify their results, but they reported that "a large number of errors in the performance of the medical examination by young physicians were noted . . ."[25]

Meanings and Implications

In considering the results of these studies, done over a period of many years, it should be noted that aside from those published as books, they all appeared in one or another of three of the most prestigious medical journals in the United States: The *New England Journal of Medicine,* the *Journal of the American Medical Association,* and the *Journal of Medical Education,* published by the Association of American Medical Colleges. The results are disturbing—for two reasons. First, these studies, using a variety of methods in a variety of settings, show that between 20 and 40 percent of instances of patient care are of less than good (or "adequate") quality. Second, the response of organized medicine to evidence like this is, more often than not, like that of Dr. Fineberg quoted at the beginning of this chapter, and that of several physicians to reports of excess surgery, as quoted in Chapter 3: a combination of extreme defensiveness with "I'm the *doctor*—how dare you question my authority?"

To be sure, there are many doctors who practice good medicine. There are also many doctors who, privately at least, are very concerned about the deficiencies in the quality of medical practice. The PSRO program which may (or may not) be at least a partial solution to the problem of quality control, is being successfully implemented in certain parts of the country. A number of quality control studies have indicated that just having someone "looking over the shoulder" has a significant positive effect on the quality of many doctors' work. However, even the physician-controlled PSRO system is being strongly resisted in other parts of the country. In any case, change has been a long time in coming and the pace of change is slow. As Senator Sam Ervin was wont to say, "How cum?"

The Code of Silence

There are several reasons. Among them are those characteristics of medical training and hospital staff work which I reviewed at the end of the last section. Then there is the "code of silence" which seems to affect many physicians: "Thou shall not squeal on thy colleague." This has several origins: "Mind your own business;" "Let him who is without sin cast the first stone;" "Medicine is an inexact science;" "So you want to get more referrals?" and perhaps the strongest inhibitor of all, the fear of the social and professional ostracism often visited upon those who dare to speak out, even if only in professional circles.

"Mind your own business" stems from the private entrepreneurial nature of American medical practice. "Let him who is without sin . . ." refers to the fact that *every* doctor, certainly including myself, has made mistakes in the past and will make them in the future. Since the *routines* for quality assessment are so rudimentary and poorly implemented generally, even though sophisticated techniques are available, quality control as now practiced in many institutions often falls back on the "*I* think" of the person doing quality audit. Thus the available response.

"Medicine is an inexact science." True enough, but a great deal is known, in fact. Processes *can* be judged and outcomes *can* be measured. This is in fact a weak excuse.

Referral of patients from one physician to another is the lifeblood of private entrepreneural practice as it functions in this country. Life can be very hard for a specialist to whom nobody refers patients, or for a primary care practitioner who finds physicians not accepting his referrals, and/or not sending his patients back to him. Finally, the social and professional ostracism which can be the lot of the physician who speaks out against erring colleagues, can be as stark and painful as that visited by his co-workers on the cop who reports police crime to higher authority.

But perhaps the most important factor in the maintenance of the code of silence is the medical license. The medical license puts the profession in a secure and powerful position regardless of the quality of its work, or so it seems. The profession's position of dominance in the health care delivery system seems unshakeable, so why should it, collectively, worry too much about quality? Thus in the final section of this chapter, we will turn to somewhat detailed consideration of the nature of medical licensing.

Medical Licensure

Although about twenty-five health professions and occupations are licensed in one or more states, the central profession in the health care delivery system is the medical profession. Medicine can be defined as that body of knowledge concerning the processes of human disease, the mechanisms of disease prevention, treatment and rehabilitation, the processes by which the human body maintains normal functioning, and the mechanisms of health maintenance. The practice of medicine is the delivery to people of the fruits of that body of knowledge called medicine. Health care delivery systems are not solely concerned with medical practice, as I pointed out in Chapter 2. They provide for payment for care, construct and operate institutions, provide employment, carry out educational and research activities, provide to some the the opportunity to make financial profits, and to others the opportunity to fulfill personal and professional needs and meet career goals. However, a major purpose of all these activities is to make it possible for medical practice to be carried on. Thus, medical practice is the focus, the raison d'être of any health care delivery system.

A study carried out in 1967 for the then existing National Advisory Commission on Health Manpower by Edward Forgotson, Ruth Roemer, and Roger Newman reviewed the statutory definitions of medical practice in the fifty states. The study concluded that the states generally agree, with some variations in wording, that medical practice means "diagnosing, treating, operating, or prescribing for a disease, ailment, pain, or condition."[26] Thus doctors control the center of the center. However, that has not always been the case.

History

An early attempt at medical licensure was that of the Royal College of Physicians in England, created in 1518 by King Henry VIII to supervise medical practice in the area of the City of London.[27] In the College's Charter its purpose was stated:

> to curb the audacity of those wicked men who shall profess medicine more for the sake of their avarice than from the assurance of any good conscience, whereby very many inconveniences may ensue to the rude and credulous populace.[28]

According to Dr. Robert Derbyshire, a leading authority on medical licensure, "the earliest law for control of the medical profession in America was drawn up in Virginia in 1639. This provided for the regulation of the fees of physicians and was apparently precipitated by the belief of the planters that they were being overcharged for the treatment of their slaves."[29] Nevertheless, regulation of medical practice progressed little for over one hundred years. Dr. Richard Shryock quotes an historian, William Smith, writing in 1757 on the state of American medical practice:

> "Few physicians among us are eminent for their skill. Quacks abound like locusts in Egypt. . . . This," he added, "is less to be wondered at as the profession is under no kind of Regulation. Any man at his pleasure sets up for Physician, Apothecary [Pharmacist], and Chirurger [Surgeon]."[30]

Early Licensing Laws

The first colonial licensing act was passed in New York City in 1760. Gradually, the several colonies, then states, passed licensing laws, and by the early nineteenth century, there was fairly general coverage. At first, states either established medical licensing boards or gave the licensing power over to state medical societies. Early standards for gaining a license included an apprenticeship with a licensed, practicing physician (the quality of the apprenticeship supervisors themselves was apparently unregulated), and passage of an examination.

With the appearance of a small but significant number of medical schools in the United States (seven by 1810), states began accepting evidence of graduation from a medical school as the requirement for licensure, especially since all medical schools of the day required an apprenticeship for admission. This in turn led, however, to a proliferation of medical schools: there were thirty-four by 1840, and another forty-seven were added between that date and 1875. The medical schools themselves were unregulated, however. The increasingly poor quality of their graduates was one factor that led to the gradual disappearance of medical licensure from most states by 1850. Another factor was the nature of medical practice itself.

The physicians who were licensed by the colonies beginning in 1760 were the scientific and political ancestors of the majority group of physicians who dominate medical practice today: the allopaths. However, they did not call themselves allopaths (and most still do not); that was an appellation applied by practitioners of competing theories of medicine which appeared in the nineteenth century. These included Thomsonianism, a home-grown naturopathy based on herbalism and botanical preparations, homeopathy, a European import based on the theory that like cures like, especially in very small doses, and eclecticism, which took a bit from this and a bit from that. The allopaths called themselves the "regulars" or the "orthodox physicians." The orthodox labelled all practitioners of competing disciplines as "quacks," "charlatans," "fakes," or members of "sects."

The truth was that no medical discipline could do very much for patients. In the first half of the nineteenth century, the understanding of normal bodily functioning was just beginning, and disease was poorly understood: pathology (the study of disease processes) was an unknown science. The major weapons in the armamentarium of the "regulars" were blood-letting, intestinal purging with emetics and laxatives, sweating, and cupping. Benjamin Rush, a leading faculty member of the oldest medical school in the country at the University of Pennsylvania, and a signer of the Declaration of Independence, popularized the use of these "thera-pies" for all sorts of conditions. His influence was long-lasting. Bleeding, although with leeches rather than lancets, was still in use at the time of the American Civil War. This period was called the Heroic Age of Medicine. The word "hero" was applied to the patients who endured the treatments, not the physicians who administered them!

Repeal

It is obvious that there were many ills on which bleeding and purging had no effect, except possibly to make them worse. The competing disciplines were neither more nor less effective. By 1850, most state legislatures had come to realize this. Since no one could do very much good, why should the "regulars" have their practice protected by state power? And so the protection was lifted.

The third quarter of the nineteenth century saw virtual chaos in medical practice. New sects sprang up like weeds; the regulars continued undaunted and new medical schools to train them sprang up like weeds too. There were true quacks everywhere, within each discipline and outside them all; there were no quality controls even over the regulars. However, beginning with the discovery and development of the science of pathology by the German scientist Rudolf Virchow in the mid-nineteenth century, the basis for the eventual development of allopathy as a truly scientific, and effective weapon against disease began to be laid down. The situation began to change, again.

Modern Licensing Laws

The degree to which the gradually developing effectiveness of allopathy actually influenced the decision-making process of state legislatures is unclear. To determine that, the debates leading to the reestablishment of licensing laws which took place in the last quarter of the nineteenth century would have to be examined, a task which to my knowledge has not been done. However, the licensing laws returned beginning around 1875. By 1898, all states had them. It was during this period, of course, that the first triumphs of bacteriology were achieved. Although those triumphs affected the health of the public principally through public health measures, not medical practice, there was an association between these triumphs and regular medicine because of the linkage, at least in Germany then the world's center for medical education, between research in pathology and bacteriology and the training of "regular" physicians. Furthermore, it was during this period that the two developments which made modern surgery possible took place: the advent of effective anesthesia, and the discovery of the principles of anti- and then asepsis.* "Regulars" were responsible for these developments too. Thus, whether or not legislators were always clearly aware of the fact, allopathy was developing a scientific basis, making it logical to develop licensing laws to both regulate and protect it.

In about half of the states, this second generation of licensing laws was significantly different from its forebears. Not only was a medical school diploma required, but passage of an examination administered by a state board of medicine was required as well. Now it is certainly true that in most states the medical society had a great deal of influence in selecting the members of the board of medicine, but at least it was no longer the state medical society simply determining licensure on its own. On the other hand, about half the states still accepted a medical school diploma alone as meeting the requirement for licensure. Since the medical schools were not regulated and since few state boards even examined them (Illinois was an outstanding exception), the "diploma mill," the medical school which provided its students with a diploma and not much else, was still popular in those states which required only a diploma for licensure. Thus there were still many abuses, and many ill-qualified doctors.

In the early twentieth century, the groundwork was laid for what were to be the last major changes in the physician licensing system as we know it today. The American Medical Association, at that time representing only a minority of physicians, dominated by academics rather than practitioners, and a relatively progressive

*Antisepsis is the practice of disinfection against disease-causing organisms; asepsis is the practice of cleanliness to prevent disease-causing organisms from appearing and growing.

voice (unlike today) began evaluating and rating medical schools. State medical boards began setting requirements for medical school curriculae, so that the school's would qualify for recognition by the boards. More states required passage of an examination in addition to a diploma. (For more detail on the history of medical education, see the next four chapters.)

In 1910, the Carnegie Foundation for the Advancement of Teaching published a report by Abraham Flexner of a study which it had sponsored on the state of American medical education. Flexner, whose Report I discuss in detail in Chapter 8, deplored a great deal of what he saw. His Report received a great deal of publicity, and it hastened completion of many changes already underway. By 1920 or so, most states required for a license, graduation from an AMA-approved school, the meeting by those schools of certain minimum academic criteria expressed in law, and passage of an examination.

In certain states, licensure was also extended to certain of the sects, homeopathy, eclecticism, and a new one, osteopathy, each with their own board at least at first; but "orthodoxy" clearly had established its preeminent position. Thus the form and substance of medical boards as they are now constituted, which we shall examine in more detail below, was established in the first quarter of this century.

The Theory of Licensure

Licensure came back into vogue, as we just saw, during a period when allopathy was developing a product of some worth to offer the public, or at least when its potential to offer such a product was being perceived. Therefore, it could be held that it was in the public interest to distinguish allopathy, "regular" medicine, from the other disciplines, to protect it from unfair competition, and to protect the public from true quackery. In the mid-nineteenth century, charges by regulars of quackery against other disciplines had a hollow ring: none of them were very effective. By the beginning of this century such charges could be given some credence: the regulars had begun to develop some useful tools in surgery, and if they could not do very much in treating many of the common infections of the day, at least they had begun to understand them and so could offer palliation with some logic behind it. Thus the theoretical basis of modern licensure was laid.

The state, through its police power, would guarantee to the medical profession a monopoly over that which it described as the practice of medicine: diagnosing, prescribing, and surgically operating. Through the profession's control of the medical schools, and its influence over the state medical boards and the licensing examinations, the profession would be guaranteed control over entry into, maintenance in, and exit from the profession of each individual member. The state would enforce the monopoly through the criminal justice system, prosecuting those persons caught "practicing medicine without a license." In return for these benefits, the profession was to guarantee that the care its members provided was of good quality. The profession averred that it could guarantee the latter using structural standards of educational requirements, work experience, and performance on examination.

According to Derbyshire, a key element in this arrangement is that the medical license is a privilege, not a right. That is, the states granted physicians the *privilege* of having a monopoly, in return for the guarantee by the profession that the care offered to the public by its members would be of good quality. In 1956, the Federation of State Medical Boards of the United States published its *Guide to the Essentials of a Modern Medical Practice Act.* The suggested preamble reads:

> Recognizing that the practice of medicine is a privilege granted by legislative authority and not a natural right of individuals, it is deemed necessary as a matter of policy in the interests of public health, safety and welfare to provide laws and provisions covering the practice of that privilege and its subsequent use, control and regulation to the end that the public shall be properly protected against unprofessional, improper, unauthorized and unqualified practice of medicine and from unprofessional conduct of persons licensed to practice medicine.

Derbyshire goes on to quote Dr. Sidney Shindell, an authority on legal medicine. Dr. Shindell noted that:

> While a medical practice act conveys special status on physicians, status is incidental to its primary purpose. Essentially its purpose is to provide a means by which society may exercise formal control over persons designated to minister to its ills. . . . Inescapable is the fact that both

the privileges and limitations of the profession are in the hands of society.[31]

Unfortunately, for many years now, courts in many states have ruled that the license is a property right of the physician who holds it, not a privilege to practice medicine granted to the physician by the people of the state through their elected representatives. The American Medical Association holds to this view as well. Bruce E. Vodicka, J.D., of the AMA Office of the General Counsel, has said:

> Since the right to practice medicine is a valuable property right under the Constitution, courts tend to construe medical practice acts strictly in favor of the accused physician.[32]

I must admit that although I have searched hard for it, I have not been able to locate in the Constitution the principle referred to by Mr. Vodicka. That may be a limitation of mine, but I do know that neither "medicine" nor "health" is mentioned in the document. Be that as it may, however, physicians facing disciplinary action from state medical boards can and do claim protection under the general due process clauses of the Constitution and can drag cases out through the courts for years, practicing all the while. The fact that state boards of medicine are inhibited from taking action by the presence of the property right/due process concept, is probably one of the two most important reasons accounting for the generally low level of state medical board activity in disciplinary matters. The other is, of course, the traditional reluctance of physicians to get involved in disciplining other physicians, for reasons I have discussed above.

I believe that the single most salutary change that could occur in state licensing laws would be the clear embodiment in the laws of the concept of the medical license as a privilege, under the ultimate control of the people, who grant the privilege. No one would want to see physicians denied ultimate access to the courts, nor would one want to see the personal rights of physicians who may be wrongfully accused of misconduct trampled roughly underfoot. But the restoration of the privilege-to-practice concept could at least give the medical boards the power to order physicians under investigation to practice under supervision, to refrain from prescribing certain drugs, to refrain from doing certain kinds of surgery, to be required to seek second opinions in certain kinds of cases, and the like, without going through lengthy court proceedings, before final determination of the case is made.

Licensing Boards at Present

Unfortunately, there are no recent surveys of the composition, powers, and functioning of state medical licensing boards. This section is based on Dr. Derbyshire's book and an USDHEW study cited in the references, both of which date from the late 60s. However, with the exceptions noted and, I am sure, a few others, I doubt that the situation has changed much since then.[33]

In each state, there is a Medical Board or its equivalent. It is to these Boards that the state legislatures delegate the powers of examination, licensing, and discipline—the three principal functions of Medical Boards. There is little evidence of accountability, either to the public or the legislature; indeed in most instances Medical Board proceedings are entirely confidential. In most states, physicians dominate the medical boards and only physicians sit on the Boards in about one-half the states.

Dr. Derbyshire studied the backgrounds of the physician-members of the boards in 1967 and developed this revealing composite picture of a medical board member:

> He is a Caucasian man, a little over fifty-eight years of age (only one woman serves on a board, that of New Hampshire); most likely a general practitioner; if not, a general surgeon or an internist. He is a leader in the medical community and well known to the members of his state medical society. He possesses no singular attributes which qualify him to judge the academic attainments of applicants for licensure, but he is sincere in carrying out his duties and may seek help in formulating his examination questions. He is a graduate of an approved American medical school and is better qualified to carry out the disciplinary duties of his office than the educational and examining functions.[34]

Furthermore, in about one-half of the states the medical societies have a direct voice in the appointment of members and there is no indication that in other states physicians of whom medical societies would disapprove are appointed.

In recent years, a few states have taken to adding lay persons with no health professional connections to their Boards of Medicine.[35] As of 1976 there were eight: California, Maine, Michigan, Minnesota, New Jersey, Ohio, South Dakota, and Washington. It is still too early to tell if putting pure "health care consumers" on medical boards will make any difference in how they function.

Medical Discipline

A medical license is generally granted once and is retained for life, barring practice of extremely poor quality, "moral turpitude," or some similar offense. Physicians in the United States rarely lose their licenses. In the period 1963–1967, Dr. Derbyshire found that nationally 938 disciplinary actions were undertaken by state medical boards. Of these, 334 involved revocation of license, while the rest involved probation, suspension, and reprimand. Nearly 50 percent of these actions were related to narcotics addiction; only seven involved "gross malpractice." A *New York Times* survey found that for the period 1971–1974, there was an average of seventy-two revocations annually, fewer than 2 percent of them for incompetency.[36]

In Chapter 3, I reviewed the evidence on unnecessary surgery. In this chapter, I reviewed the evidence on the general level of quality of medical practice in our country. The incidence of malpractice litigation is increasing, and although it does not seem to be directly correlated with poor quality care, it does indicate, at least in part, public dissatisfaction with some of the work of some physicians. There are around 300,000 physicians in active practice in the United States. In the face of the volume of poor care that evidently exists, the level of disciplinary action of medical boards appears to be inordinately low.

Boards rarely lift licenses for incompetency or "gross malpractice," which is bad enough. But they don't even seem to be doing their job in winnowing out physicians who have illnesses serious enough to compromise their ability to practice. The incidence of alcoholism in the general population has been estimated at 5 percent; the incidence of narcotics addiction at 0.5 percent. There is no reason to believe that the incidence of these conditions is lower among doctors than it is in the general population; indeed it may be higher particularly for narcotics addiction, which Dr. Derbyshire refers to as an occupational disease of medical practice. These data mean that there may be as many as 15,000 practicing physicians who are alcoholics or narcotic addicts. Yet in the period 1963–67 a total of only 440 disciplinary actions were taken by state medical boards on account of narcotics addiction; 41 on account of alcoholism. Less than one-half of these actions were revocation of license.

Thus the monitoring of the work of licensed physicians and the disciplining of those who stand in need of it, for whatever reason —incompetence, illness, "moral turpitude," or fraud is not carried out as well as it could be. There are several reasons for this. The boards are dominated by the profession itself, the profession being ruled in part by a "code of silence" which I discussed above. The state medical societies, most of which view as prime functions defending the profession against any and all criticism and sanctifying the physician (see Dr. Fineberg's statement at the beginning of this chapter), make or strongly influence the gubernatorial appointments to most medical boards.

A natural reluctance on the part of medical board members to become involved in the long drawn out litigation which occurs in many cases owing to the legal interpretation of the medical license as a property right, is understandable. From Dr. Derbyshire's composite picture of the average medical board member it can be concluded that few of them are experts in clinical medicine, academic medicine, quality assessment and control, or the law. Medical boards often operate with small budgets and have limited investigatory staff. Private physicians challenging a board ruling in the courts can often afford to hire expensive legal help while a board is often forced to rely on the already overworked legal staff of the state health department's general counsel or the office of the state attorney general.

Even when a medical board disciplines a doctor in its own state it may participate in the process of loosing him upon the unsuspecting citizens of another. For example, in 1976 a New York State physician lost his license for sexually molesting female patients. While proceedings were pending against him, in a case that was building over a six-year period, he applied for a license in Michigan. The doctor's application was routinely endorsed, citing him as "an ethical practitioner and of good moral character," by the state Board of Regents (which handles medical discipline in New York) and his county medical society, one month before his license was revoked and five months after formal proceedings had started against him.[37] For some unknown reason, eight months after his license was revoked, the American Medical Association still listed him as a physician in good standing in that state.

Finally, boards in many states are limited in the kinds of penalties they can assess. Only half provide for anything other than revocation or suspension of the license. When one's primary responsibility is the protection of the public good and welfare, consideration of a single individual's ability to earn a living should be only a secondary consideration. For many board members, however, it seems to be primary: "How can we take away Dr. Y's means of livelihood" (particularly when Dr. Y has a $100,000 mortgage, a vacation home, a boat, three cars, and four children who first require braces and then a college education)?

If graded penalties existed, perhaps board members would be more active in disciplining physicians and really getting into quality control work (in which they presently engage very little). Possible graded penalties, and perhaps penalties is too strong a word, include: the requirement of practicing under supervision, limiting surgical privileges, limiting prescribing privileges, requiring second opinions for surgery, requiring continuing medical education. Much of this, of course, would involve hospital staffs as well as individual physicians. To be able to invoke such penalties, Medical Boards would have to know that hospital medical staffs would and could provide such supervision for a member in need of it. However, hospitals could be required to demonstrate such capabilities, through state hospital licensing laws and hospital codes.

Medical Licensing and Physician Dominance of the Health Care Delivery System

I have pointed out on more than one occasion how the physician dominates the health care delivery system in the United States. Medical care, the treatment of sick people, is the centerpiece of our health care delivery system. The central elements of medical practice are making the diagnosis, prescribing drugs, and surgically operating. The licensing laws give physicians sole control over, in a sense ownership of, these three functions. (The picture would certainly be different if the centerpieces of the health care delivery system were activities in health maintenance and disease prevention.) And whoever controls medical practice controls the keystone of the arch, as I have said before. For example, insurance companies generally determine their own policies regarding benefits, coverage, premiums, and the like (subject to government regulation in certain instances), but they cannot sell health insurance policies if there is no medical practice to buy. The boards of directors of voluntary hospitals determine hospital size, location, and facilities (again subject to government regulation), but if medical practice is not carried out on their premises, their powers come to nothing. Finally, a local government agency may decide what kind of medical service it wants to offer, but it is dependent upon medical practitioners to supply that service, and if it cannot pay the going physician's rate, it cannot provide the service.

It is not that difficult to teach people how to take medical histories and perform physical examinations. In addition to medical students, many thousands of nursing and physicians' assistant students are being taught these skills today. Once one has done enough histories and physicals, the process of drawing diagnostic conclusions from one's findings becomes fairly straightforward, except in cases of relatively rare problems. Nevertheless, by law, only physicians are permitted to make diagnoses.

Likewise, for many common health problems, determination of the correct drug therapy is a fairly straightforward process, yet only physicians are allowed to prescribe drugs. It may even be legally dangerous for non-physician health care providers to recommend non-prescription drugs to patients, even though the patient could choose such drugs himself. A similar analogy can be drawn for simple surgical procedures like sewing up severe cuts and lancing boils. Appropriate skills in this area can be taught to nonphysicians, and are taught to military medical corpsmen, for example (who also are taught how to make many diagnoses and to prescribe certain drugs for certain well-defined conditions).

My point is not that only physicians are capable by knowledge and training of diagnosing, prescribing, and surgically operating, under any circumstances. (Under certain circumstances, which can be well-defined and quality controlled, others can be taught them too, in less time and for a lower cost. I shall discuss the data on the quality of the performance of non-physicians in certain areas of "medical practice" in detail in Chapter 12.) It is that the licensing laws, written in the main over sixty years ago, *permit* only physicians to diagnose, treat, and surgically operate. Thus it is the licensing laws, rather than something innate in the physician himself, which gives him the hammerlock he has on that which is defined as the "practice of medicine." In the next four chapters, I shall review the history of the system this country has developed over the years for educating these all powerful beings.

SECTION *III*

Medical Education: Historical Development and Present Status

7

To 1910

Medical schools and what they do are of critical importance in determining the structure and function of the health care delivery system. The medical schools select the people who will become doctors. The schools then provide all of their training and education to the level of the M.D. degree. The medical schools also have a significant influence on postgraduate training and education. Doctors have control over the keystones of the health care delivery system as it operates in this country: the processes of diagnosing, prescribing, and surgically operating. This control is confirmed and maintained by the licensing system. Further, in economic terms, doctors make the majority of decisions affecting the expenditure of resources in the health care delivery system. Thus the doctors dominate the health care delivery system. By this chain of logic, the importance of the medical schools to the health care delivery system and the fact that they bear a major responsibility for the way it is structured and how it functions should be obvious. To fully understand the present situation, it is useful to have some historical background.

The history of American medical education revolves around the year 1910. In that year, The Carnegie Foundation for the Advancement of Teaching published a report entitled *Medical Education in the United States and Canada* written by an educator, Abraham Flexner. The Flexner Report, which I shall discuss in detail in the next chapter, marks a watershed generally considered to divide the history of American medical education into two distinct eras: "pre-Flexner," and, as one might expect, "post-Flexner." Of course, when the situation is examined closely, it is found that the demarcation was not nearly as sharp as conventional wisdom would have it seem. The changes in medical education which generally carry the label "Flexnerian" began about fifty years before the Report was written, and did not conclude until about twenty years after it appeared. Nevertheless, the Report is a remarkable document containing a great deal of wisdom and 1910 is a useful landmark; so I will use it as such.

Early Days

The first doctors arrived in the North American colonies with earliest English settlers, at the beginning of the seventeenth century. From that time to this day, doctors trained in other countries have come to these shores to live and work. However, in the seventeenth century, the passage to America was not easy to make, and the physical and intellectual life was not particularly attractive for a university-trained physician from Great Britain or the continent. Thus an apprenticeship training system developed. A model for it already existed in Europe, especially for the training of surgeons and apothecaries (druggists).

Apprenticeship

An apprentice was ordinarily indentured to an established practitioner for a stipulated period of time, up to eight years being a common term. In addition to learning (so he hoped) about the profession of medicine from his senior, the apprentice was expected to perform certain duties around the house, like grooming the horses, cleaning the stables, and general handiwork, especially during the early years of his term. The apprentice, or his family, paid the senior a fee in addition to providing free labor. At the end of the term, the senior would issue a certificate testifying that the apprentice was now fully capable of independent practice. Although indenturing disappeared after Independence, apprenticeship remained an important feature of American medical education until the end of the nineteenth century.

In England, medical practitioners were divided into three distinct groups: the physicians, the surgeons, and the apothecaries. Into the eighteenth century many surgeons also engaged in barbering, the trade from which surgery descended. Although apothecaries engaged in some general medical practice (an important although unofficial function of pharmacists in many developing countries, and Japan, to this day), their principle function was dispensing drugs. In pre-Revolutionary America, however, these distinctions did not generally hold. Most doctors prepared and dispensed their own drugs.

As manufactured drugs (rather than homemade remedies), began to make their appearance from Great Britain towards the end of the eighteenth century, many physicians opened their own drug stores. Doctors also often practiced surgery, without being either specialist surgeons or barbers. An important factor in the development of the generalist approach to medical practice was the predominately rural character of the country, which had only three major urban centers at the time of the Revolutionary War: Boston, New York, and Philadelphia.

European-trained physicians began to emigrate to the colonies with some regularity in the eighteenth century, as distinct urban centers with some people of wealth began to make their appearance. (Apparently per capita income levels were as important a factor in physician migration patterns in the eighteenth century as they are today.) Nevertheless, homegrown apprenticeship-trained physicians outnumbered them, and the apprenticeship system as it developed in this country tended to produce generalists rather than specialists.

The First Medical Schools

As I pointed out in the last chapter, regulation of medical practice in the American Colonies was sporadic until well into the eighteenth century. Various political jurisdictions passed various laws attempting to establish controls, but they were apparently ephemeral, as well as ineffective. The 1760s saw the occurrence of two significant events: the passage in New York City of a licensing law which not only endured but which was followed by the appearance of licensing laws in most of the other colonies, then states,[1] and the creation of the first medical school.

Although my undergraduate alma mater, Columbia College, likes to credit its colonial ancestor, Kings College, with the creation of the first medical school in North America, most historians give that honor to the College of Philadelphia. It inaugurated the first American medical school on November 14, 1765. The principal faculty members, William Shippen, Jr., and John Morgan, were both recent graduates of the medical school of Edinburgh University, already a popular school for Americans wishing to study medicine abroad. Graduating in the first class, in 1768, was Benjamin Rush, the proponent of "heroic medicine" (remember, it was the patients who were the heroes), whose theories and practices influenced American medicine well into the nineteenth century.

By 1813, the United States had seven medical colleges: at the University of Pennsylvania (formerly the College of Philadelphia), Harvard, Dartmouth, the University of Maryland (the medical school was its first college), Yale University, the College of Physicians and Surgeons in New York City (a non-university institution which absorbed the Kings College, later Columbia College, medical school, reuniting with Columbia College in 1860), and the College of Physicians and Surgeons of the Western District of New York. Five of these were university-based. The schools all required an apprenticeship for admission but had few other admission requirements, provided series of lectures over a two- to three-year period, usually for three to five months a year, plus some demonstrations of technique, usually in anatomy. The lecture series were often not graded in difficulty or complexity; that is, one set did not necessarily build upon what was taught in preceding sets. Thus, the student did not as a matter of course begin with relatively simple material and proceed to more difficult subjects.

The Decline of Medical Education: 1810–1870

The licensing laws, or lack of them, has had an important influence on the development of medical schools since the early nineteenth century. Early licensing laws had generally given state medical societies the right and power to examine persons certificated from apprenticeship programs and grant licenses to those persons passing the examinations. Towards the end of the eighteenth century, some states began adding to the eligibility requirement for licensure that of graduation from a medical school. By the 1820s, however, most states had moved to the position that a diploma from a medical school was the only requirement for licensure. Examinations were dropped: the candidate need only present his diploma and receive his license. However, there was no regulation of the medical schools. They could teach whatever they wanted to, setting their own standards. That was the rub.

The Proprietary Schools

Entrepreneurs saw an opportunity in this situation and grabbed it. The proprietary, i.e., private, profit-making medical school made its appearance. Many of them seemed to say to the aspiring physician: "The diploma is all you need to be licensed to practice medicine? We will supply it to you. Whether we will give you anything in the way of knowledge, training, or education to go with it is another matter entirely!" Throughout the nineteenth century indeed, there were many schools which gave their graduates little else than a diploma. As the state licensing laws disappeared in the 1840s in the face of the ineffectiveness of "regular" medicine and the rise of competing medical disciplines, the schools could offer only the prestige of the diploma and the possible advantage it might bring to its holders competing in the medical marketplace as an incentive to take their courses. Completely unregulated and beholden to no authority, they competed with each other and for student fees by making their programs easier and easier, and shorter and shorter. Nevertheless, even in the absence of licensing laws, by mid-century there was apparently a good market for medical education.

Flexner states that during the nineteenth century, 457 medical schools opened in the United States and Canada. To be sure, some of them were quite short-lived. Between 1810 and 1840, 26 new medical colleges were founded and by 1876 another 47 had been established.[2] Since income was at stake, the competition between schools was really fierce. Sometimes there were vigorous struggles between faculty groups in a single school over control of the school, and its revenues. Kaufman describes a particularly colorful event:

> One of the most memorable episodes of intrafaculty rivalry occurred in 1856 and revolved around a faculty dispute over control of the Eclectic Medical Institute of Cincinnati. The dispute became so hot that it actually led to open and violent warfare between the two factions. At one point there were two armies of students and faculty members confronting each other with knives, pistols, bludgeons, and blunderbusses. The faction that held the building faced a siege by the opposing forces. According to reports, the tall and bewhiskered Professor Joseph Rodes Buchanan, a leading exponent of phrenology, urged his troops to the battle crying, "On my lads." Finally the siege was broken when a six-pound cannon was located and used to defend the building; the sight of the cannon dispersed the forces. The rest of the battle was fought in court.[3]

The quality of the education offered in such an institution presumably was not too high, and indeed Kaufman cites a great deal of evidence from contemporary sources showing that it was very low: no laboratory experience, no clinical experience, few case demonstrations, poor lectures and lecturers, no equipment, no libraries, and so on.

Early Attempts at Reform: 1825–1870

The first recorded convention to discuss the quality of medical practice and medical education and how to improve them was held in Northampton, Massachusetts, in 1827.[4] It was attended by representatives of the state medical societies and the medical colleges of New England. The convention proposed a set of minimum standards for the education and examination requirements of licensure. The convention decided that a bachelor of arts degree was desirable for candidates for admission to medical school; that a minimum of three years of study in medical school with no more than six weeks vacation per year should be required (four years for those without a baccalaureate degree, who still had to present evidence of a good preparatory education), and that each candidate for licensure should have to pass exams in anatomy, physiology, surgery, theory and practice of medicine, materia medica (a mixture of pharmacology, the study of drug action, and pharmacy, the preparation of drugs), chemistry, and midwifery, and defend a dissertation.

These standards were high, so high in fact that they were never adopted. There was no way to enforce them. Licensing laws did not at that time deal with medical school curriculae, and the laws were already on their way out, in any case. Schools could choose not to adopt the standards and most of them did so choose. The easier schools attracted the students, while the more difficult ones, the ones with higher standards, lost them. Since in those days schools were entirely dependent upon student fees for their economic survival, in the absence of external regulation no school could afford to maintain high standards.

This sequence of events, the calling of a convention to discuss the quality of medical education and adopt resolutions prescribing reform measures, resulting in no measureable change, was repeated with some regularity throughout the nineteenth century. Sometimes, not even the convention got off the ground. In 1836, the Medical College of Georgia called a national convention, to meet in Washington, D.C. No one came. A convention met in Ohio in 1835 and again in 1838 with the object of improving medical education. Its recommendations, including a graded curriculum, beginning with basic sciences and concluding with clinical work, led to naught. It is interesting to note that the basic science/clinical-science juxtaposition, providing for sequencing but separation as well, is one of the basic principles of contemporary medical school curriculum design. It was a fresh and needed idea—in 1838. An 1840 convention scheduled for Philadelphia failed to attract any attendees as did the 1836 Washington effort. A convention did finally meet in New York in 1846, attended by 119 delegates from sixteen states. This meeting had no immediate effect on the quality of American medical education, but it did lead to the establishment of the American Medical Association.

Early Days of the AMA

In the beginning one of the AMA's principal concerns was with the quality of medical education. (A second was fighting the "quacks," "charlatans," and sects.) It developed a set of minimum standards for preparatory work and medical education, higher than the level met by most schools at the time, but lower than those adopted by the Northampton convention twenty years earlier. However, there was still no reason for any schools to meet even the AMA's standards. By 1850, no state had an enforceable medical licensing statute, and many had no pertinent laws at all. A medical college diploma might give its holder an advantage over his competitors; that, and a concern for one's potential patients, were the only forces motivating a person wanting to be a physician to go to a medical school. Because this was the case, the schools had the only remnant of "licensing power" which was left to anyone: they could choose *not* to grant a diploma to a particular candidate. However, concerning their standards, the AMA could only exhort, cajole, and pass resolutions.

In 1860, the AMA adopted a new set of minimum standards, including the requirement that medical schools and professorships be privately endowed so that they would not be dependent on student fees for their income. No medical college not meeting the standards could be represented in the AMA (which provided for medical school voting representation until 1874). The Civil War came, however, and in its aftermath, the situation deteriorated even further. It got so bad that in 1869 an AMA president actually asked for *federal legislation* to raise the standards of medical education. Most schools had virtually no requirements for pre-medical education. They provided a few short courses of lectures for a few months a year, during two years or so. There were often no labs, no dissection, no patient contact, and so on, as had been the case in many schools for the preceeding fifty years or more. By 1875, some observers concluded that medicine could no longer be considered a "learned profession."

Reform Begins: 1860–1900

The Graded Curriculum

In 1859, Lind University in Chicago established a new medical school.[5] The University was supported by Sylvester Lind, a wealthy businessman who endowed both it and the medical school, in line with the AMA's minimum standards of 1860. The school was thus not dependent on student fees and could afford to set minimum educational standards higher than those of its competitors in Chicago. When Mr. Lind lost his fortune in 1863, the medical school became the independent Chicago Medical College, still maintaining its former standards. Lind/CMC required a good preparatory education and was the first school to adopt a graded, sequenced, curriculum. It was fairly short, but it did follow some logical progression. The CMC managed to attract students, survived, and merged into Northwestern University in 1891.

In 1870, Harvard Medical School adopted a broad reform package: a graded curriculum over three academic years of nine months each, with oral and written examinations required in every department. Until that year, Harvard had been just about as slovenly as the rest of the medical schools of the country, but the University's new President, Charles Eliot, was determined that reform should occur. It did, despite resistence from the older faculty members. The school's enrollment dropped precipitously, but the reforms were maintained. Within a few years, Pennsylvania, Syracuse, and Michigan had joined in the reform movement.

Knowledge and Licensing

There were several reasons for these changes. In the 1850s, Virchow and his colleagues in Germany had begun to develop the science of pathology. By the 1870s the development of the science of microbiology was in full swing. Medical schools finally had something real to teach about disease and its diagnosis, even if they still had little to teach about its treatment. Secondly, licensing laws were being reenacted in certain states. By 1898, all states had them. As I pointed out in the previous chapter, about half the states had readopted the old system of requiring only a medical school diploma for licensure, with no enforceable provisions for regulation of the schools. However, half of the states also required passage of examination. This had an indirect effect on the schools in these states, because they now had to prepare their graduates to pass state examinations. Attendance at an (unregulated) medical school would no longer guarantee the student a license: licensure, in half the states, at least, had become separate from medical education. The circle had turned full: the situation was now what it had been when the first licensing laws were enacted towards the end of the eighteenth century.

The Medical Schools Begin to Organize

In 1876, the American Medical College Association was formed, by some of the "better" schools in the country. Again as had been done so many times before, a set of minimum standards, including a graded, three-year curriculum, was adopted. Meeting the standards was made a requirement for membership. However, most of the original members could not meet the standards while staying competitive with the non-conforming proprietory schools. The mandatory standards were downgraded at the 1882 Annual Meeting, and the Association did not meet again until 1889.

The Johns Hopkins

In 1893, the first modern American medical school opened, the Johns Hopkins in Baltimore.[6] It was a privately endowed school, so it could operate independent of student income. It was planned to be an integral part of a new university. A university hospital was designed specifically for the use of the school. It had a core of full-time faculty. It saw as one of its principal functions the carrying out of medical research. It also viewed itself as a resource to the nation and the world for training medical educators and researchers. It would be very selective in choosing its students. The training of "mere practitioners" would be left to the other schools. It had a graded four-year curriculum, with two years to be spent in the pre-clinical "basic" sciences of anatomy, physiology, chemistry, pathology, pharmacology, and microbiology, and two years spent doing clinical work "on the wards" and "in the clinics" of the university hospital. The design of the medical school was heavily influenced by developments which had taken place during the previous twenty-five years or so in Prussia. The idea of requiring extensive hospital work with bedside teaching for medical students, in a hospital directly connected to the medical school was a new one to the United States. The model for the university hospital itself was the English voluntary one which can be traced back to the founding of Guy's Hospital in London in 1725.

The Hopkins was extraordinarily successful. Within twenty years of its opening, each of sixty American medical schools had three or more Hopkins graduates on their faculties. Hopkins became the model for the medical school as it still functions, by and large, in this country today. However, the changeover, obviously drastic if one compares the Hopkins system with what existed in most American medical schools at the time, did not occur voluntarily, or by accident. The change did not occur because men of intelligence and good will surveyed the situation, got together, and voluntarily agreed to improve. Voluntary efforts had been underway for three-quarters of a century and most met with dismal failure. (Hopkins was in fact an outstanding exception). Major change occurred primarily only because the power of government was enlisted in the cause.

Today the licensing laws determine and maintain the position of the physician at the top of the health care delivery system. During the period 1890–1920, the licensing laws were a major force in changing the face of American medical education. In fact, if the power of the government had not been utilized by the reformers, it is doubtful that the reforms would have taken place, at least at that time, and to the extent they did.

The Medical Schools and the Licensing Boards

In 1890, the American Medical College Association met after a lapse of eight years.[7] It renamed itself the National Association of Medical Colleges, later and permanently, the Association of American Medical Colleges. For the umpteenth time a reform-minded convention adopted a set of minimum standards for medical schools, covering requirements for admission, a graded curriculum, minimum time in residence, and examination before graduation. This effort at standard-setting would probably have met with as much success as the first effort in 1827, if the reformers in the schools had not moved to join forces with the licensing bodies.

In 1891, the National Confederation of State Medical Examining and Licensing Boards voted to require that at least three years of medical school be a minimum standard for eligibility for licensure—whether or not a state required examination or a diploma alone for licensure. Even though the National Confederation by no means had complete control over its constituents, the effect was electrifying. By 1893, over 95 percent of schools had three-year curriculae. Content was, of course, not regulated, and a great deal of medical education was still of poor quality. Nevertheless, the sequence of events showed what the power of the government could do for a reform movement which had been essentially ineffective for three-quarters of a century.

For example, in 1894 the AAMC resolved that to be a member, a medical school had to adopt the four-year course. The AAMC promptly suffered a 22 percent decline in membership. In 1897, with fifty-four members, it could count only about one-half of the "orthodox" schools in its fold, about one-third of all schools. The state boards were not moving further; half of them still required only a diploma for licensure. The next move came from the practitioners.

The American Medical Association Pulls Itself Together

In 1900, the American Medical Association could count only a minority of American physicians among its members. Nevertheless, it was still the leading national organization representing practitioners of "regular" medicine even though its leadership was drawn largely from academic circles. In 1901, the AMA underwent a major structural change (it had experienced several since its founding), which resulted in the organizational pattern we recognize today.[8] It became in essence an organization of organizations, the latter being the state medical societies. At the same time it made membership available to any physician joining a local medical society recognized as a constituent member of a state medical society. This had not previously been the case; physicians had had to join the AMA directly, a complex process. Thus, while making governance indirect, for the first time the AMA made membership generally available.

Although individuals belong to the AMA, they are not directly represented in its decision-making process. Instead, members of local medical societies elect only their own governing bodies, which then elect delegates to state medical society governing bodies, which in turn elect the majority of members of the ruling body of the AMA, the House of Delegates, which, finally, elects the AMA Board of Trustees. The AMA thus became responsible principally to one constituency, the ruling bodies of the state medical societies, whereas previously a wide variety of constituencies had had voices in the leadership. Through the state medical societies, the AMA clearly now represented the practitioners. Following the organizational reform, the membership in state medical societies doubled in seven years: in 1908 it stood at 70,000, almost 50 percent of the total number of doctors. Membership in the AMA also equaled about 70,000, up from around 10,000 in 1900.

The AMA had always been interested in medical education reform, that being the movement that gave birth to the organization in the first place. The concern had been primarily with the quality of the product. However, the doctor already in practice had another concern: the number of competitors he had. In 1906, there were over 121,000 doctors in the United States, about one for every 675 persons. There were 162 medical schools, graduating 5,364 new physicians, twenty-six years earlier there had been only 100 schools, which produced 3,241 graduates.[9] In 1906, the field was overcrowded. Since there were a significant number of obviously poor medical schools, one logical outcome of any significant education reform would be to close them down. There was an obvious coincidence here between moral concern over the quality of medical education and practice and the self-interest of limiting future competition. The mix was powerful, and its existence certainly was an important factor in the establishment of the AMA's Council on Medical Education in 1904.

The Council on Medical Education

The reorganized AMA decided to move with renewed vigor in medical education reform. In 1902 a committee on medical education was created. Its work lead to the permanent establishment of a Council on Medical Education in 1904.[10] The CME's first chairman was Professor Arthur Dean Bevan of Rush Medical College in Chicago (which happened to be the site of the AMA's recently established national headquarters), and its first secretary was Nathan P. Colwell. They remained in office until 1928 and 1931 respectively, by which time the required reforms had been essentially accomplished.

The task of the CME, according to Kaufman, was "to secure the adoption of higher standards, to investigate the 'character of work done by each medical school,' and to inform the colleges of the AMA requirements."[11] Rosemary Stevens notes that:

> As a first move, the council that year adopted its own 'ideal standard' for schools: preliminary education of university entrance level; a five-year medical course (one year of physics, chemistry, and biology, two years of laboratory sciences, two years in the clinical branches); and a sixth year as an intern. These standards were much higher than those required for membership in the Association of American Medical Colleges. At the same time the council realistically also set minimum standards: four years of high school for admission; a four-year medical course; and satisfactory performance in a state licensing examination (this being known through the lists of state board results by schools already being published in the

Journal). Thus the existing movements of publicity and regulation were combined.[12]

The CME then began doing studies. In its first survey, in 1906, the CME ranked schools on the basis of the percentage of its graduates failing state licensing exams. In more than one-quarter of the schools, more than 20 percent of graduates could not make the grade. In 1907 the CME reported the results of a national survey of 160 schools based on visits to them by Dr. Colwell and a Council member. In the public release, schools were not named, but it was stated, according to Kaufman "that of the 160 schools, 'only about 50 percent are sufficiently equipped to teach modern medicine,' 30 percent 'are doing poor work,' and 20 percent 'are unworthy of recognition.' " Kaufman further notes:

> When Arthur D. Bevan, the chairman of the council, made his 1907 report, he noted that when the council made its inspection, it "found schools which are absolutely worthless, without any equipment for laboratory teaching, without any dispensaries, without any hospital facilities, some which are no better equipped to teach medicine than is a Turkish-bath establishment or a barbershop." In addition, Bevan declared: "Many schools are conducted for the purpose of preparing a student to pass a state board examination and not with the object of making him a competent practitioner."[13]

Each school privately received a copy of its report. The CME adopted a letter-grade ranking system: *A* for acceptable, *B* for doubtful, and *C* for unacceptable. There were 82 *A* schools, 46 *B* schools, and 32 *C* schools. However, all of this would have meant little if not for the relationship which was developing between the AMA and the state licensing boards. The medium was the state medical societies, which now were the principal constituents of the AMA. As Dr. Stevens states the state medical societies were "encouraged to stimulate educational reform: Dr. Bevan asked them to see that 'the right sort of men' were appointed to the licensing boards. Thus the licensing boards became, in effect, if not formally, the council's agents." Thus the reform movement really got underway. Stevens notes: "These activities [of the CME, the state medical societies, and the medical boards] stimulated the states to effect some reform, if only (as Dr. Colwell subtly suggested to them) to avoid being dumping grounds for poor-quality physicians."[14] Schools began merging, raising standards, or simply going out of business. Between 1906 and 1910, the number of medical schools dropped from 162 to 131.

By 1907, Bevan and Colwell had decided that the time had come to go public. However, they felt that a study done by the CME and/or the AAMC would not be considered to be impartial or objective. And so it was that they turned for assistance to the Carnegie Foundation for the Advancement of Teaching and its president, Henry S. Pritchett. Pritchett, an educator himself, agreed to support the study. To carry it out he chose another educator, Abraham Flexner. Thus the Flexner Report was born.

8

The Flexner Report

According to the report of the United States Commissioner of Education in 1899, there were in that year 23,778 medical students and 4911 medical graduates. Between 1875 and 1899 the increase in the number of medical students was 177 percent. But not alone upon statistics do we depend for confirmation of the crowded state of the profession. The fact is so patent and alive that much of the editorial space of leading medical journals is devoted to a discussion of the condition, its cause and its cure.

That a majority of the profession is incompetent and unworthy, is not subject to statistical proof. To the unprejudiced medical observer of the profession of almost any locality, the truth is patent that very many of its members are persons of inferior ability, questionable character and coarse and common fiber. The little esteem in which the profession is held by laity and government atteests its unworthiness. Patients whose number is legion throw themselves from its arms into the embrace of quackery, and we must admit that the support is often as effective in the one case as in the other . . . Granted that the wisest and most conscientious often stumble, to any one possessed of medical skill witnessing the mistaken diagnoses, inefficient and ofttimes barbarous, treatment, and the unconscionable fleecing of a credulous public by members of the profession, is borne in the conviction that, like the traveler on the Jericho road, he has fallen among thieves . . . Unquestionably the cause of professional degeneracy lies in the education requirements made for entrance to the profession; and hence the question resolves itself into one of medical colleges, their number, their location and their standards. . . ."

—Inez C. Philbrick, A.M., M.D.

Abraham Flexner was born into an upper-middle class German Jewish family in Louisville, Kentucky, in 1866, just after the Civil War. In 1883, he became an undergraduate student at the then brand-new Johns Hopkins University in Baltimore. He completed his baccalaureate work in two years. In 1890, he opened a private secondary school in Louisville. It became quite successful. He was able to put one brother, Jacob, through medical school, and another, Simon, to work in the pathology laboratories at Hopkins. Simon eventually became the first director of the Rockefeller Institute.

In 1905, Abraham sold his school and went to Germany for two years. During that time he wrote *The American College,* his first book. Upon his return, the president of Johns Hopkins, with whom he had remained in close contact over the years, introduced him to Dr. Pritchett of the Carnegie Foundation. Pritchett decided that Flexner, an expert in educational theory and practice, rather than either a physician or a medical educator, was the man to undertake the job that Bevan and Colwell had asked the Foundation to do: study the medical education system in the United States.

Although Flexner did not appear to be committed in advance to supporting the AMA-CME position, he certainly was heavily influenced by what he knew first-hand of German medical education. Further, in advance of beginning the study, he spent a great deal of time at the Hopkins medical school, itself modelled after the German example and still in 1910 dominated by a German-trained faculty. Thus he was armed in advance with a particular conception of what the ideal medical school would look like.

Flexner was meticulous in his work. He personally visited every medical school in the United States and Canada in 1908–1909. He went so far as to examine academic records of individual students concerning both performance in medical school and their preparatory education. The Flexner Report was published by the Carnegie Foundation in 1910. It received a great deal of publicity in the popular press. It has had a profound effect on American medical education since that time. However, on the one hand it was not quite as influential as many observers have since made it out to be, and on the other, the medical school design which has come to be called "Flexnerian" bears only a modest resemblance to what Flexner actually recommended in his Report.

Causes of Reform

Change in American medical education was already well underway in 1910. Medical education reform had been advocated by various interests, leading medical educators and practitioners among them, since 1825, as we saw in the previous chapter. There was ample objective evidence for the need for reform. It is fascinating that the content of reform proposals varied little throughout the nineteenth century, except that they became somewhat more elaborate as scientific knowledge increased. The recommendations always dealt in the main with preparatory education, the graded curriculum, laboratory work, clinical work in medical school under supervision, and the like, an eminently rational approach. Nevertheless, not too much happened until two particular events which I described in the previous chapter occurred. First, with the rapid increase in the number of physicians occurring from 1880 onwards, it came to be in the interest of the practitioner himself to do something about quality control (even though he might have to do something about the quality of his own work), because that would help to limit competition. Second, the reorganization of the AMA in 1900–1901 which gave the state medical societies control of its governance structure was a key event. On the one hand it made the practitioners the AMA's major constituency, thus rapidly increasing its membership; on the other hand, it gave the AMA a direct line to most state licensing boards, through the state medical associations. This coalescence of interests and modes of operation is what quickly led to change.

Flexner's Influence on Reform

We saw in the previous chapter that the number of medical schools began dropping in 1907, coincident with the first efforts of the CME to police medical education. Also, some of the remaining schools, particularly the non-proprietary ones, began tightening up, on both their educational programs and entrance requirements. Thus the Flexner Report, as Banta clearly points out, did not start the reform movement. However, it did catalyze, strengthen, and publicize, it. The Report provided a clear factual description of the deficiencies, while presenting an organized prescription for change. Furthermore, in its aftermath, Flexner was very influential in persuading private foundations to put their money into medical education, supporting those schools that changed in the "right" way.

Flexner's Findings

The Report has two parts. The first presents Flexner's summary views of the state of education in the various segments of the medical curriculum. He interlards the several chapters with program recommendations, although there is one chapter concerned only with his proposed consolidation of existing schools and his ideal geographic distribution of schools. There are also separate chapters on medical education for women and "Negroes." Part II presents the specific findings for each school visited.

General

Flexner found in American medical education a great deal to criticize. However, other than his particular concerns with educational technique, his observations were not new. (New were the specificity, the detail, the extensive proof, the naming of names, and the publicity.) Flexner criticized deficient student preparation; low admissions standards; the lack of a scientific basis for medical education; the lack of equipment and laboratory exercises; the lack of adequate, supervised clinical experience; relatively small, part-time faculties engaged in extensive private practice and in the proprietaries engaged in education for the purpose of making money. Flexner also sharply criticized the extensive use of lectures and didactic teaching methods, coupled with an examination system which rewarded rote memorization.

A few quotes will illustrate these points (page references to the Report are given in parentheses).

- On admissions standards:

  "What is your honest opinion of your own enrollment?" a professor in a Philadelphia school was asked. "Well, the most I would claim," he answered, "is that nobody who is absolutely worthless gets in!" (p. 35)

- On the standards of laboratory work in some schools:

  ". . . school positions are valued as professional stepping stones [by the faculty], not as scientific opportunities; laboratories are often slovenly and, except during class hours, entirely abandoned. (p. 81)

- On proprietary medical schools:

> For many years a school of this sort was a veritable gold mine to its owners. Fees were divided outright, or invested in buildings which the faculty owned. Once in a while the income was split: a large share went to the teachers, the rest was devoted to carrying mortgaged buildings held by the trustees. These structures themselves were not infrequently erected in pursuance of business policy. (p. 81)

- On the quality of some "teaching" hospitals and their medical staffs:

> Such institutions are mere boardinghouses for the sick. Physicians call there as they call at a private house, seeing twenty patients in the former instance, a single patient in the latter. . . . The visiting staff of physicians is appointed through favor, pull, or bargain, and the schools make the best of it. A small clique occasionally controls the situation. Conspicuous fitness cannot be the sole or main consideration. (p. 112)

- On the limitations on direct clinical experience, this time in obstetrics.

> . . . the very worst showing is made in the matter of obstetrics. Didactic lectures are utterly worthless. The manikin is of value only to a limited degree. For the rest, the student requires discipline and experience. The safety and comfort of both patients—mother and child—depend on the trained care and dexterity of the physician. The practice is a fine art which cannot be picked up in the exigencies of outpatient work, poorly supervised at that. Principles, methods, technique, can be learned and skill acquired only in an adequately equipped maternity hospital. . . . Difficulties and limitations in such matters sit lightly on most of our medical schools. (pp. 117–18)

- On didactic teaching:

> Out-and-out didactic teaching is hopelessly antiquated; it belongs to an age of accepted dogma or supposedly complete information, when the professor "knew" and the students "learned." The lecture indeed continues of limited use. It may be employed in beginning a subject to orient the student, to indicate relations, to forecast a line of study in its practical bearings; from time to time, too, a lecture may profitably sum up, interpret, and relate results experimentally ascertained. Textbooks, atlases, charts, occupy a similar position. They are not, in the first place, a substitute for sense experience, but they may well guide and fill out the student's laboratory findings. In general, the value of recitation and of the quiz is in proportion to their concreteness and informality. Outside the workshop there is danger of detachment and rote. (pp. 60–61)

Specific

In Part II of his Report, Flexner had some choice words for specific medical schools.

- On the two schools in Alabama:

  The foregoing account makes it clear that really satisfactory medical education is not now to be had in Alabama. The entrance standards are low; the schools are inadequately equipped; and they are without proper financial resources. (p. 186)

- On the California Medical College in Oakland:

  Laboratory facilities: The school occupies a few neglected rooms on the second floor of a fifty-foot frame building. Its so-called equipment is dirty and disorderly beyond description. Its outfit in anatomy consists of a small box of bones and the dried-up filthy fragments of a single cadaver. A few bottles of reagents constitute the chemical laboratory. A cold and rusty incubator, a single microscope, and a few unlabeled wet specimens, etc., form the so-called "equipment" for pathology and bacteriology. (p. 190)

- On the Jenner Medical College in Chicago:

  Clinical facilities: Clinical facilities are practically nil—one or two night clinics being all that the school claims to offer. The school once had access to Grace Hospital, a private institution of thirty beds; but it has recently been turned out for failure to pay for the privilege. The dispensary attendance varies from two to ten, four nights weekly. No particular rooms for dispensary purposes are provided: "patients are taken right into the rooms where the classes are."

  An out and out commercial enterprise. The instruction is plainly a quiz-compend drill aimed at the written examinations set by the state board of Illinois and of other states. (p. 62)

- Medical education as a whole in New York State was taken to task:

  New York has a double duty and a double opportunity in medical education. It must in the first place produce most of its own physicians and a considerable share of those who practise in neighboring states, which, like New Jersey, are without medical schools. Its eleven medical schools have so energetically done their part in this matter that New York itself and all the adjoining states are suffering from plethora. There is, therefore, no section of the Union which is at this moment readier for an upward step: population is comparatively well distributed, communication is easy, roads are good, educational facilities abundant, and doctors superabundant. . . .

> But New York may be fairly asked to do more than produce doctors, however excellent the type. Its vast hospital and university resources should make it the Berlin or Vienna of the continent; a genuinely productive contributor to medical progress; the center to which, in the intervals of a busy life, physicians will repair to freshen their knowledge and to renew their professional youth; to which the young graduate from the interior—from the schools of Pittsburgh, Ann Arbor, Madison, Iowa City—will look for the extension of his scientific and clinical experience.
>
> [However] little has as yet been done to realize this opportunity. The postgraduate schools are of very limited scope; the great New York schools have been in the main clinically unproductive . . . (p. 275)

• Hopkins of course came out very well:

> Laboratory facilities: These facilities are in every respect unexcelled. As the institution has been from the beginning on a graduate basis, teaching and research have been always equally prominent in its activities.
>
> Clinical facilities: The Johns Hopkins Hospital and Dispensary provide practically ideal opportunities. The medical staff of the hospital and the clinical faculty of the medical school are identical; the scientific laboratories ranged around the hospital are in close touch with clinical problems, immediate and investigative. The medical school plant is thus an organic whole, in which laboratories and clinics are inextricably interwoven. Recent foundations have greatly augmented the original hospital plant in the direction of psychiatry, pediatrics, and tuberculosis. Three hundred and eighty-five beds under complete control are now available.
>
> The dispensary is largely attended, and is admirably conducted from the standpoint of both public service and pedagogic efficiency. (p. 235)

There were a few other schools for which Flexner had some kind words: the University of Michigan, the University of Pennsylvania, the Jefferson Medical College, the Medico-Chirurgical College of Philadelphia, the University of Maryland, the College of Physicians and Surgeons of Baltimore, Rush Medical College (Chicago), Western Reserve, Washington University of St. Louis, Tulane, McGill, Toronto, Columbia, Cornell, Harvard, and Tufts. In general, however, Flexner's diagnosis was of serious illness.

Flexner's Recommendations

Numbers

Flexner was convinced that as well as there being severe quality problems, there was a severe problem of over-production of physicians as well. Relying solely on doctor-population ratios for determining need, but doing some very meticulous calculations, Flexner concluded that the annual output should decrease from about 4500 to 3500, and that the number of schools should be cut drastically, from 150 to 31. (Flexner's figures on the number of medical schools are somewhat different from those of the AAMC *Report* cited above.)

Program

Flexner also made a series of program recommendations: (1) that a minimum two years of undergraduate college work be required for admission to medical school; (2) that a four-year curriculum be adopted, with two years in the basic medical sciences being followed by two years of supervised clinical work on both inpatient and outpatient hospital services; (3) that regular laboratory teaching exercises be introduced; (4) that the quality of instruction be improved through the use of full-time faculty; and (5) that the medical schools be brought into the framework of the universities. These were the recommendations which were generally adopted, as we shall see below, some with good effect, some with bad, some misinterpreted. However, Flexner made a whole series of other recommendations as well, most of which have generally been ignored. It is useful to review them.*

*In the text I will simply summarize this set of recommendations and comments, as I have done the others, supplemented by some short quotations. However, since these parts of the Report tend to be more obscure, or to have been obscured, I am placing more extensive quotations in Appendix I where interested readers can consider them in some detail. In the text I will refer to these appendix items as I. a., I. b., and so forth.

On the Social Role of Medicine and the Importance of Prevention

Near the beginning of his Report, Flexner commented on the importance of preventive health activities to society, the social responsibility of the medical schools, the inappropriateness of profit-making in either medical practice or medical education, and the role of the state in regulating both:

> The overwhelming importance of preventive medicine, sanitation, and public health indicates that in modern life the medical profession is an organ differentiated for its own highest purposes, not a business to be exploited by individuals according to their own fancy. (I. a.)

Flexner described the importance of social medicine, that is, the role of medical practice in the social structure, and the importance to the physician, and thus to the patient, of the understanding of those relationships:

> . . . the physicians' function is fast becoming social and preventive, rather than individual and curative. (I. b.)

Flexner felt that public health practice is part of the *work* of both the physician and the medical school:

> . . . the laboratory sciences all culminate and come together in the hygienic laboratory; out of which emerges the young physician, equipped with sound views as to the nature, causation, spread, prevention, and cure of disease . . . (I. c.)

Flexner also discussed the science-service gap, or, as it is colloquially known today, "the problem of technology transfer."

> Society reaps at this moment but a small fraction of the advantage which current knowledge has the power to confer. That sick man is relatively rare for whom actually all is done that is at this day humanly feasible—as feasible in the small hamlet as in the large city, in the public hospital as in the private sanatorium. We have indeed in America medical practitioners not inferior to the best elsewhere, but there is probably no other country in the world in which there is so great a distance and so fatal a difference between the best, the average, and the worst. (p. 20)

On the Role and Responsibility of the State in Regulating Medical Practice and Medical Education

Flexner advocated an activist role for state governments in setting minimum standards for entry to medical school, through the state licensing boards. In fact, he felt that medical education reform in general would not come about without government intervention:

> Inevitably, the way to better medical education lies through fewer medical schools; but legal enactments on the subject of medical education and practice will be required before the medical schools will either give up or relate themselves soundly to the educational resources of their respective states. (I. d.)

In considering the social responsibility of the physician, Flexner commented on the resultant right of the state to regulate, i.e., "interfere with," those institutions which train the physicians:

> The right of the state to deal with entire subject [of medical education] in its own interest can assuredly not be gainsaid. The physician is a social instrument. . . . Practically the medical school is a public service corporation. (I. c.)

He went on to discuss the issues of freedom which would arise from such interference:

> The community through such regulation undertakes to abridge the freedom of particular individuals to exploit certain conditions for their personal benefit. But its aim is thereby to secure for all others more freedom at a higher level. (I. f.)

Flexner felt that in the main state boards of medicine should influence schools of medicine indirectly, through standards applied to individual applicants for licensure. However, in cases where direct intervention was needed, Flexner heartily endorsed it:

> The law that protects the public against the unfit doctor should in fairness protect the student against the unfit school. (I. g.)

This recommendation was, in fact, one of the less well-known ones which was implemented. (Most of the rest were not.) State boards of medicine were involved with the business of defining medical school curriculae to a rather high degree of specificity between 1910 and 1925. Between 1925 and 1930, the Association of American Medical Colleges and the Council on Medical Education managed to get them to discontinue this practice. Since that time, medical schools have been largely self-regulated (see Chapters 9 and 11).

In discussing the means of evaluation available to state boards of medicine, Flexner put little trust in written examination. He believed strongly in what is now called "competency-based evaluation." Not only would this approach correctly evaluate individual condidates, but it would also evaluate schools:

> If the written examination were relegated to a subordinate position, the weight of the test would fall upon the applicant's ability to do things; schools incapable for whatever reason of training students in the necessary technique would be rapidly exposed through the annual publication of statistics proclaiming their failure. (I. h.)

Finally, Flexner believed in uniform state licensing laws enforced by a single agency. (Recall that national licensing had been proposed by an AMA president in 1869.) Since Flexner believed that medical licensing agencies should control schools as well as individuals, the body created would be a powerful one indeed:

> Perhaps the entire country may some day be covered by a national organization engaged in protecting the public health against the formidable combination made by ignorance, incompetency, commercialism, and disease. (I. i.)

On Teaching Methods, Curriculum, and Organization

Flexner discussed the problems of teaching medicine, particularly the basic medical sciences, in the rote-memory, didactic mode, which stressed the importance of examinations, featured in most medical schools in his day. A modern version of this educational approach which stresses memorization of facts rather the learning of the ability to solve problems is featured in many medical schools today. (I. j.)

A bit later on he followed these observations with a comment on the importance of general education to the physicians, especially in relation to his developing social role:

> . . . the social role of the physician will generally expand, and to support such expansion, he will crave a more liberal and disinterested educational experience. (I. k.)

Although only in a footnote, Flexner advocated that instruction in the history of science and medicine be part of the regular medical curriculum:

> Nothing would do more to orient the student intelligently than a knowledge of the history of medical science and teaching. It is a great pity that some effort is not made in the better medical schools to interest the student in the subject. A proper historical perspective would render impossible such opposition to improved medical teaching as is now based on conscientious but mistaken devotion to outgrown conditions. (p. 52)

To Flexner the teaching of the scientific method was the most important task of the medical school, for both the future investigator and the future practitioner:

> The main intellectual tool of the investigator is the working hypothesis, or theory, as it is more commonly called. . . . Upon this he acts, and the practical outcome of his procedure refutes, confirms, or modifies his theory . . . This is essentially the technique of research: wherein is it irrelevant to bedside practice? (I. 1.)

Flexner saw the importance of teaching basic science to medical students in a manner which makes it clinically relevant.

> . . . undergraduate [medical] instruction will be throughout explicitly conscious of its professional end and aim. In no other way can all the sciences belonging to the medical curriculum be thoroughly kneaded. An active apperceptive relation must be established and maintained between laboratory and clinical experience. Such a relation cannot be one-sided; it will not spontaneously set itself up in the last two years if it is deliberately suppressed in the first two. There is no cement like interest, no stimulus like the hint of a coming practical application. (p. 59)

Flexner stressed the importance of teaching medicine in an ambulatory care setting.

> The backbone of the structure [for clinical teaching] is the clinic in internal medicine. (I. m.)

One of the widely-hailed modern innovations of our time is the geographically spread-out school: basic science teaching in one place; clinical teaching elsewhere.[1] Encountering the administrative and practical difficulties inherent in this arrangement, Flexner had little use for the idea. (I. n.)

On Faculty and the Place of Research

Flexner had a clear idea of why it was important for medical school faculty members to undertake research.

> . . . practitioners of modern medicine must be alert, systematic, thorough, critically open-minded; they will get no such training from perfunctory teachers. Educationally, then, research is required of the medical faculty because only research will keep the teachers in condition. A non-productive school, conceivably up-to-date today, would be out-of-date tomorrow; its dead atmosphere would soon breed a careless and unenlightened dogmatism. (p. 56)

Research in medical school, then, is clearly to be supportive of the teaching function, its most important feature. According to Flexner, teachers should do research not as an end in itself, but in order to keep themselves up to snuff in the classroom. However, Flexner also saw a definite role for the non-investigator teacher of particularly high quality. (I. o.)

As to modes of paying medical school faculty members, particularly clinical ones, Flexner would have frowned sternly on the modern "geographic full-time" system. (I. p.) Under geographic full-time, clinical faculty members receive only part of their income from the medical school. They earn the balance in private entrepreneurial fee-for-service practice. There are about as many arrangements for regulating the private practice of faculty members, and sharing the income, as there are medical schools.

Finally, on the Purpose of Medical Schools

In contrast with the never-ending debates over the relative importance of patient care, teaching, and research in medical school today, Flexner had a clear idea of the medical school's principal function. He was brief, and to the point:

> Of course the business of the medical school is the making of doctors; nine-tenths of its graduates will, as Dr. Osler holds, never be anything else. (p. 56)

Flexner confirmed this view by suggesting that the best way to evaluate medical schools is through outcome measures:

> In the end the final test of a medical school is its outcome in the matter of clinicians. (p. 105)

The True Flexnerian Model for Medical Education

A careful reading of the Flexner Report reveals a design for a good medical education system which is quite different in many respects from the one which has developed in the sixty-five years since the Report was published. In summary, a Flexnerian system of medical education would have the following features.

Preventive medicine would be stressed and the work of government public health departments would be integrated with that of the medical schools. The concepts of the social nature of the physician's work and the social responsibility of the physician would be among the most basic tenets of the educational philosophy. Because of the social nature of medical practice, the state would have the right to evaluate and control not only the work of individual physicians, but also of the medical schools which create them. In line with the concept of the social responsibility of the medical profession, a great deal of attention would be paid to closing the science-service gap and raising the quality of the work of all physicians to that of the best ones.

The most important task of the medical educational process would be to teach the understanding and use of the scientific method. Thus the didactic-lecture/rote-memorization method of teaching, and examinations would be of limited utility. Lectures would be used primarily for introductions to and summations of subject areas. Examinations would be used more as learning experiences than as measures of performance. The problem-solving method of instruction, i.e., the practical use of the scientific method, would be widely employed. To the greatest extent possible, basic medical science teaching would be integrated with and made relevant to clinical teaching. The use of the problem-solving method would, of course, greatly facilitate this integration.

Understanding the social role of the physician and the social nature of medical practice would be important parts of the curriculum. Thus by implication, epidemiology, biostatics, health care delivery systems analysis, medical history, ethics, behavioral science, and sociology, political science, and economics as they apply to health and health care delivery would occupy central places in medical education, rather than being at or beyond the fringe as they now are. In considering the educational prerequisites for medical school entry, equal attention would be paid to student preparation in the natural sciences, the social sciences, and the arts.

The principal responsibility of medical schools would be to train practitioners. There would be a profession of medical educator. Research by them would be encouraged, as a means of keeping their minds fresh, but it would also be recognized that there is such a thing as a "pure teacher." Medical educators would be evaluated primarily on the basis of their performances as instructors. The bulk of biomedical research would be carried out in institutes designed and founded for that purpose. Full-time medical faculty would be employed on a salaried basis only. "Geographic full-time" would not be permitted.

Teaching medicine in ambulatory care settings would be stressed, since that setting more closely approximates the one in which the majority of practitioners work than does the inpatient side of a university hospital.

Outcome evaluations would be used to the greatest extent possible in measuring the work of medical schools. That is, their effectiveness would be determined by the quality of their work and the social utility of the physicians which they produced. Flexner would begin an evaluation of the work of a medical school by examining what it does in its ambulatory services, not what it does on the inpatient side. Furthermore, his three principal evaluative criteria would be: continuity of service by the instructors, continuity of care afforded to the patients by the students, and availability to the students of the clinical laboratory.

The performance of physicians would be evaluated principally by measures of competence in doing their work, rather than by written examination. State boards of medicine would adopt uniform licensing laws, and possibly would be replaced by a single national agency. Whatever its nature, the regulatory agency(s) would deal directly with the medical schools as well as with the products of their work. To quote Flexner, the principal reason to regulate both physicians and medical schools would be to "protect the public health against the formidable combination made by ignorance, incompetency, commercialism, and disease."

This is quite a radical prescription. To implement it widely today would require a national political upheaval of titanic proportions, if not a revolution. This is to say nothing of the educating and reeducating which would be necessary to train medical school faculties which could teach in the true Flexnerian mode. However, it must be remembered that the Flexner Report did not reflect the musings of some idealistic dreamer. Flexner came from a solid, middle class family in Louisville, Kentucky. His brother Simon became Director of the the Rockefeller Foundation. Flexner's study was supported by the Carnegie Foundation. The author was mainstream, and the Report was intended to be the same.

Flexner was obviously interested in producing a better brand of physician. His prescription is in fact logical and internally consistent. It rests on the bedrock of two basic postulates: that the scientific method is the foundation of any effective medical practice and that medicine is part of the social fabric and has a fundamental social responsibility, principally related to the maintenance of the health of the population. Everything else flows from these two precepts.

What Happened to the Flexner Report and Why

Reforms Adopted

At the beginning of the section on Flexner's recommendations, I summarized the principal ones which were adopted. They dealt with admissions standards, length and grading of the curriculum, standards for pre-clinical and clinical work, attachment of the medical schools to the universities and improvement in the quality of faculties and the instruction they provided.

Interestingly, the two features which are often referred to as the bedrock of "Flexnerian Reform" or the "Flexnerian System," are nowhere to be found in the Report, at least in the form in which they are usually described. The first is the lock-step, two-plus-two, basic science–clinical-science curriculum. The other is biomedical research as a principal function, for its own sake, of a medical school. Flexner did feel that there was a natural progression to be followed from basic science to clinical science. He did specify that the first year should be concerned with "anatomy, including histology and embryology, [and] physiology, including biochemistry," and that the second year should cover "pharmacology, pathology, bacteriology, and physical diagnosis."[2] He did feel that the third year should be spent "in the clinics" and the fourth year "on the wards." However, he did *not* specify the lock-step character of the curriculum as it appears in most medical schools (virtually all until about fifteen years ago), and he did specify that there should be a high degree of interdigitation between basic science and clinical learning.[3] Significant amounts of clinical correlative work in the preclinical years have been introduced in only a minority of medical schools, and only in the last fifteen years or so. Faculty resistance to this concept, especially among basic scientists, appears to be very high. Furthermore, Flexner heartily condemned the teaching approach to basic science instruction still used in many medical schools: didactic lecturing, rote memorization, and frequent examination.

Research Policy

As for biomedical research, Flexner did say: "In short, research, untrammeled by near reference to practical ends, will go on in every properly organized medical school; its critical method will dominate all teaching whatsoever; . . ." But the end of that sentence is: "but undergraduate instruction will be throughout explicitly conscious of its professional end and aim."[4] Flexner, as I also showed in the previous section, viewed the role of research in medical schools as *supportive* of the educational function, not the other way round. Faculty members were advised to do research to be able to remain sharp as teachers. The present place of research in medical schools as a dominant function, as the principal preoccupation of many faculty members, as the main yardstick for measuring faculty performance in relation to advancement, was not a Flexnerian prescription at all. In fact, biomedical research did not become a significant activity at many medical schools until after World War II when significant amounts of Federal money to support biomedical research became available, as we shall see in Chapter 10.

The Hopkins Model

It has always been thought that Flexner was enthralled with the Johns Hopkins model, and what he simply wanted to do was make over all medical schools in the likeness. Flexner was certainly deeply impressed with Hopkins, particularly with the placing of medical education in the university, and the emphasis on teaching the scientific basis of medical practice. But although he didn't say so directly, there were obviously many features of the model which he could not have liked: the divorce of treatment from preventive medicine, the separation of basic science from clinical teaching, the lecture method of instruction, and so on. The Hopkins system was not new, having been in operation more than fifteen years. True Flexnerian reform would have affected Hopkins almost as much as it did those schools that closed.

The truly worst schools, those which sold diplomas, had no equipment, had qualitatively and quantitatively wretched staffs, and so on, did close. Other schools merged. Still others were "up-graded." However, the up-grading was not to the true Flexner model, as derived from the careful reading of the Report reviewed above, but to the Hopkins (and to a certain extent Harvard) model, which approximated the true Flexner model only in certain limited ways.

Thus the Flexner Report was and still is distorted by the controllers of the medical education system. Bits and pieces were extracted, and the rest went by the wayside. But why did this happen? In the Progressive Era, with the major foundation support that was being made available, why were the medical schools not swept into an experience of really major change? At this point, I can attempt an answer to that question based only partly on fact. The rest is surmise. I hope that future researchers will be able to ascertain more facts and either place my thesis on a firm footing or replace it with something better.

Why What Happened, Happened

To understand the direction the reforms took, one must understand the priorities and motivations of the major affected interest groups: the owner/operators of the proprietary (generally poor quality) medical schools, the scientific medical establishment in the university-related medical schools, the mass of practicing physicians, the public at large, and the major corporations. I will review these motivations and priorities very briefly, and, as I said above, hope that future research will elucidate them more clearly.

The End of the Proprietary Schools

The interest of the owner/operators of the proprietary schools was clearly in keeping them open and operating at a profit. However, as David Banta has pointed out, reform was already underway. Even without Flexner, proprietary schools would have had to make improvements in faculty and facilities. The changes cost money, so much that they could not afford to keep up. The proprietary interests of most of these schools were simply trampled underfoot by the other affected groups. The AMA took clear aim at the proprietary schools through the Council on Medical Education. The CME had developed a four-rank rating system for medical schools: *A+*, the very best; *A*, good; *B*, in need of improvement; *C*, clearly unacceptable.[5] By 1914, thirty-one state medical boards were refusing to recognize diplomas from Class *C* schools. In 1915, the AMA House of Delegates directed the CME to automatically rank proprietary schools as Class *C*. Although some of the better representatives of the profit-making schools did survive, either on their own or through merger, as non-profit institutions, the proprietary medical school was eliminated from the American scene by the Flexner Report and its aftermath. This development certainly satisfied the interests of those who were concerned with reducing the number of medical graduates being produced each year.

The Interests of the Scientific-Medical Establishment

The principal interest of the scientific medical (sci/med) establishment, the group which dominated the best medical schools, and which was leading the struggle to put medicine on a scientific basis, was to entrench itself and ensure its power. In the mid-nineteenth century, allopathy had been no more effective in treating human ills than its major competitors: homeopathy, Thomsonianism, naturopathy, and electicism. In the late nineteenth century, allopathy acquired new rivals in chiropractic and osteopathy. By the turn of the twentieth century however, allopathy was beginning to become scientifically effective with discoveries in bacteriology, asepsis, and anesthesia. Thus, allopathy was on its way to putting the other sects out of business, or at least severely restricting their influence, for reasons of scientific progress.

However, to make sure of this, the sci/med establishment within allopathy had to clean its own house and establish its hegemony over allopathic medical education. The real message of Flexner meant nothing to this drive, but the Hopkins model certainly did. So the Hopkins/Flexner reform, which actually meant reform for everyone else besides those which already looked like Hopkins, was strongly pushed by the sci/med establishment. After all, when everyone else either looks like you, or at least wants to look like you, you have to feel that your leadership position is pretty secure.

The interest of the sci/med establishment in the Flexner Report was not to change itself, which the Report really advocated, but to use parts of the Report to solidify its leadership of allopathic medical education and position itself for the final assault on the competing sects. Thus was born the myth of the "Flexnerian Model." The two-plus-two curriculum, the upgraded admissions standards, the introduction of a great deal of basic science instruction, were certainly in Flexner's Report, but represented only a small part of his recommendations, as I have shown. The sci/med establishment really selected-out the Hopkins Model, but I suppose the Flexner name sounded better. And thus it was that a distortion and careful selection of Flexner's proposals really served the interests of the sci/med establishment very well.

The Practitioners

For the mass of practicing allopathic physicians, the name of the game was reduction in numbers. Although there were quite a few sects, for some reason which I don't understand, the allopaths always clearly outnumbered them, even when the main allopathic treatments were purging and bleeding. The practicing allopaths were very concerned, however, about having too many of their own kind about. Flexner advocated reducing the annual output of physicians by about 25 percent, with a still-growing population. The practitioners could have cared less about the rest of the Report, except for the proposals to strengthen the licensing boards and quality control in general, which they likely found rather threatening. However, the reduction in the future output of the medical education system suited the interests of the practitioners very well, so that piece of the Report received their strong support.

The Public Interest

The interest of the general public at the time consisted in eliminating true quackery, in eliminating incompetence among allopaths, and in expanding scientific medicine. True Flexnerian reform would have served the interest of the people far better than what really happened. However, Flexner's arguments on social responsibility, teaching methods, and the like were very sophisticated, and not one of the professional or corporate interest groups supported them. I am not familiar with the organized public interest groups of the time, but if they were involved with this issue at all, they were apparently content to go along with the interests of the two principal professional groups, which certainly seemed to represent steps in the right direction.

The Corporate Sector

Finally, we come to the corporate sector. Howard Berliner, a perceptive student of Flexnerian reform, sees "the interest of the industrial capitalists in scientific medicine . . . as a need (a) to legitimate the existing social structure in light of the prevailing scientism present in the general social consciousness, and (b) to subordinate the means of reproduction of the productive sector of society (i.e., medical care institutions), to capital accumulation."[6] The corporate sector has always had an interest in maintaining the health of its workers at least to a level at which absenteeism from the job due to illness is not a significant problem. For that reason, the corporate sector played a major role in the success of the Sanitary Reform movement in the nineteenth century. It was logical for it to support a reform which seemed to promise improved health for the workers, while at the same time not costing all that much.

The Introduction to the Flexner Report was written by Henry S. Pritchett, President of the Carnegie Foundation. Although Flexner developed the sophisticated, socially responsible model for medical education described above, Pritchett concentrated on a few simple points: (1) there were too many doctors; (2) the main reason for this was the existence of the commercial (profit-making) schools; (3) didactic teaching abounded, but as laboratory teaching became more necessary the poorer and smaller schools could not afford to keep up; (4) many medical students, particularly the poorer ones, were inadequately prepared; (5) teaching hospitals were necessary for proper medical education. Pritchett hammered away particularly at the commercial schools, did not discuss any needs for reform of the schools already university-based, and introduced Hopkins as the specific model to emulate.[7]

He and his corporate colleagues then proceeded to put their money where their mouths were, through their private foundations. As Rosemary Stevens points out: "The total foundation commitment to medical education up to 1938 has been estimated at $154 million; most of this went to the leading private schools. Foundations were thus the most vital outside force in effecting changes in medical education after 1910, and, for a long time, they took the place of government suport."[8]

Ideological Problems

Finally, in trying to understand why the real Flexner Report was not implemented, but why what might be called the Flexner Myth was, one has to examine the ideological problems involved. Flexner, in talking about the social responsibility of the physician, was talking about a people-oriented health care delivery system. In talking about medical schools in which the main job was to turn out practicing physicians, he was talking about the subordination of self of people who really wanted to be researchers or superstar consultants to the needs of teaching. Real teaching requires a tremendous amount of giving on the part of the teacher. In talking about the role of the state in the regulation of the medical education system, Flexner was talking about one which would be responsible to the needs of the people for health care delivery. In coming down so hard on commercialism in medical education, and on private practice among medical educators, Flexner was attacking profit-making in the medical education system, if not in the health care delivery system in general. In stressing the role of prevention in medicine, and the close relationship which should exist between medical schools and government departments of public health, Flexner was by implication outlining a limited role for private practice in the health care delivery system.

Will the Real Abe Flexner Please Stand Up?

In summary, the sci/med establishment selected out of the Flexner Report those pieces which appealed to it and quietly rejected all of the rest. As one reads their encomiums over the years, it is obvious that the sci/med establishment has continued to do this, creating the Flexner Myth.[9] The corporate class actively supported the sci/med establishment. Although the practitioners were apparently not directly involved in the original decision-making process (the AMA not being in their hands in 1910), they certainly benefitted over the years as the number of schools, and the number of doctors, fell. The owner/operators of the commercial schools got the short end of the stick. (A few of them may have wondered why the corporate giants turned thumbs down on profit-making in medical education when it was so acceptable to the corporations in their own fields of production.) Finally, the general public benefitted, but not nearly as much as they could have if the Report had really been implemented.

If the real Abe Flexner could stand up, and if his total package of recommendations could be implemented today, with a few additions concerned with team practice and leadership, the result would be a system of medical education with a high degree of social relevance. In fact, I have drawn significantly on Flexner's thinking for the reform recommendations I have to offer in Chapter 13. Sometimes there is nothing newer than something old.

9

Years of Consolidation: 1910–1945

In the years immediately following the publication of the Flexner Report, the process of shrinking the number of medical schools, which had begun in 1906 pursuant to the early efforts of the Council on Medical Education, continued (see table 9.1.). From a peak of 162 medical schools in 1906, the number had fallen to 76 in 1930, and 10 of those offered pre-clinical instruction only. The physician-population ratio declined as well. It had stood at 147 per 100,000 in 1910. By 1930, the ratio had fallen to 126 per 100,000. Furthermore, since specialization was beginning to develop in earnest by the latter year, the effective competition among physicians fell by an amount even greater than the fall in the doctor-population ratio. In 1931, 75 percent of physicians were in primary care (general practice, internal medicine, pediatrics). (By 1945, that proportion had fallen to about 60 percent, while the physician-population ratio had risen slightly, to 134 per 100,000.) Finally, by 1930, competition had been reduced not only by the fall in the physician-population ratio and the rise in specialization, but also by the virtual elimination of the competing disciplines, with the exception of a few osteopaths and fewer still homeopaths, through strict application of the licensing laws.[1] One of the major goals of the medical education reformers had been achieved.

Improving Quality

In the reformers own terms, quality was improved as well. By 1925, every medical school required four years of high school and two years of undergraduate college education for admission. By 1945, virtually all medical schools required four years of college, or three years from a college which would grant the student a B.A. degree after completion of one or two years of medical school. By 1925, curriculae had generally fallen into the pattern which has been labelled Flexnerian, but is really Hopkinsonian since it lacked

Table 9.1. **Numbers of Medical Schools, Graduates, and Doctors, and Doctor-Population Ratios, Selected Years, 1906–1930.**

Year	Medical Schools	Graduates	Doctors	Doctors per 100,000 pop. (Approx.)
1906	160	5,747	121,484	142
1910	131	4,440	135,334	147
1915	96	3,536	143,787	143
1920	85	3,047	145,707	137
1925	80	3,974	147,010	127
1930	76	4,565	154,472	126

Sources: Association of American Medical Colleges, *Final Report of the Commission on Medical Education,* New York, 1932, Appendix, tables 60 and 104; U.S. Department of Commerce, *Statistical Abstract of the United States, 1974,* Washington, D.C., 1974, table 2.

Flexner's recommended flexibility and clinical relevance in the pre-clinical years: two years of basic science (anatomy, physiology, and biochemistry in the first year, pathology, pharmacology, and microbiology in the second), followed by two years of clinical work. In 1915, in an attempt to deal with lax licensing standards still used by some state licensing boards, an independent, voluntary examining body called the National Board of Medical Examiners had been formed to administer one standardized test for all medical graduates. By 1925, many states had recognized it in lieu of their own examinations, and others were raising their own standards to meet those of the NBME.[2]

The Role of the Foundations

Key to many of these changes were the private foundations, particularly John D. Rockefeller's General Education Board. Abraham Flexner, whose brother Simon was, you will recall, Director of the Rockefeller Foundation, became a member of the GEB in 1913. Major grants primarily for faculty support, with a requirement for matching funds, went to schools adopting the Hopkins model: Johns Hopkins itself, the University of Chicago, Washington University in St. Louis, Rochester, Iowa, Cornell, and Vanderbilt.[3] Successful reform in these institutions was copied at Columbia University, Minnesota, Michigan, Wisconsin, and Missouri. Hopkins had been supplying medical faculty to the better schools for some years, and the availability of money to those schools which would follow the Hopkins model, virtually ensured its replication around the country.

The Hopkins Model for Faculty

Johns Hopkins had been created by a small group of determined and intelligent men. The designer, really creator, of the hospital which became the model for the "university hospital" around the country was a reformer of military medicine, John Shaw Billings. The university's president was Daniel Coit Gilman, who believed that the road to reform of medical education lay in integrating it within the university. The leading medical faculty members were the dean, William H. Welch, a pathologist, a brilliant internist, William Osler, an innovative surgeon, William Halsted, and Franklin Mall, the professor of anatomy. Although they all agreed on the necessity of reform, there were disagreements about how to get there.

Osler, who wrote the first modern American textbook of medicine, believed in clinical relevance, bedside teaching, and the use of part-time clinical faculty for teaching. Mall, a basic scientist, was interested neither in teaching nor in clinical medicine. He felt that it was research work which qualified one for advancement in medical education, either in basic or clinical science. He was heavily influenced in this regard by his own German training. He also believed that all medical school faculty should be full-time.[4]

Full-time or Part-time?

Both Mall and Osler were thrust on the horns of a dilemma which remains unresolved to this day, a dilemma, and basic contradiction, created by the existence of private entrepreneurial fee-for-service medical practice and the lucrative income it can afford to the competent physician, particularly one with a medical school appointment. Osler felt, quite rightly, that practicing clinicians have an important role to play in teaching clinical medicine. Mall felt that having a private practice would conflict with one's teaching responsibilities, and in any case, practitioners couldn't do research. However, medical schools had a hard enough time finding money to pay their basic scientists, much less could they afford to support clinicians on salary, particularly at a level anywhere near what one could make in private practice. This situation lead to the establishment of two institutions which still exist in virtually all American Medical schools, and which still lead to serious conflicts.

The first is the "geographic full-time" system. Clinicians are physically at the medical school all the time, but spend some of it doing private practice in an office provided to them by the school. There are various arrangements for sharing the income generated, between the doctor, his department, and the school. (See also Chapter 11.) Conflicts of interest are definitely introduced by this system in which faculty private income is funding, in part, medical education.

The other institution which leads to conflict is the double pay scale, a lower one for basic scientists and a higher one for clinicians (all schools now have at least some clinical faculty on full-time salary). This means that an anatomist teaching medical students gets a significantly lower salary than a surgeon teaching the same students (possibly) the same material. The surgeon is paid on the "clinical scale," plus his private practice income, while the anatomist is paid on the "basic science" scale. The only factor influencing the level of the "clinical scale" is the private medical marketplace.

Both Osler and Mall were right in certain respects. Osler wanted active clinical faculty; Mall wanted full-time faculty who could concentrate on the medical school work. The existence of the private practice system did not allow for a successful resolution of the conflict in either direction. Although many part-time clinicians are successful teachers, many others are distracted by practice demands; not enough money will ever be available to put all clinical teachers on salary, as long as the private medical market place determines the scale. In 1906, Osler left Hopkins for a prestigious position at Oxford University in England. In 1913, a few full-time clinical chairs were established at Hopkins with a GEB grant, under Mall's influence, however. In a 1911 letter to the then president of Johns Hopkins criticizing the Flexner Report, Osler recognized the true meaning of what this step would mean in terms of the school's orientation:

> To say, for example, as contrasted with the instructors in the laboratory side the clinical staff has been on the whole less productive and less devoted is simply not true. . . . We chance the sacrifice of something that is really vital, the existence of a great clinical school organically united with the profession and with the public. . . . I fear lest the broad spirit which has characterized the school should narrow, as teacher and student chased each other down the fascinating road of research, forgetful of those wider interests to which a great hospital must minister.[5]

Part-time clinicians have never been swept out of medical schools; nor could they be, economically. However, with Mall's influence over the full-time clinical positions which did exist at Hopkins, research achievements became the key to advancement, in the Hopkins Model medical school. Nevertheless, as we shall see below, research did not become a major factor in the work of most medical schools, nor something very many of them seemed interested in doing (see the 1932 AAMC report on medical education discussed below), until significant amounts of money became available to support the activity after World War II.

Controlling the Medical Cirriculum

I pointed out above how, beginning in 1906, the AMA's Council on Medical Education worked with the state medical boards to raise standards for medical licensure, thus indirectly affecting medical school programs and quality. Recall that Flexner recommended that if this approach to raising standards didn't work, the state medical boards could and should get into the business of regulating medical schools directly. He justified this kind of action on the basis of the social role of medicine.

The state medical boards did in fact do just that. They involved themselves heavily in curriculum design, setting out regulations to the extent that a school, even one of recognized high quality, that wanted to experiment a bit stood in danger of losing its approved status from one or more state boards. This kind of rigidity was fine with the sci/med establishment when the aim of the AMA, and of the Association of American Medical Colleges, which always had represented the better schools anyway, was to get rid of the marginal schools, particularly the proprietaries. Once that goal had been achieved (the job was virtually complete by around 1920), the remaining schools began to champ at the regulatory bit. "Government interference" was perfectly appropriate when it served the purposes of the leading schools; it being no longer needed, the remaining school now wanted to be relieved of the burden. Listen to the AAMC itself, representing its position in 1925:

> The various efforts of the profession, educators, and licensing bodies to elevate and standardize medical education have largely eliminated the proprietary and commercial schools, and have established certain minimum requirements which are regarded as necessary for proper training. While these regulations of various kinds have been largely responsible for the elevation of the standards of training, they have led to great rigidity and a considerable amount of overregulation. At no period in history have there been such rapid additions to knowledge regarding disease and health. The medical faculties as well as the licensing bodies have endeav-

ored to keep abreast of this growing body of knowledge by adding requirements and examinations and, in consequence, have created great overcrowding of the curriculum. . . .

There is now need for a sounder basis of action on the part of the regulatory bodies and the various organizations concerned with both general and medical education in formulating requirements for licensure and training.[6]

They certainly were forthright.

In 1925, the AAMC approached the Federation of State Medical Boards (FSMB) and asked for a moratorium (the AAMC called it a "truce") on further curriculum regulation and the suspending of curriculum controls altogether for several years. In 1929, the FSMB passed the following resolution:

Resolved, That in each State the medical practice act and its administration conform as far as possible to the educational principles of the Association of American Medical Colleges.

The following year, the FSMB gave in entirely to the AAMC, amending its constitution and bylaws in the following manner:

In all matters of premedical education, courses of study, and educational requirements for the degree of Doctor of Medicine or its equivalent, the Federation recognizes the Association of American Medical Colleges as the standardizing agency for this purpose.

The Federation regards as its proper function (a) the determining of fitness for the practice of medicine, and (b) the enforcement of regulatory measures.[7]

State boards did retain some standards for minimum total time required in medical school and for certain basic courses, but for the most part, the AAMC now regulated itself in the matter of cirriculum. The AMA continued to rank schools, by a variety of criteria. In 1942, the AMA and the AAMC jointly established the body which presently accredits medical schools, the Liaison Committee on Medical Schools. Medical schools are not licensed by the states and are regulated by the Federal government only in limited areas, primarily by indirection, i.e., if you don't do task *x*, you won't get *y* dollars. By and large, they are subject to self-regulation, a process open to abuse. I shall discuss the current status of medical school accreditation in Chapter 11.

Specialization

In 1930, about 75 percent of all physicians were primary care providers, mainly general practitioners. Nevertheless, the prestigious Commission on Medical Eudcation, which had been organized in 1925 by the AAMC, was concerned about the problem:

> Partly because of the skill required in the use of certain instruments, undue emphasis has been given to the various specialties, a number of which have been developed around technical procedures. There has been an extensive subdivision of labor in the field of practice. . . . This subdivision of labor, however, has gone beyond the actual needs of the community and most patients. . . .
>
> The tendency to partition practice into organs, systems, and techniques, with consequent dispersion of responsibility for the patient as a whole, not infrequently turns out to be unnecessary, costly, and misleading. . . . Because his efforts are often confined to a single phase of medicine, the specialist looks too frequently upon the problem of the patient solely from the aspect of his specialty, rather than from the needs of the patient as a whole.[8]

Once again, private entrepreneurial practice, with its built-in opportunities for high income, particularly in the specialties, was a powerful stimulus to specialization.

Specialty Boards

Despite the AAMC's caveat, specialization proceeded apace, nay accelerated. (Fifty years later, the proportions are reversed: at least 75 percent of all physicians are specialists.) The 1930s saw the explosive growth of a phenomenon called Specialty Boards. They constitute a type of voluntary certification in which a group of like medical specialists get together, set standards and criteria for the specialty as they define it, establish examination, educational, and experience requirements for certification, and then proceed to administer them. They are successful to the extent that board-certified specialists are chosen by the public for the named services, and hospitals limit privileges to carry out named categories of work to board-certified specialists.[9] Recently, insurance companies and Medicare/Medicaid have set higher fees for specialists for a variety of tasks and services.

The first specialty board was established in 1916, the American Board for Ophthalmic Examinations, renamed the American Board of Ophthalmology in 1933. The otolaryngologists (ear, nose, and throat specialists) broke away from the formerly combined board in 1924, setting up the American Board of Otolaryngology in 1924. Obstetrics and gynecology followed in 1930, pediatrics in 1932. Orthopedic surgery, colon and rectal surgery, anesthesiology, and general surgery followed suit in 1934–1937. By 1940, there were fifteen specialty boards.

Motivation

Why the rush to specialize, particularly in the light of the AAMC's own warnings on the subject? One motivation was economic, of course. It is likely that it is not a coincidence that the majority of specialty boards were formed during the Great Depression, when the majority of physicians were scrabbling for a living, just like almost everybody else. Freymann has a lovely quote from Herodotus (485–425 B.C.) demonstrating that specialization is nothing new. Upon visiting Egypt, Herodotus noted that:

> . . . every physician is for one disease and not for several, and the whole country is full of physicians; for there are physicians of the eyes, others of the head, others of the teeth, others of the belly, others of the obscure diseases.[10]

Whatever the reason for Egyptian specialization, Freymann observes that an important motivation for modern specialization is the nature of medical knowledge, or the lack of it. He quotes an English physician, H. Miller, writing in the *Lancet* in 1966:

> The fact is that medicine consists of few well-lit islands of scientific certitude, surrounded by a boundless ocean of shadowy uncertainty and ignorance.

Freymann himself then goes on to say:

> With their new scientific training, physicians knew that the best way to perform an experiment was to limit variables. Since a human being presents an infinite number of variables that are poorly standardized and almost impossible to control, it was better science for each doctor to

occupy a little island of knowledge and certitude and learn as much as possible about a few variables. Furthermore, educational psychologists have shown that the acquisition of knowledge increases power and diminishes insecurity, but that any uncertainty diminishes power and increases insecurity. Everyone clings to the knowledge he possesses for security. These were the reasons for specialization.[11]

Not only does specialization bring psychological security and higher incomes, but for people who are not bothered by constant repetition of the same kinds of work tasks, specialization is also easier than general practice. Once the body of knowledge in your specialty has been mastered, that's it. You have one area to concentrate on—for the rest of your life. Although the better ones do, the specialist really does not have to bother remembering that huge body of knowledge which is medicine, nor does he need concern himself with patient complaints outside of his neatly compartmentalized area.

Of course, from the public's point of view, specialization itself is desirable, so that those persons who have difficult and/or complex illnesses can be properly taken care of. The problem is not specialization itself, but the proportion of physicians who are specialists. For example, consider surgery. Manual skills of any sort are honed to their finest point—and kept there—only by constant repetition. As we saw in Chapters 3 and 5, there is in fact too much surgery in this country, and even with that there are too many surgeons who do too few operations per week to possibly maintain a high level of skill. The solution to this particular problem is, however, the same as for specialism as a whole: fewer specialists, who do more of the work for which they are specifically trained.

Control in Specialization

The specialty board system led to some control of the quality of specialty training programs in hospitals, but despite the AAMC's anti-specialization plea, none over numbers. In 1933, the AAMC, FSMB, National Board of Medical Examiners, and several other organizations formed the Advisory Board for Medical Specialties. Among other things, it was to approve the creation of new specialty boards. The AMA's Council on Medical Education claimed this prerogative, however, and refused to join the club. In the end, the CME and the ABMS agreed to work together in sanctioning new specialty boards. The CME kept for itself the power to review and approve the hospital residency training programs which turned out the specialists.[12]

The CME has never made an effort to limit the number of residency positions available. It only reviews the educational content of residency programs. If the standards are met, the residency is approved. There is no effort to relate the total number of residency positions in a particular specialty to any projected national needs for that kind of specialist. Hospitals like to claim that residency training programs are entirely educational in nature. Their protestations to the contrary notwithstanding, however, most hospitals create residency positions to meet service, not projected educational needs. That is, a hospital will devote so and so many beds to surgery, and will need so and so many doctors on its own paid staff to handle the load, i.e., assisting its private physicians and handling its own directly-admitted patients. One result of this system was that the available number of hospital residency positions far outstripped the number of graduates of American medical schools. This led directly to the importation of large numbers of foreign medical graduates to fill the residency positions—and meet service needs. Federal legislation passed in 1976, the Health Professions Educational Assistance Act, sharply limiting the number of foreign medical graduates who may enter the country, will eventually cause major changes in the ways hospitals conduct their business.

Since 1972, residency reviews have been supervised by a new body, the Liaison Committee on Graduate Medical Education, with representatives from the AMA, the AAMC, the renamed American Board of Medical Specialties, the Council of Medical Specialty Societies, the American Hospital Association, and in token roles, the federal government and the general public.[13] Although its procedures are more complex than those followed previously, the LCGME shows little inclination to get into specialty distribution planning, preferring to leave the matter to "voluntary action."

There are screams of anguish from the medical education (med/ed) establishment every time a federal legislative proposal to regulate specialty distribution is made. A current federal requirement regulating, and forcing an increase in, the number of primary care residencies (but not touching distribution among the specialties) got through Congress only over the determined opposition of the med/ed establishment. In this area, voluntarism has been tried for fifty years. It has failed miserably. Yet proposals from within certain segments of the med/ed establishment that the LCGME itself strictly regulate residency training position numbers in relation to national needs before the federal government finally does it, meet with the same screams of anguish, from the same elements who decry "government interference" so strongly. They seem to want to continue business as usual, even though the health care needs of the people are not being met. An eventual political and economic calamity for the medical profession appears to be in the making.

The AAMC's 1932 View of Medical Education

As we have seen, the origins of American medical education reform can be traced back to the first adoption of the graded curriculum by the Lind University Medical School in Chicago in 1859. Harvard was the first major medical school to adopt the graded curriculum, in 1870. In 1893, the prototype of the modern American medical school was established at the Johns Hopkins University. However, medical education reform did not take place in any significant measure until the first decade of this century when there occurred the coincidence of private practitioner interest in controlling competition, scientific advance, AMA reorganization to represent first and foremost the state medical societies and their private practitioner constituents, and large corporation concern with medical care.

The changes initiated during the beginning of the 1900s, catalyzed by the Flexner Report, had been consolidated to a great extent by 1925. In that year, the Association of American Medical Colleges organized a Commission on Medical Education. Its *Final Report,* published in 1932, makes for interesting reading, even today. Since so many of its observations and recommendations are still relevant almost a half-century later, I will briefly review the major ones here, sometimes quoted, sometimes summarized, in the order in which they appear in the *Report.*

- "The Commission has believed from the beginning that an emphasis on educational principles in medical training and licensure can be secured only by modifying the point of view and broadening the interests of those responsible for medical education and licensure, not by recommendations, statistics, new regulations, further legislation, or manipulation of the curriculum." (p. 3)
- "The immediate need was to secure relief, if possible, from the restraint and burden of external regulations, particularly those of the various state licensing bodies regulating the details of medical training, and to stimulate the experimentation in medical education." (p. 4)
- It was recognized that the product of medical education should bear some relationship to the needs of the community for medical service. (pp. 5, 12)
- "Medical education should emphasize to students the influences of urbanization, industrialization, and present-day conditions of living which are important in the causation, treatment, and prevention of disease. . . . it is important that the physician be acquainted with the social, economic, and other environmental factors which have an influence on the individual and his health." (p. 14)
- The Commission recognized and stressed the problem of the science-service gap ("technology-transfer"), just as did Flexner. (pp. 18–19)
- As noted above, the Commission was particularly concerned with the problem of overspecialization and warned against it on several occasions. (pp. 23–24, 114–19, 172)
- The Commission noted that the population was aging (they predicted correctly that by 1975, 25 percent of United States residents would be fifty or older), and called attention to the increasing importance of chronic disease. At the same time, it noted that the increased life expectancy which had been observed in the previous fifty years had been due almost entirely to reduction in childhood mortality. (p. 25)
- The Commission stressed the importance of prevention in clinical practice (pp. 26, 30–31) and in medical training. (pp. 60–62)
- The Commission noted that physician incomes were not high. (p. 36) Indeed, high incomes for a *majority* of physicians are a relatively recent phenomenon. Competition served to hold incomes down into the 1920s, and the Great Depression kept them that way. The mean net annual income of nonsalaried physicians was $5200 in 1929, but had dropped below $3000 by 1933.
- Even in 1932, when the doctor/population ratio was down to 126/100,000, and the medical disciplines competing with allopathy had either been put out of business entirely or vastly reduced in

relative numbers and influence, the Commission felt that there was "an oversupply of physicians." (p. 64) This concern was reiterated. (p. 93)

- "Legally the practice of medicine . . . is a monopoly. . . . The intent of this monopoly is not to create benefits for the medical profession, but to protect the public." (p. 89)
- The problems of geographic maldistribution were well recognized. (pp. 104–113)
- As noted above, the AAMC wanted, and got, the discontinuation of state medical board interference in medical school curriculae. (pp. 165–69)
- Turning to medical education itself, the Commission noted some of its then-current defects:

> [There is] instruction in too many subjects in too great detail. . . . [and] great overloading of the curriculum. The dependence upon sheer memory tends to defeat the development of a scientific attitude and point of view.
>
> Teachers, graduates, and students agree that topics are presented too frequently from the standpoint of the special interest of the teacher and from the aspect of technical details.
>
> There is widespread opinion, however, that an unreasonable amount of time is consumed in meaningless laboratory work as a method of education.
>
> The chief criticism of the clinical instruction is that it is often focused upon the rare and serious diseases. . . . The presentation of many such problems . . . gives the student an erroneous idea of the medical problems in the community at large. (pp. 174–75)

- The Commission outlined its conception of a good medical school program:

> [It] is exemplified by the discontinuance of the rigid class system and uniform time and course schedules which require every student to complete exactly the same courses in the same time, and the substitution of small sections; personal contacts between students and teachers in the clinic, hospital, and laboratory; use of tutors, counsellors, and preceptors; reasonable freedom for reading, thinking, and elective work; emphasis upon achievement rather than attendance; reduction of lecturing to a minimum; encouragement of independent work; stimulation of scientific curiosity; use of comprehensive instead of departmental examinations; and postponement of specialized training until after completion of the basic preparation.
>
> The present concept aims to develop sound habits as well as methods of independent study and thought which will equip the student to continue his self-education throughout life. . . .

The medical course, partly because of the requirements for licensure, has been concerned more with the factual matter a student had memorized at the time of graduation than with the development of intellectual resourcefulness and sound habits and methods of study. Too great an emphasis has been placed on description and the memorizing of many details and facts which, though they are of little permanent significance, are of immediate value in passing the examinations and in meeting the requirements of licensure to practice. (pp. 177–78)

- As did Flexner, the Commission stressed the importance of clinically correlating basic science instruction and of teaching clinical medicine in an ambulatory care setting. (pp. 181–97, 209–211)
- The Commission returned to the subject of preventive medicine and its basic science, epidemiology: "Both curative and preventive medicine are dependent upon an understanding of the importance of the same environmental factors. Efforts to create an artificial separation of these two fields of medicine are unsound." (p. 220) The Commission pointed out that most clinicians know little about preventive medicine and recommended that preventive-medicine teaching be integrated into clinical teaching. If felt similarly about teaching the social aspects of medicine:

The principles guiding the economic and social factors in medical care should be emphasized to medical students. The presentation of these principles should be made a part of the regular instruction in the clinical subjects, not as courses detached from the main body of medical knowledge. (p. 229)

- The Commission also concerned itself with the problems of teaching and teachers in medical schools:

The extent to which the profession of education appeals to men and women of ability and promise is determined largely by the inducements and attractiveness of the field. At the present time it is probably true that mastery of the clinical subjects and ability to teach are not sufficiently considered in the selection of the personnel of some faculties, and little attention is paid to the preparation of medical teachers in the art of teaching. The great emphasis in selection is placed upon ability and interest in, or willingness to do, research, in which outstanding ability is rare. Too much emphasis is placed upon this single requirement, important as it is.

In the clinical divisions the responsibilities for the care of patients, both in the hospital and outpatient services, demand a high order of clinical ability and interest in problems of medical practice and community health. These responsibilities are not alone the application of the medical sciences to disease in the nature of clinical physiology, but require a keen insight into a large variety of human, psychological, emotional, economic, social, and environmental factors which often

> determine successful diagnosis, treatment, and prevention. . . .
> If clinical teaching is to attract and hold teachers of the caliber and ability which it requires, and provide a corps of younger instructors from which the senior members of the staff may be recruited, there must be a fuller recognition of the freedom and dignity which such work should command. (pp. 244–45)

Although the Commission was very concerned about "government interference" and "the oversupply of physicians," its general view was a progressive one even for today. It stressed the importance of prevention, what we would call "primary care," and the social aspects of medicine. In its conclusion, it noted that "most sickness and disability are due to only a few causes, and often they are preventable." The Commission recognized that teaching students to be physicians is a profession in itself. Its prescription for medical curriculum form and content is still advanced—and still quite correct: flexibility; deemphasis of lectures, memorization, and examinations; teaching the scientific method; clinical correlations; emphasizing the common not the rare; and so on. To the best of my knowledge, this approach has yet to be introduced in more than a handful of schools—fifty years later.

The Depression and World War II

The medical education system remained fairly stable through the Depression. There were about 4500 to 5000 graduates per year in the period 1930–1940, from 76 (then in 1933, 77) schools. Elton Rayack cites evidence showing that the AMA played a significant role in this situation. The AMA and the Federation of State Medical Boards were both very concerned about the "overproduction of medical men." The AMA talked about "professional birth control." An AMA President discussed the threat "to the economic welfare of the future practitioner" of this "overproduction."[14] The AMA brought strong pressure to bear on the medical schools to reduce intake. Acceptances did in fact fall between 1933 and 1939. Interestingly enough, either because the students who made it into medical school were better, or because medical schools became less severe in grading, medical school output actually rose slightly during that period. Of course, it can be surmised that the economic situation of the country also inhibited medical school expansion.

World War II brought about an effort on the part of the schools to expand their production. By squeezing the curriculum and shortening vacations, one whole extra class of 5000 graduates was produced during the peak war years of 1943–44. The long lead time for training doctors did result in a war-effort–related total of almost 6400 graduates in 1947, but by 1949, the total was back to 5100 or so. By the next year, however, there were two new schools.[15] An upward climb in medical school output began again, leading eventually to a doubling of output in the succeeding twenty-five years. It is to a consideration of the post-War era that we turn in the next chapter.

10

Years of Expansion: 1945–1976

1945–1965: Building the Research Base

The Schools Move to Expand

Coming out of the wartime situation, perhaps with a taste of what it was like to be bigger and more important, certainly with larger cash flows, the medical schools started looking for additional money.[1] Before the war, the bulk of their income had come from tuition, endowment income, and foundation grants (which often went to build up endowments rather than to direct expenditure). During the war, significant federal financial support became available to medical schools for the first time, for accelerated physician training programs. After the war, these funds dried up, at the same time that inflation was growing.

The medical schools recognized their developing plight quickly. Writing in 1946, Dr. Raymond B. Allen, then Dean of the medical school of the University of Illinois in Chicago, said:

> The medical schools of this country will need to double their budgets for teaching and research by 1960 in order to take full advantage of the wartime momentum of medical research which has discovered so much and brought to light enough promising leads to keep many workers busy for years to come. It is not to be expected that the advance of medical science will continue at its present rapid rate unless significantly larger budgets are made available to medical schools.[2]

At a Congressional hearing in 1949 the philanthropist Albert Lasker said that "the heads of the greatest medical schools in the United States" had told him that they were "on the verge of financial collapse." Dr. Alan Gregg, Director of Medical Sciences for the Rockefeller Foundation (no less) said: "Unless our medical schools receive substantially larger sums for their essential expenses, we shall not in the future have the care which modern medicine could provide."[3]

Meanwhile, there was a lot of to-ing and fro-ing about doctor-population ratios. Recall that in 1910 the figure was 146 per 100,000 population. In 1930, it was 125 per 100,000. By 1945, it has risen to 134 per 100,000, at which level it remained for the next five years. (The ratio fell off slightly to 132 in the fifties, reaching a post-war low of 130 in 1960.) Although in percentage terms the net decrease from 1910 wasn't that great, it must be remembered that most of the competing medical disciplines had been knocked out of the field. The remaining competitor of any significance, osteopathy, which retained full medical practice rights in many states, had 5 percent as many practitioners as did allopathy in 1950, 4 percent in 1970.[4]

After World War II, the AMA said the doctor-population was adequate. Other interests, in the medical education establishment, in government, and among the general public, said it was not.

Either could have been right, and both could have been right, or wrong, at the same time. Recall that I showed in Chapters 3 and 5 that doctor-population ratios tell us very little about available medical services except when they are *very* low, as in many underdeveloped countries. Doctor-population ratios do not take into account what doctors are actually doing and how many other health professionals there are and what they are doing; they do not reflect geographic and specialty distributions; they do not reflect the fact that under fee-for-service, private practice doctors to a great extent create their own demand; and so forth. Thus the argument raged (and still does) around a relatively meaningless statistic.

At that time the major thrust nationally to assist the medical schools was for federal financial aid to medical schools. Several bills to provide such aid were introduced in the 81st Congress (1949–50). Proposals to pay for "the costs of instruction, including support of faculty salaries and operating facilities, grants for construction and equipment of schools, and federal subsidy of scholarships" were incorporated into the Wagner-Murray-Dingell National Health Insurance bill of 1949.[5] Although the AMA recognized that the schools had financial needs, it bitterly opposed federal aid, arguing that expansion was unnecessary and any possible "federal interference" unthinkable. The AMA did support private aid to medical education and was instrumental in forming the nonprofit National Fund for Medical Education. The NFME never raised very large amounts of money, but interestingly enough in recent years has become a major supporter of innovative projects in medical education.

For the first time in history, the AAMC parted company with the AMA on a significant issue. The AAMC summarized its position as follows:

1. There is a definite need now for federal aid to medical education provided the educational and administrative policies can continue to rest in the hands of the medical colleges without political interference and with the maintenance of academic freedom.
2. Such aid should not interfere with private and state aid.
3. Aid to students should have a need qualification. If there is any indentured service, it must have an escape clause. Scholarships should be awarded to those already admitted to medical schools.

> Many educators prefer aid in the form of loans, others prefer gifts instead of loans, in view of the long training period.
>
> 4. Attention must be given to the maintenance of standards in the present medical school operations . . . [While incentives for expansion are not opposed, incentives] for new students should not be so attractive as to cause expansion beyond facilities at too rapid a rate.[6]

As part of its hard-fought victory over the proponents of national health insurance, the AMA also defeated the supporters of federal aid to medical education. By so doing, the AMA indirectly caused the only major change which has taken place in American medical education since the time of Flexner: the creation, and then ascendancy leading to domination over medical education, of a Medical Research Establishment.

Research Takes Over, for a Very Good Reason: Money

A Research Imperative?

You will recall that in his Report Flexner had strongly recommended that unless they were particularly outstanding teaching experts, medical school faculty members should undertake research, to keep themselves fresh and to make sure that their teaching did not become dull and dated. In other words, research was to be undertaken in medical schools to support their principal function: teaching. Now it happens that, according to Freymann, Flexner was strongly influenced by Hopkins' Professor of Anatomy, Franklin Mall, who himself was heavily influenced by his own German training in the 1880s, in which research by medical faculty members was viewed as an important end in itself. Mall felt, in fact, that research output was the only reasonable basis for evaluating faculty performance, whether in the basic science or clinical arena. This thinking did not make its way into Flexner's Report. However, it was certainly an important element in the Hopkins Model which was so widely emulated (rather than the true Flexnerian Model). Furthermore, Mall's research orientation may well have influenced Flexner's policies when as a member of Rockefeller's General Education Board after 1913 he handed out so much money to American medical schools.

By 1930, a relatively significant amount of research was being undertaken by medical school faculty members. Nevertheless, the absolute amount was small, as was the overall influence of research on medical education. Despite Flexner's best efforts, many schools still depended in large measure on part-time faculty members who otherwise practiced private fee-for-service medicine. In 1954, fifteen medical schools still had no full-time faculty whatsoever. Although exact figures are not available, the average school probably had fewer than forty full-time faculty members in 1930. (Twenty years later, the number had risen to only fifty, according to Freymann.)[7] With this small average number of full-time faculty members, research could be a significant activity only in the few schools which had large faculties. Nevertheless, the schools certainly managed to train physicians.

Thus there was no magical relationship between medical education and research. That relationship was in the Prussian model on which Hopkins was based, but in his analytical work Flexner discussed it only as a support for the teaching function. The word "research" doesn't even appear in the index of the Flexner Report. The AAMC wasn't particularly concerned with the research function as a *necessary* part of the medical education process either. The word "research" does appear in the index of the Commission on Medical Education's 1932 Final Report, once. It refers to a passage discussing research as an activity which the occasional very bright medical student might want to undertake, as an elective. After World War II, as we saw above, when the AAMC first went looking for federal money to support medical school operations, it did not ask for research money. It did not describe research as the missing essential in the educational process. No, it simply asked for direct federal support of medical school operations.

Nevertheless, the research function has taken over most American medical schools as a, sometimes the, principal activity. This happened, beginning forty years or so after the Flexner Report, not because of any impelling logic, but because increasingly large amounts of money, particularly federal money, became available to support it. And this happened, in large measure, because the AMA prevented the development of direct federal-aid-to-medical-education programs.

The NIH and Medical Faculty

The vehicle for the transmittal of federal research money to the schools was the National Institutes of Health.[8] In 1887, a bacteriologic research lab had been set up in the United States Public Health Service. This government research activity gradually expanded, and the unit became the National Institute of Health in 1930. In 1937, a National Cancer Institute was established in the NIH, with a significant new function: it could give financial grants to nonfederal institutions. Little happened during the war. However, immediately afterwards, an interesting alliance developed between a group of influential Congressmen led by Senator Lister Hill of Alabama and Representative John Fogarty of Rhode Island, and a group of research-minded, wealthy, private citizens led by one Mrs. Mary Lasker, wife of the philanthropist, Albert Lasker.

In 1944, $150,000 of an NIH annual budget of $2.5 million went to support extramural research (research carried on outside the NIH). Growth began immediately after the war. By 1947, the NIH research budget was $8.3 million. By 1955, it was $70 million, and one-third of medical school income was from research grants, primarily federally funded. These grants went directly to individual scientists, thus establishing a new independent interest group within the medical schools. It was not until 1960 that some research money was made available to institutions as well.

By 1958, there were over ten thousand medical school faculty members, double the number ten years before. The number more than doubled again in the next ten years. By that time, nearly half of medical school faculty members received some federal money. One-third received half their pay or more from the federal government, 15 percent were totally dependent on federal support, and the federal government was spending over $600 million per year in medical schools, primarily on research. The growth of research in medical schools was further aided by the passage in 1956 of AMA backed federal legislation providing matching grants for the construction of medical school research facilities. The AMA had only feebly supported, and the Eisenhower Administration killed, a bill which would have provided support for construction of medical school teaching facilities. Research was okay with the AMA;

they just didn't want more doctors. As Rayack points out, research does (or can) increase the *demand* for medical practitioners, while direct aid to medical education does (or can) increase *supply*.[9] The former exerts an upward pressure on physician incomes; the latter a downward pressure.

Distortions

Providing federal financial support for medical schools through the medium of research grants introduced any number of distortions into the medical education system.[10] The NIH and its leadership were not blind, of course. They recognized that at least some research money was supporting educational activities. Some of the consequences of that fact were certainly predictable, even in the early days of rapid growth of financial support in the mid-fifties. But the NIH leadership seemed unable, or unwilling, to do anything about it.

There was a very wide range of support levels among the schools. In general, the rich ones got richer while the poor ones didn't make out very well. Those schools which had some research activity going at the time the whole process got underway were in the best position to attract grant support. Then the process became self-perpetuating. The best way for a school with little or no research activity to get into the act was to attract (steal) a top researcher-grants man from another school, preferably along with his entire team from senior associates to lab technicians. At times it seems as if the national research community could really benefit from the free-agent drafts and anti-tampering rules which have been so well-developed by the professional sports leagues.

Since grants went primarily to individuals rather than to institutions, in many of them duchies were created around the top researchers, or at least around the top grant-getters. The academic reward system was revised, as is only to be expected, to benefit the researcher/grantsmen. They developed self-perpetuating hierarchies within their own realms, and of course became very important role models for students and house staff. On the other hand, deans' offices and the university presidents liked the "overhead money," (a surcharge on the grant for "general support expenses"), kept pushing the percentage up, and didn't ask too many questions as long as that overhead kept flowing in.

Nationally, the NIH set up a grants review system which was free of "government interference" to a significant degree. Most decisions on grant awards were made by peer-review "study sections," relatively free from outside political influence. Study sections, which review grant applications and make recommendations to the NIH, are made up of experts in the field in which the proposed research will be carried out. Study section members are often beneficiaries of NIH grants themselves, and the persons applying for the grant in question may well have sat on the study section when the present study section member was applying for *his* grant. Although the NIH does its best to avoid and control direct conflict-of-interest and one-hand-washes-the-other situations, the research community is so small in many fields that at least informal, very often benign, conflict-of-interest is bound to occur at least sometimes. Thus, the study section system has elements of the incestuous: members of study sections tend to be top researchers, while it is the top researchers who tend to attract the grants.

With money rewards going to research, teaching became submerged at many institutions. Publish or perish became a strictly enforced rule for promotion and tenure (permanent job) decisions. Most young academics abided by it if they knew what was good for them. Loyalties of federally-supported researchers were in general not to their schools. They were loyal to their chief and/or the National Institute which was funding them. By 1970, there were about ten National Institutes, most of them for disease categories. As Freymann says: "Deans discovered that there were only three areas of over-all concern to their faculties—the size of the student body, curriculum planning (these two gave them control over their teaching load), and parking."

As clinical departments, as well as basic science departments, began to avail themselves of research grants, research became the key to advancement in them as well. "Shades of Franklin Mall!" as Freymann says. Thus even in the clinical departments, research or grant-getting ability, not skill in patient care, to say nothing of teaching, became that which was striven for. In some schools, it is difficult to distinguish clinical and basic science departments on the basis of their work output. The M.D's are distinguished from the Ph.D.'s only by their higher salaries (the so-called "clinical scale"). Thus teaching became downgraded in the clinical as well as the basic science departments, with primary clinical teaching responsibilities for medical students in some schools often left to the least experienced teachers or clinicians: the house staff.

Ultimate Outcomes

The medical schools have followed Willie Sutton's advice: they went where the money was. There was nothing malicious about this; it was only natural. They needed money after the War; the federal government was the only real resource available; the AMA blocked the direct aid the schools had wanted; the schools went for what was available. Neither, however, was there anything magical about it. The Medical Education Establishment now would have us believe that research is the necessary bedrock of medical education, that "poor quality" would result from either a divorce of biomedical research from medical education, or a sharp reduction in the research effort, or a reorientation of it towards applied research. However, no argument was ever made before the massive federal research support effort started that it was necessary for the creation of quality medical education, nor is there much evidence that the quality of the product the schools are turning out is particularly high. In fact, the evidence I cited in Chapters 3 and 6 indicates that the opposite is the case.

As Freymann says:

> With a seemingly inexhaustable supply of federal funds, research became a goal in itself—a juggernaut with its own massive momentum, its own raison d'être, racing on, oblivious of its only justification: to serve mankind. And because a generation of doctors had grown up in this atmosphere, the same philosophy had come to pervade much of the health care system.

A Matter of Accountability

The most unfortunate aspect of the whole experience was that the medical schools flubbed the dub, so to speak. In their first experience as a recipient of federal money, in ever-increasing amounts, they missed a golden opportunity to demonstrate public responsibility and accountability. Not only were they getting money, but they were largely self-governing in terms of spending it. The study-section–peer-review system for making grant awards, in combination with a friendly, facilitative NIH bureaucracy, a benevolent, trusting Congressional leadership, and a powerful citizens' lobby, put a large measure of self-determination in the hands of the medical schools.

The medical schools could have set biomedical research priorities in terms of national health needs as measured by epidemiological methods. They could have given significant attention to making sure that the fruits of research were made available to the largest number of people at the earliest time. They could have made sure that medical school teaching was not downgraded but was maintained as at least an equal partner with research. They could have distributed the money more evenly among their members, consciously helping the poorer schools. They could have shown concern over the increasing problems of subordination of institutional and public needs to those of individual faculty members. They could have dealt with the substitution of research activity for patient care as the major goal and function of many large clinical departments. They could have responded positively to the concern with the direction and policies of the biomedical research effort expressed in some Congressional quarters as early as 1961 by Representative L.H. Fountain.[11] The medical education establishment in fact did none of these things, but instead created, in Freymann's term, "a juggernaut with its own massive momentum" for which "research became a goal in itself." A major opportunity was missed. Yet the medical schools still demand complete self-governance in using the federal money now being given them for direct support of operations. Previous experience must give one pause for thought.

It should be understood that I am not against biomedical research, per se. Research is the only way our body of knowledge is enlarged, and progress comes only with an enlargement of our body of knowledge. Since the war, our nation's biomedical research effort has produced a number of significant scientific advances. However, I am against a research effort which is only rather modestly responsive and accountable to the taxpayers who are footing the bill. I am also against a research effort that so distorts our medical education system that in many quarters has largely forgotten its original primary function: the education and training of physicians who are ready, willing, and able to meet the broad range of needs of our people for health care.

1965–1977: Era of Growth

Medical Schools Expand—in Number and Size

The number of schools had remained stable at 77 from 1933 through 1948. That year there were 5543 graduates. In the next fifteen years, 10 new schools were created, primarily by state governments. Existing schools expanded so that the 13 percent growth in the number of schools was accompanied by a 31 percent growth in the number of graduates, to 7,264 by 1963. In the next ten years, 27 new schools were created, a further 31 percent increase, for a total of 114.* By 1975, there were 12,714 graduates, a whopping 75 percent increase over 1963! Another 11 medical schools were in the planning stages. The really big years for growth in the number of schools were 1967, 1968, and 1971 (five each), and in the number of graduates, 1974 and 1975 (over 1000 each).[12]

Again, was this magical, was it imperative, or was it a response to a stimulus? As with the burgeoning research effort, it was neither of the first two, and it was the third. And again, the stimulus was money. In the late fifties, two federal government reports, called Bayne-Jones, and Bane, after their principal authors, had warned that the country was facing a serious doctor shortage.[13] Their conclusions were based primarily on estimates of doctor-population ratios. Those conclusions echoed those of two other government studies done at the beginning of the decade.

Legislative efforts to provide direct federal aid to medical education had in fact continued through the fifties but a combination of a Republican administration and determined AMA opposition made sure they came to nothing. In the late fifties, the AMA began

*Of these, 107 were fully accredited, 5 were provisionally accredited, and 2 were two-year schools.

to change its position, recognizing that there was, or at least might be, an impending doctor shortage. Nevertheless, the AMA remained as frightened as ever of "federal interference," much preferred "private initiatives," grudgingly supported a onetime only shot of construction aid, and vigorously fought any incentives for enrollment expansion. To proposals for student loans and scholarships, AMA opposition was as determined as ever. The AAMC, on the other hand, strongly supported renewed legislative efforts to enact a medical education aid program which had accompanied President Kennedy's accession to the White House. In 1963, the AMA suffered its first major legislative defeat in many a moon.* A law was passed providing money not only for construction but also for student loans. AMA losses mounted. In 1965, student scholarships were added, plus, for the first time direct aid to the schools for general educational purposes, related to the number of students enrolled, and having a requirement for expansion. The ball was now rolling. The results were outlined above. Once again, the medical schools were responding to money.[15]

Actually, the new money was coming along none too soon. After increasing more than twelve-fold between 1955 and 1963, the rate of expansion of NIH appropriations began slowing down. Between 1967 and 1971 it was virtually flat, responding to the exigencies of the Vietnam War and the change of Federal Administration in 1969. Between 1968 and 1970, research grants to medical schools actually declined—13 percent in current dollars and 23 percent in real dollars taking inflation into account.[16] However, there was money for medical school expansion, not only federal money but, in an economic boom period created by war expenditures, state money as well. So while some schools were suffering severely, especially those relying heavily on "soft" research money for faculty support, others were being established and expanding, especially those with "hard" tax-levy funds from state governments.

*The last previous significant loss had been in the early twenties when federal aid for state maternal and child health care programs was approved by Congress, the Sheppard-Towner Act.[14] The AMA eventually managed to kill the program in 1932.

The 1970 Carnegie Commission Report

In 1970, the Carnegie Foundation sponsored another report on medical education, this time through The Carnegie Commission on Higher Education. The report, called *Higher Education and the Nation's Health,* focussed most sharply on the need for additional health manpower, both physician and non-physician.[17] The Commission concluded that there was severe shortage of physicians and that the shortage would get worse even with the expansion then already underway or on the books. Although the Commission gave a cursory look at the health care delivery system and even made a few brief recommendations for change, its conclusions were based primarily on the old standbys: doctor-population ratios.

The Commission did not consider what doctors do, the fee-for-service system, and so on. In a fairly short report, they devoted a few pages to describing some changes in medical school curriculum and content which were actually taking place. Both Flexner and the Commission on Medical Education had spent a great deal of time on curriculum, both describing and prescribing. Both earlier Reports were concerned with the necessity of relating the *content* of medical education to the needs of the people. The 1970 Carnegie Commission seemed more concerned with numbers, and money.

The 1970 Report completely misinterpreted the Flexner Report on the role of biological research in medical education. "The Flexner model," the 1970 Report said, "based on Johns Hopkins, Harvard, and, before them, German medical education, called for emphasis on biological research. Science was to be at the base of medical education." The second sentence is true. The first confuses Flexner, Hopkins, and Germany. Between both sentences, the Commission equates the basing of medical education on science with emphasizing biological research. That is not a necessary equation at all. Recall that Flexner said that the role of research in medical schools was to support teaching and keep the teachers fresh. He also said that medical education should be based on scientific *knowledge* and that the most important thing to teach medical students was the scientific method. Neither of these views of Flexner means that biologic research must be emphasized in medical schools. Indeed, as we have seen, it was not—until research money became available in large amounts after World War II. Furthermore, having a large biomedical research establishment in a medical school is no guarantee that medical students will be taught the scientific *method,* the educational process with which Flexner was principally concerned. In fact, people immersed in doing research can become much more interested in teaching about the outcomes of that research ("facts") than they are interested in teaching scientific methodology. The research-based model of medical education is not in actuality Flexner's, but the Mall/Hopkins model.

Nevertheless, while misnaming it, the 1970 Report did correctly criticize the research-based medical school. It noted that some medical schools relating strongly to health care delivery issues in their communities and some which made basic science teaching more clearly a university function were developing. The Report gave them its blessing, but did not recommend change for the others. The Report encouraged multi-disciplinary teaching and practice, recommended that opportunities for minority-group members and women in medical school be increased and that there be more allied health personnel, particularly physicians' assistants. It suggested shortening the medical curriculum and dealing with physician manpower geographic-distribution problems by a combination of voluntarism and incentives. It called for improved health manpower planning.

However, the 1970 Report was primarily concerned with growth. It recommended new medical schools and health-sciences centers. It called for the creation of 126 new entities, termed Area Health Education Centers. These institutions, some in areas with no health-sciences centers, would be responsible for important activities in graduate and continuing health-sciences education. Finally, the Report called for increasing and regularizing federal financial support for health-sciences education. Increases were forthcoming; regularity was not.

The 1971 Health Manpower Legislation and Its Aftermath

A renewal of Federal support for health manpower came in 1971 (P.L. 92–157). It aided not only schools of medicine, but also dentistry, osteopathy, veterinary medicine, pharmacy, and podiatry. Capitation grants (general support funds related to the number of enrolled students) were increased and for the first time made available to all schools, not just those expanding rapidly. They were tied to modest expansion of enrollment and to some curriculum innovation. However, this marked the first time that federal money was made available to all schools to support general operations. In 1968, the AMA finally reversed its long-held position and come out in support of direct federal aid to the medical schools.

Responding in part to an important report, *The Graduate Education of Physicians,* which an AMA sponsored commission chaired by John S. Millis, Ph.D. had produced in 1966, there were special funds to support the development of programs in family medicine. There was also construction money, provision for student loans and scholarships, postgraduate training support, money for Area Health Education Centers, and special project grants to support innovation in medical education.

However, the appropriations didn't always match the authorizations, and Nixon-Administration-spending didn't always match appropriations. Nevertheless, from 1971 on research grants started going up again, and in 1973 a new funding mechanism was added: the project-specific contract. By 1975, in real dollars, the total of awards to medical schools, $874.5 million primarily in grants and contracts, was 44 percent above what it had been in 1967. However, from 1971 new traumas had been added to the sometimes realized, ever-present, threat of a real reduction in funds: artificially low presidential science budgets, congressional increases, "tilts" towards one or two diseases (Nixon liked a "War on Cancer"), vetoes, overrides, recissions, impoundments, court cases, fund releases, and so on. The same applied to health manpower funds. However, the more medical schools became dependent on capitation payments to maintain their basic operations, the more annual changes in federal aid hurt. It was like being on a roller coaster ride—blindfolded: you never knew when you were going to be up and when you were going to be down. Although in the end, the actual changes in funding were relatively small for the most part, the uncertainty each year was great.

Content Changes in an Era of Expansion

The rapid expansion in the number of medical schools between 1965 and 1972, twenty-four new schools appeared in those seven years, a 27-percent increase, provided the first major opportunity for innovation in American medical education since the time of the Flexner Report. What actually happened, not much of which was real in terms of change in product outcome, is very instructive.

Curriculum Change

There were several major changes in the curriculum. About 30 percent of the schools, some new, some old, adopted a "systems" approach to teaching basic science material, originated at the Western Reserve medical school in 1952. In it the traditional departmental courses given in the first two years are completely or partially scrapped in favor of teaching some or all of the material by organ system. Thus instead of taking separate courses in anatomy, biochemistry, physiology, and pathology, the student studies the cardiovascular *system,* the respiratory *system,* the musculoskeletal *system,* and so on in all of their aspects. This approach, especially when it includes clinical correlations is intended to make the material "stick" better in the minds of the students. In schools in which the teaching work is given high priority and in which great attention is given to make sure that the teaching from the different disciplines is truly integrated, it seems to work well. In others, with less careful coordination and supervision, interdigitation of the formerly separate courses rather than their integration is what happens. In any case, over two-thirds of the schools stuck with the old Hopkins method of teaching basic science, with departmental courses. Basic science faculty members seem to be most happy with that approach because it is the one they know.

Most schools scrapped the "on-the-wards-in-the-third-year/in-the-clinics-in-the-fourth-year" plan for one set of third-year "clerkships" in the major clinical disciplines, arranged to include both inpatient (mostly) and outpatient experiences. The fourth year became entirely elective at many schools.

In the early 1970s a myth was accepted throughout the land that the substitution of a three-year curriculum for the traditional four-year one would increase the total output of medical school graduates. It did—for the one year in which a converting school graduated two classes at the same time. Obviously, the number of doctors produced in any one year is related only to the number of students admitted to that class when it began its medical education, whether that was four or three or two or five years prior to graduation. In most schools, three-year curriculae were created not by reducing the amount of material required to be learned (that would have called for the agreement of fifty state licensing boards and the National Board of Medical Examiners), but by eliminating elective time, shortening vacations, lengthening school days, and generally packing full the available time. Student and faculty stress mounted. It was realized that the output of physicians did not increase permanently. Many schools which switched over to a three-year curriculum have now switched back to a four-year one. Some have retained a three-year option for particularly bright, aggressive students.

Programmatic Change

The 1970 Carnegie Report called attention to "the *health care delivery* model [medical school]. [I]n addition to training, [it] does research in health care delivery, advises local hospitals and health authorities, works with community colleges and comprehensive colleges on the training of allied health personnel, carries on continuing education for health personnel, and generally orients itself to external service. . . ."[18] This is a great idea, even though it is not new. In the language and terms of reference of his era, Flexner enunciated this approach as one which he thought all schools should adopt. It would make medical education relevant to the needs of the people, and would make a very expensive enterprise into a valuable resource in meeting the health *care* needs of its community. This concept strikes fear into the hearts of staunch defenders of the Mall/Hopkins basic science faith, like D.W. Seldin.[19] Several schools put this model on paper during the era of expansion. A few, like Michigan State and the Peoria and Rockford clinical campuses of the University of Illinois are still attempting to carry it out.

At most schools that intended to do it the idea met a quick and sorry end, snowed under by tradition and a few other things. Implementation of this concept is not easy. In addition to pretty plans on paper, it takes time, dedication, the right manpower, money, diplomacy, keeping one's eye on the ball, and above all the recognition that health care delivery system analysis and planning is a profession in itself, not something that any individual clinician or other amateur can do. Not an easy combination to put together. Few schools did. This concept, enunciated beautifully for hospitals as well as medical schools in Dr. Freymann's book, is a particularly hard one for most medical school faculty members to swallow. It is the precise opposite of the inner-directed non-socially responsible or responsive, biomedical research model under which most of us were trained. Faculty resistance was, and is, fierce. Only where core faculty are carefully selected to have the right philosophy, and/or the leadership is determined to implement the ideas, not just write about them, can success be achieved.

Interdisciplinary education was another watchword of the expansionist era. Like the health care delivery model, it appeared in the plans of a number of schools, written up beautifully in some cases, and in the same way, it didn't make it in most schools. Over the years, a number of observers, like the 1970 Carnegie Commission, have concluded that one good mode for providing health care is in teams of doctors, nurses, social workers, and other professional and in some cases nonprofessional health care providers, with vastly different hierarchical and interpersonal relationships than now exist among most health professionals. In particular, the doctor has to learn that he or she is not always appropriately King of the Hill. It is logical then to conclude that a good way to create health professionals who can work in teams is to train them in teams, in an interdisciplinary mode.

In most instances this concept ran aground even more quickly than did the health care delivery model of medical education, for many of the same reasons. However, to make the chances of success even more remote, faculty resistance to this idea was even more ingrained than it was to the previous one. Physician-dominance is deeply rooted psychologically in most physicians. The idea is implanted from day one of training, in most schools, consciously and unconsciously. It is an idea that is much older than the sanctity-of-research notion. It is built into nurse's training as well, and I have found that a number of nurses who say that they want to do interdisciplinary educational work with physicians just can't handle it when push comes to shove. Male chauvanism plays an important part here. Again, it takes very special people, very special leadership, and very special administrative skills to make this one work.

I have shown elsewhere in this book that primary care services are seriously deficient in the United States. One approach to the problem developed in the sixties was the idea of a new academic discipline, "family medicine." Family medicine grew out of general practice, dropping surgery and in some cases operative obstetrics (delivering babies), to concentrate on providing medical care for adults and children. Family medicine also provides an identifiable academic discipline with which those thousands of general practitioners around the country who have been increasingly isolated by the increasing specialization and research orientation of most medical schools can identify. Family medicine intends to concentrate on family care and to have a particular concern for the social, economic, and behavioral aspects of illness.

This is one innovation that has succeeded in most schools. Most schools have departments of family medicine if for no other reason than that there is special federal, and in many cases state, money to support them. They are still working to completely define their role and place. Internal medicine and pediatrics have certainly not surrendered the primary care turf to family medicine. (Obstetrics-gynecology and even surgery would also like to be considered "primary care" specialties, especially when money is attached to the term.) Few family medicine departments do much research. Some faculty members, drawn straight out of many years of private general practice, have trouble adjusting to the academic role. In some cases, they line up with the most reactionary elements in the school, harking back to their own educational experiences thirty years before, rather than with the more progressive ones. Most importantly, the clinical role of family medicine needs to be more clearly defined. Is it just general practice upgraded? If a family practitioner does nothing more than provide basic primary care, how is he or she different from a well-trained physician's assistant or clinical nurse practitioner? Is a more productive role perhaps that of team organizer and leader, professional and patient educator, problem-solver, diagnostician, applied epidemiologist and health care planner? This situation should sort itself out in the next decade or so.

Conclusion

There were no major changes of substance in American medical education in the 1965–75 era of expansion—besides expansion. Medical education did not become people-oriented except in a couple of isolated instances. The research function, which for all its trials and tribulations actually increased its take significantly during the period, remained dominant, and the hospital remained the focus of clinical teaching. An analysis of change and attempted change teaches one three lessons: (1) it is very easy to change the label on the jar without changing what is in the jar—and call it change (a favorite American approach to reform); (2) the inertial resistance to change in American medical education is enormous; and (3) comparing the 1965–75 experience with the 1905–1915 experience, it can be concluded that real change in medical education is most likely to take place when such change would be to the benefit of a significant number of practitioners.

The last is a fascinating conclusion, particularly when one considers the isolation of most practitioners from the medical education process. But one only has to look at the experience with the attempted changes of the era of expansion to see its validity. By the mid-sixties most physicians were doing well economically and some were feeling quite overworked. Thus expansion of the doctor supply, the most important effect of the era of expansion, didn't bother them. The one internal reform that succeeded, the establishment of departments of family medicine, was in the interest of thousands of general practitioners, and actively opposed by few other practitioners. As for the other changes, practitioners either couldn't have cared less (systems teaching), or would be actively opposed in many instances (the health care delivery model, except where it encompassed private fee-for-service practice). I shall return to a consideration of the road to change in the last chapter.

1976—A Pivotal Year?

Legislation

In 1976, another Health Professions Educational Assistance Act (P.L. 94–484) was passed. A complicated and complex law, I will only briefly review it here. It extended capitation payments, something the medical schools wanted badly, of course. It also extended student scholarships and loans, the National Health Service Corps (the agency created in 1971 to provide young physicians to work in under-served areas), and several other programs. However, this time the payoff by the medical schools for capitation money was not expansion, but increased attention to primary care. Over a three-year period, certain national standards for the proportion of first-year residency positions which are of the primary care type (defined as internal medicine, pediatrics, and family medicine), have to be met, rising to 50 percent by fiscal 1980.

Furthermore, in order to be eligible for capitation payments, during a three-year period beginning in 1978, the schools had to agree to accept into their third year any American citizen who had completed two years of medical studies abroad and who had passed Part I of the National Board of Medical Examiners examinations, covering the basic sciences. This last provision really stuck in the craw of the medical education establishment, which denounced "government interference in the academic process." "In 1977, they managed to get federal legislation making the provisions for taking U.S. Foreign Medical Students (USFMS) into third-year classes somewhat more acceptable. Again, however, I find "government interference" a weak argument, coming from the medical schools. They are all for "government interference" when money is attached to it and when what they are asked to do is either what they want to do anyway or at least doesn't seriously conflict with their established programs.

Nevertheless, I think that the public must be concerned with the recent proliferation of private profit-making, thoroughly unregulated medical schools, especially in the Caribbean. These schools are designed specifically for American citizens who have failed to gain admission into an American medical school. It is not that difficult to train people to pass licensing board examinations. However, in training to be a *physician* there is no substitute for clinical experience—one of the strongest suits of most American medical schools and one of the weakest areas of most proprietary schools in neighboring countries. We may be approaching a situation akin to that of the 1890–1910 period with its proliferation of "diploma mills." The modern equivalent of them will be "Board-passing mills." Serious policy, legal, and political questions are raised by this development. I do not have space here to consider them, but they must be attended to.

During the legislative process leading up to passage of the bill the medical schools, joined on some issues by the AMA, managed to eliminate other proposed requirements that they considered even more painful. (The original USFMS provision had caught the schools completely off-guard, having been slipped into the bill unnoticed during the final House-Senate Conference before passage.) Key Congressmen had wanted all residency positions to be approved by the government and assigned by specialty, numbers to be determined rationally in terms of national needs. They had wanted to require that some medical training be done away from the schools (so-called "remote-site"), so that students would perforce get a taste of ambulatory care, community hospitals, and/or rural or central city work. There had been sentiment for a requirement for work in an underserved area for all medical school graduates, not just those working off a loan payoff, as allowed by previous legislation. The medical education establishment won on all of these points.

In another provision which did get through, P.L. 94–484 almost entirely closed the door to the entry of foreign-born foreign medical graduates to residency-training positions in United States hospitals, by changing both the educational requirements for entry and the immigration laws. This was at least partly in response to a new feeling on the part of many observers, among whom the AMA is *not* prominent, that we now face an impending oversupply of physicians by the 1980s. The doors had been opened to FMGs by changes in the immigration laws around 1965. Hospitals created new residency positions right and left to deal with internal staffing problems but not with national educational needs. There were far more positions available than American schools could fill, and hospitals welcomed FMGs with open arms. By 1973, however, FMGs were accounting for about 45 percent of all newly licensed physicians in the United States. The best place to deal with oversupply was obviously there.[20]

Another Carnegie Report

In 1976, another Carnegie Foundation report on medical education came out, this one by the successor agency to the Carnegie Commission, the Carnegie Council of Policy Studies in Higher Education.[21] It was entitled, significantly, *Progress and Problems in Medical and Dental Education: Federal Support Versus Federal Control.* It amazes me how quickly reversals of positions can be made, and with such aplomb too. In 1970, Carnegie had issued dire warnings of an impending physician shortage. By 1976, they were issuing dire warnings of an impending oversupply. Again, it must be understood that this commission like all of its predecessors, relied almost entirely on physician-population ratios to come to its conclusions. To this end, they recommended shutting the door on FMGs, accomplished by P.L. 94–484, and sharply curtailing medical school expansion, achieved by a combination of federal law and sharp cutbacks in state spending.

But is the real concern of the Carnegie report physician oversupply? I think not, based on an analysis of its principal recommendations. After describing a picture of change in medical education that is more rosy than real, the Council sharply criticized such proposals as required remote-site training and residency-position controls as amounting to "unwarrented interference with academic decisions of the schools and a degree of federal control over allocation of health manpower that goes far beyond interference in any other field."[22] (Yet "federal interference" to restrict entry of FMGs, which will adversely affect the operations of many hospitals is all right, of course.) Then the Council recommended that federal financial support be stabilized and predictable. They recommended that geographic maldistribution be dealt with voluntarily.

Primary care programs should be encouraged by incentives, not be required by controls. (Remember that the Commission on Medical Education warned on overspecialization in 1932.) The Council recommended stabilization of biomedical research support, and did propose an increase of support for research in health manpower training and health care delivery problems. Finally, they blamed many current health problems on "life style."

The real aim of this report is to get the federal government to continue to throw money at the medical schools—evenly—while urging it to get out of the schools' collective hair and to continue to allow the schools to follow the policies they have followed for so many years, which generally have not met broad social needs for health care, merrily spending taxpayers' money as they see fit.

I believe that the history of the next ten to twenty-five years of medical education in this country will be chiefly concerned with this issue of public accountability and public responsibility of those institutions which are principally supported by the public's dollar.

11

Medical Education Today

. . . medical education has, paradoxically, become less a preparation for becoming a medical practitioner and more a preparation for becoming a medical student. Repeatedly, students are provided with experiences that appear to have been designed to help them learn how to take lecture notes, to study for examinations, to say things that please and satisfy their teachers, to restrain any tendency to express strong opinions, to work obediently at activities they are not convinced are either important or relevant, and, in general, to follow instructions. All of this is fine preparation for being a medical student in a conventional medical school. It is, of course, not only irrelevant to being an independent and creative practitioner,

it is contrary to the very requirements of being a mature professional. In this sense, medical education has provided repeated confirmation of a derivative of the Peter principle: we immerse students in the skills of being followers in preparation for careers as leaders.

—*Hilliard Jason, M.D., Ed.D.*

These institutions [the American medical schools] have given the country the best educated physicians in the world.

—*Robert G. Petersdorf, M.D.*
President, American College of Physicians
Philadelphia, PA

The doctors should fear arrogance
more than cardiac arrest.
If they are too proud,
and some are,
then they leave home on horseback
but God returns them on foot.

—*Anne Sexton*
From her poem "Doctors"

Basic Data

The major sources of data on medical education in the United States are the American Medical Association and the Association of American Medical Colleges. Each year the last issue of the *Journal of the American Medical Association* is an "Annual Report: Medical Education in the United States" for the preceding academic year. There is summary data for all medical schools and, in an appendix, data by school. There is also data on graduate medical education, medical education programs sponsored by government agencies, and graduate education in public health.

In its *Journal of Medical Education,* the AAMC publishes "Datagrams," presenting data on a wide variety of single topics. Some, such as "Medical Student Enrollment," are published on a recurrent basis. Others report the results of special one-time studies of such topics as women in medical schools (August, 1976) and medical school faculty ethnicity (January, 1976). In this chapter, I rely mainly on the "76th Annual Report, Medical Education in the United States: 1975–1976," *JAMA,* December 27, 1976, and several recent *JME* Datagrams. Some other data are referenced in the Notes.[1]

Number of Schools

As of October, 1976, there were 112 fully accredited medical schools in the United States and the Commonwealth of Puerto Rico. Two of these offered only the first two years of (basic science) instruction, with their students being required to transfer at the end of that time into the third year of a four-year program. There were also four provisionally accredited four-year schools: the University of South Dakota (in the process of changing over from two- to four-year status), Wright State University in Ohio, the Uniformed Services University of the Health Sciences (which faced possible closure by the Carter Administration), and the University of South Carolina at Columbia which was scheduled to open in September, 1977.

Geographic Distribution

New York State has the highest number of fully accredited schools (12). Other states with relatively large numbers of schools include California (8), Illinois and Pennsylvania (7 each), Texas (6), and Massachusetts, Missouri and Ohio, (4 each). In New York, California, Illinois, Texas, Missouri, and Ohio, two or more separate medical schools operated by the state's university are included in the total. The following states have only one medical school each: Arizona, Arkansas, Colorado, Hawaii, Indiana, Iowa, Kansas, Mississippi, New Hampshire, New Mexico, North Dakota, Oklahoma, Oregon, Rhode Island, South Carolina, Utah, Vermont,

Washington and West Virginia. Puerto Rico also has one school. Only in New Hampshire (Dartmouth) and Rhode Island (Brown), are the schools not operated by the state's university. The states without medical schools are Maine, Delaware, Montana, Wyoming, Idaho, and Alaska. Nevada has a two-year school, only. About 60 percent of medical schools are publicly owned and operated, almost entirely by state governments. The balance are in the private sector, although about 85 percent of them receive some aid from their respective state governments.[2]

Types of Institutional Relationships

As a major result of the Flexner Report, most medical schools are part of a university. A few are still independently incorporated institutions. In an increasing number of universities, the medical school is part of a group of schools, called a "health sciences center," which trains health care providers. In most universities with medical schools and/or health sciences centers the necessarily complex relationships produce various points of strain. Medical education is almost unique among the disciplines of higher learning in that, as a necessary part of the educational process, the institution itself delivers the product it is teaching, i.e., medical practice, to the public. This does not apply to schools of law or architecture. For example, although individual faculty members in such schools often practice their professions, law schools do not defend clients, nor do most schools of architecture design buildings. Schools of medicine, however, through their own and affiliated hospitals and outpatient services, do provide direct patient care.

Provision of patient care carries unique responsibilities, imposes high personal financial liability (*very* high in some cases), and requires skills on the part of at least some of its practitioner/teachers which do not carry much academic weight in the conventional sense. Thus the university's academic review committee on faculty promotion may not recognize achievement in the same way that its medical school committee might. If the former can overrule the latter, tension can arise. Furthermore, high medical school faculty salaries, related to private, fee-for-service practice, can cause resentment on the part of university faculty. Finally, there are intra-health sciences center rivalries between doctors, dentists, nurses, social workers, and the allied health professions, related to hierarchical status, sexual chauvanism, academic responsibilities, and income differentials.

Faculty

In 1976, there were about 40,000 full-time members in United States medical schools, producing an incredibly low overall student–full-time-faculty ratio of 1.4 to 1. In addition, there were over 78,000 part-time faculty members, of whom about 70,000 served on a voluntary basis. Of the latter group, almost 95 percent (66,000) were clinical faculty.[3] (This latter figure means that 20–25 percent of all active medical practitioners in the United States, depending upon exactly who is counted by the reporting institutions as "clinical faculty," are on medical school faculties.) Thus the total number of faculty members is over 115,000. In terms of individuals, although not in terms of full-time equivalents, as we shall see below, faculty actually outnumber students by slightly better than 2 to 1! About 27 percent of all full-time faculty members are in basic science departments (anatomy, biochemistry, microbiology, pathology, pharmacology, and physiology). About 6 percent of all full-time faculty positions are vacant.

With a full-time faculty-student ratio of 1 to 1.4, and an over-all faculty-student ratio of more than 2 to 1, it is quite clear that a great deal of faculty time must be spent doing work other than education. (See also below under "The Costs of Medical Education.") In addition to teaching and clinical practice, medical school faculty also engage in research (this goes for clinical as well as basic science faculty) and administrative work.

However, little research has been done on the important question of how medical school faculty members actually spend their time. In the early 1970s, one large-scale attempt to study this matter was made by an Institute of Medicine committee which produced some very important data on the costs of health sciences education.[4] Their study of how faculty use their time relied on daily logs filled out by faculty members themselves for relatively short periods of time. Because of the methodological problems inherent in this approach, cited by the committee itself, the results, which I will consider in some detail below, must be viewed with care. Nevertheless, in examining the medical education system, the seeming profligacy with which expensive faculty time is spent, even considering the importance of research and clinical practice to the medical education process, must be taken into account.

Paying Faculty

There are few medical schools which provide the whole incomes of more than a handful of their clinical faculty members. Instead, the so-called "geographic full-time" system is used. Geographic full-time exists in reality in many institutions of higher education which do not pay salaries anywhere near the going rate for private sector practitioners of the several university disciplines, but it is not quite so highly institutionalized as it is in medical schools. Under geographic full-time, a system which you will recall was attacked with vigor by Flexner, the faculty member is physically present in the institution all of the time, but earns part or all of his or her total income in private entrepreneurial fee-for-service practice. In most schools there is a limit on what can be privately earned, related by a formula to the base salary provided by the institution. The formulae, billing systems, methods for using excess private income, and degree of compliance with whatever system is in force vary widely from school to school.

The principal advantage of the geographic full-time system for the medical schools is that their operating budgets do not reflect the full and true cost of operations, part of the cost being borne in part by faculty members' private patients. The geographic full-time system does enable medical schools to have on their faculties many members who would otherwise be solely in private practice, and thus it exposes students to a wide variety of practitioners whom they might not otherwise see. Among its disadvantages are the facts that the availability of private practice income creates a conflict-of-interest situation for many medical school faculty members (should I teach or make money today?), and that private practice is in effect subsidizing medical education.

Students

In the 1975–76 academic year, there were over 56,000 students enrolled in American medical schools. Although more than 13,500 students were graduated in that year, over 15,000 entered the first-year class. Since the average attrition rate for medical students is below 2 percent, we can expect to be producing over 15,000 doctors annually by 1979. Slightly over 1 percent (687) of students in American medical schools are from other countries. Although the exact total of Americans attending medical schools in other countries is unknown, on the basis of the number taking an examination at the end of the second year, passage of which enables the student to apply for admission to the clinical years of an American medical school (third and fourth), it can be estimated that over 6,000 Americans are going to medical school abroad.[5]

State of Origin

Medical schools, even the private ones, tend to accept students predominately from their own or neighboring states.[6] Ninety-two percent of students in state-operated medical schools are from the state of location. Fifty-five percent of students in privately-owned medical schools are from the state of location, and a majority of privately-owned schools take a majority of their students from their state of location.

Female Enrollment

In terms of sex distribution, the percentage of women among medical students has been gradually increasing over the years.[7] In 1929, 4.5 percent of all medical school acceptees were women. By 1950, the proportion was 5.3 percent; 1960, 7.0 percent; 1970, 11.3 percent; and 1975, 23.7 percent. In 1975–76, one-fifth of the total enrollment was female. As the AAMC "Datagram" for August, 1976 points out:

> The dramatic change, in the rather brief time span since 1970, in the number of women seeking careers in medicine reflects both the changes in societal attitudes and in women's perception of career opportunities.

These changes were also supported by the passage of federal legislation prohibiting sex discrimination in any federally funded education program.

Minority Enrollment

The representation of Black Americans, American Indians, Mexican Americans, and Mainland Puerto Ricans* in American medical schools has always been very low, until the mid-sixties amounting to 1–2 percent of total enrollment.[8] (The majority of Black American physicians have been trained in the two predominately black medical schools: Howard in Washington, D.C. and Meharry in Nashville, Tennessee.) In the four years I was at Harvard Medical School, 1958–62, there was not one black student there, in any of the classes. With the development of the civil rights movement, this situation has begun to change. Since 1972, the percentage of first-year enrollment represented by the named minorities has ranged between 8.6 percent and 10.0, while total minority enrollment has gradually increased from 6.6 to 8.2 percent. In 1974–76, there was a decline in the percentage of the named minorities in the entering classes, from 10 to 9. This may reflect the current rash of "reverse-discrimination" suits of which the Bakke case was the most prominent (usually based on the concept that the only criteria for admission to medical school should be college grades and test performance), the 1974–75 recession which hit the generally lower-paid named minorities harder than others, the rising tuition costs, and the increasing difficulty all medical students have experienced in obtaining adequate financial assistance. As Barbara Caress, a staff member of the Health Policy Advisory Center in New York City, has pointed out, it certainly does not reflect continued concern among medical schools for increasing minority student enrollment.

There have been two major arguments made in support of increasing minority student enrollment. One is that minority populations are generally medically underserved and minority-group physicians are needed to take proper care of them. The other is that racial discrimination has meant that minority group members have not had equal opportunities to become

*These are minority classifications used by the AAMC in their analyses.

doctors. To me, the first argument is seriously flawed. First of all, it is really racist to say that minority group doctors are needed to take care of minority group people. The statement implies that non-minority group doctors cannot be trained to meet the needs of minorities, and (perhaps) that minority group doctors should *only* serve minorities, thus being "ghetto-ized" as professionals. Second of all, there is some evidence (anecdotal at least), that not that many minority-group doctors actually end up practicing among the poor, medically-under-served members of their own minority groups in any case. Rather, like any private entrepreneurial fee-for-service practitioner, they tend to serve those persons who are most able to pay, or who have health insurance.

The stronger argument for admitting larger numbers of minority group members to medical school is the inequity in opportunity which has existed in the past. Opportunities to obtain professional education have not been equal for minority group members. If our society is to begin to make up for these past inequities, special consideration will have to be given to the admission of minority group candidates to medical school.

Supporters of the Bakke position argue that this approach is unfair to non-minority applicants for the obviously limited number of places. They say that under affirmative action, pro-minority admissions programs, "less-qualified" persons are admitted to medical school in an "arbitrary and capricious" manner. However, no one has shown that present admissions standards for most schools, which rely heavily on grades and test performance, are either non-arbitrary, or good predictors of future physician performance (see "Admissions Process" below). Admissions criteria which can predict the potential of the applicant to be a good physician still need to be developed. In the meantime, social justice demands that minority-group persons be given special assistance to gain admission to, and stay in, medical school.

Social Class

Grace Ziem, a faculty member at the Johns Hopkins School of Health Services, is not the first observer to note the fact that:

> Physicians in the United States have historically been selected predominately from families with business and professional occupations.[9]

In summarizing Ziem's work, Caress points out that:

> While only 24 percent of the labor force held managerial, professional jobs, fully 64 percent of those admitted to medical school in 1973 came from such families. Over two-thirds of the students admitted to medical school in 1975 came from families with incomes over $15,000 a year and 40 percent reported family incomes over $25,000. Yet only 14.1 percent of U.S. families earned $25,000 [per year] or more.[10]

Factors accounting for this situation include the high cost of medical education; for most applicants the necessity of having a high quality secondary and college education, often expensive in themselves, in order to gain admission to medical school; the social influence of the whole educational system in individuals' career choices; and the limitations on upward mobility imposed by the whole social structure of our country, which while less strong than in, say, Great Britain, still are very much present.

Admissions

The Process

Admissions to most medical schools are decided upon by a body called the Admissions Committee, an element in the faculty governance structure.[11] In response to student interest in participating in school operations, in recent years, many faculties have placed one or more students on the committee as well. The job of the committee is to consider and evaluate the group of applicants, and make the choices for admission. Most committees use several different criteria in their evaluations. Among them are college grade-point average, extra-curricular activities and life experience, performance on a standard examination taken by virtually all medical school applicants called the Medical College Admission Test (MCAT), and personal interview.

Little basic research has been done about how medical school admissions committees actually function. Anecdotal information suggests that the average admissions committee relies on grade-point averages and MCAT scores more than it does on other criteria in making its choices. However, most of what evidence is available indicates that there is little if any relationship between either college grade-point average or MCAT scores and future clinical performance as a physician.[12] At most schools, interviews are undertaken and interview results are considered in the final decision-making process. However, GPA and MCAT scores are frequently the only criteria used to decide who gets interviewed.

The current situation, in which applicants outnumber available places by almost three to one (see below), has made the admissions process a psychological meatgrinder for the applicants, the admissions committees, and the medical school admissions offices which do the administrative and staff work for the committees. The competition for medical school places is keen. It is thought that some persons who would in fact make fine doctors don't even bother to apply to medical school because of the competition that goes on during the pre-medical years. The pressure is also heavy on the admissions committees. Since the members know how prized the places are, a great deal of agonizing and many long hours of work go into the selection process. Sometimes attempts may be made by parents, political figures, alumni, major donors, and other faculty members to influence the admissions process in relation to a particular applicant. I believe that such efforts are not often successful, but they certainly are made and contribute to the pressures faced by admissions committee members.

Discussions sometimes become heated. Just as do the other two major academic committees, curriculum and academic standing, admissions committees often find that disagreements over whether or not to admit a particular student have nothing really to do with that student's qualifications or lack thereof, but rather concern basic philosophical and ideological conflicts between committee members over what a good physician is and how he or she should be trained.

Numbers

During the academic year 1976–77, there were 42,155 applicants for admission to American medical schools in the fall of 1977. Of them, 15,774 were admitted, a ratio of 2.67 applicants per place.[13] This is down from a high of 2.83 applicants per place in 1973–75, but up from a low of 1.7 applicants per place in 1960–62. Because of the increasing competition, each student is applying to a relatively large number of schools in order to increase his or her chances of getting in somewhere. There were 8.8 applications per applicant in 1976–77. This is up from a low of 2.9 applications per applicant in 1958–60. This ratio means that admissions committees must process astronomical numbers of individual applications to fill a relatively small number of places: 372,-282 in 1976–77. Popular schools with 100 places may receive 4,000 applications for them.

The explosion in the total number of applications has been unwittingly aided and abetted by something called the American Medical College Application Service (AMCAS). About three-quarters of the medical schools use it. Under AMCAS, the applicant fills out just one common application form. For each subscribing school the form is sent to, the student pays a prescribed, relatively small fee. In my day, each school had its own form, which had to be filled out individually. Since the forms were usually long, required their own copies of one's academic records, and customarily asked for an essay on "why I want to become a doctor," an inhibition to filling too many applications was present.

I do not believe that the acceptance distribution pattern within the applicant pool has been examined. However, it probably has the following appearance. During each academic year, medical school applicants are accepted in waves. There is one group of applicants whom most every school would be happy to have. When the first acceptance notices go out, some of the best students may receive four or five of them from different schools. As acceptees at more than one schools make their choices, new places open up, and more acceptance notices are sent out. The process continues until all places are filled. There are probably about 7,000 students in the "first wave," receiving three or more acceptances each. I would guess that there is another group of about 20,000 applicants in whom no one is interested. They are not invited for interviews at any schools. This means that the remaining 8,000 acceptances are made from a pool of about 15,000 people, most of whom are probably more or less equally qualified. Some skewing is caused by state schools which admit few out-of-state residents, particularly those schools in small states, but this tri-modal distribution of applicants is probably what exists.

The Power of Admissions Committees

Since the attrition rate for medical students is very low (1.5 to 2.0 percent between 1969 and 1976), most students admitted to medical school are assured of receiving the M.D. degree. Virtually everyone receiving an M.D. degree in this country goes on to obtain a medical license. Thus medical school admissions committees are choosing our future doctors. Because doctors have such an important role to play in determining the shape of the health care delivery system, admissions committees in fact can be considered an important influence on that system. Yet there is neither public accountability nor public influence in the workings of most admissions committees. I know of one medical school, McMaster in Hamilton, Ontario, Canada, in which local citizens are involved in the admissions process, primarily in judging character and personality, and there may be others. However, the practice is not common.

Furthermore, it is not even true in every school that the faculty has clearly agreed upon what kinds of doctors they want to train. Thus they are not able to give the admissions committee some clear guidelines for choosing the persons to be admitted. Again the question has not been studied to my knowledge, but it is my guess that the actions of some admissions committees are guided not by clear, carefully developed policies related to a philosophy of medical education and medical practice, but rather by the randomly mixed personal predilections and prejudices of the individual committee members. When the power of admissions committees is recognized, and the degree of their indirect influence on the health care delivery system is understood, I think that it can be recognized that a mode of work which does not include clear guidelines, if in fact I am right that it does not, is not the best way to do things.

Curriculum

Although there have been many changes in detail, and some in emphasis, there have been few major changes in the curriculae of American medical schools since the period of standardization following the publication of the Flexner Report. What major changes there have been have only occurred in a minority of schools in any case. The standard curriculum requires four years of study after the B.A. degree.* Generally, the first two years of medical school are devoted to "basic science" while the last two are the "clinical years." This "two plus two" pattern is generally termed "Flexnerian." It is true that Flexner did advocate a two plus two approach with "basic science" coming first. However, Flexner's concept of what would be taught during the basic science years has not been generally followed. Flexner advocated teaching the scientific *method,* not simply a collection of scientists' *facts.* Furthermore, there is a rigidity in the curriculae of many American medical schools which Flexner strongly warned against.

Although in the early seventies, the three-year curriculum was at least an available option in almost one-half of American medical schools for reasons discussed in the previous chapter, by 1976, only five schools had a mandatory three-year curriculum, while nine had a three-year option. The three-year curriculum is decreasing rapidly in popularity because, 1) it does not produce more doctors than the four-year one and 2) its institutions was not accompanied by an easing of the requirements either for the M.D. degree or for licensing.[14] Thirteen schools offer a six-year post high school program, although only in a handful of schools, such as Boston University, do a significant number of students take it. The number of schools offering such a program at all has decreased sharply in recent years.

*You will recall that although the bachelor's degree is a requirement for admission to most schools, a small minority of students do enter medical school after three years of college and then, receiving credit for work done in medical school, earn the bachelor's degree at some time during their medical school experience. There are a few medical schools which have comprehensive six-year B.A.–M.D. programs which a student enters directly from high school. In the medical education field, the pre-M.D. medical school experience is referred to as "undergraduate," even though in the university sense, it is graduate education. In medical education, "graduate training" refers to the internship and residency years in the hospital which follow receipt of the M.D. degree.

The Basic Science Years

In the majority of schools, the three principal courses in the first year are anatomy, physiology, and biochemistry and in the second, pathology, microbiology, and pharmacology. These are Flexner's "basic six." They are also the only six basic sciences which are specified in the medical school Accreditation Guidelines of the Liaison Committee on Medical Education (see the last section of this chapter, "Organization, Regulation, and Quality Control"). Anatomy is sometimes divided into gross and microscopic anatomy. Physiology is sometimes divided into cell biology and general physiology. Biochemistry is sometimes called physiological chemistry. Parts of microbiology, pathology, and pharmacology are occasionally taught in the first year. In recent years, separate short courses in such subjects as genetics, embryology, epidemiology and biostatistics, health care delivery, and so on have been added in. Traditionally, an introductory course in taking case histories from and performing physical examinations on patients has been given in the latter half of the second year. In some schools, this course is begun earlier, occasionally in the first year, to provide "early patient contact" for medical students, most of whom are yearning to "lay on hands." Nevertheless in the majority of schools, the basic pattern established early in this century built around the "basic six" holds.

"Systems Teaching"

In about thirty schools, at least some of the basic science instruction is provided in what is called the "systems mode." In this approach, originated at the Western Reserve University School of Medicine during the 1950s, basic science material is taught by body system, circulatory, respiratory, gastrointestinal, and so on, rather than by separate departmental courses. In a few schools, such as the University of Connecticut, the systems mode is used from the beginning of the first year. The more common pattern is to spend most or all of the first year in teaching by department in a "core curriculum" before switching into systems.

Although systems teaching has been in use for about twenty-five years, there is very little literature on it, aside from a few early papers published by Western Reserve faculty. Thus little is known about how it actually works in the schools which use it. It is, of course, possible to truly integrate teaching by several concerned departments around one organ system. Common educational objectives can be worked out, class session outlines can be carefully discussed to avoid duplication and make sure that everything is covered, joint evaluation and program revision can be carried out and so on. On the other hand, there is a strong temptation to avoid the time-consuming attempt at true integration (many faculty meetings are required), and fall back on simply interdigitation. That is, when the heart is the subject, the several concerned departments just come in serially and do their thing on the heart, without relating to each other very much at all. I experienced the latter approach when I was a medical student. (The school in which I trained has since given up systems teaching and gone back to departmental teaching.) Simple interdigitation is not particularly productive. If curricular change is not carried out secondary to a change in the concept of the desirable end product of the educational process, then it is only curricular tinkering, not basic alteration.

Dr. Robert Kane, editor of the *Journal of Community Health,* and his colleagues have put this concept very well:

> Curricula in medical schools across the country have been in a state of constant ferment. In seeking beneficial change, many medical schools have concentrated attention on the sequence of courses. Too often proposals urge a rather arbitrary new structure, such as organ systems or early clinical experience, which represents only a repackaging and renaming of old information. The same lecture or the same ideas may be delivered through a different department or some other individual or perhaps at a different time. Yet changes, to be significant, must not be dictated by fashion, whim, or even desire for improvement; they must be solidly founded on a clear concept of the desired outcome in terms of the expected behavior of the student after he has successfully completed the medical school curriculum and enters practice.

Teaching Techniques

Again, it is primarily anecdotal information from faculty colleagues and students, and personal experience, on which I must rely for this description. Medical school teaching is little studied. However, it appears that in the classroom at least we have advanced little since the days of Flexner. The emphasis in many courses in many institutions is on didactic lecturing, fact acquisition, and memorization. The present examination system rewards people with good memories, especially those who are skilled at taking examinations. Flexner advocated teaching the scientific method as the basis of medical practice, beginning in the basic science years. Apparently few schools do that, choosing instead to teach bodies of knowledge in each of the basic sciences, as they exist at the time the particular course is taught. Only one problem resulting from this approach to teaching is that in many cases, by the time the student gets into clinical practice four to eight years later, the "state-of-the-art" in the rapidly changing field of biomedicine has changed anyway, and many of the "facts" he or she has learned are useless.

Another major problem in basic science teaching is clinical irrelevance. Although in some schools, teaching objectives for the basic sciences are related to the needs of clinical practice, in many they are not. One would think that in devising a course in anatomy, biochemistry, or physiology, careful thought would be given to the question: what does the practicing physician need to know about the field, and what does he or she need to know most importantly? However, that is not always done. I remember in my microbiology* course, the final exam concerned in major part, the physiology of a bacterium which did not cause a known human disease. It happened that the organism was popular in the department at the time for the study of bacterial genetics.

The Clinical Years

The third and fourth years of the conventional four-year medical education program are spent in clinical training. The classical,

*The science of the study of microorganisms: bacteria, viruses, and others.

"Flexnerian," pattern was to spend the third year "on the wards" in a hospital or hospitals, and the fourth year "in the clinics," (outpatient services). The student would rotate among the various specialties as they were represented in his or her particular hospital. In some schools this pattern still exists, with basic inpatient experiences in internal medicine, surgery, pediatrics, obstetrics-gynecology, and psychiatry being obtained in the third year, and parallel outpatient experiences occurring in the fourth year. In many schools this situation has changed however, with single departmental clerkships combining inpatient and outpatient experiences being given in the third year, the fourth year being turned over entirely to electives.

In either format, in most schools the student clerk is simply attached to the medical team as the most junior member of the hierarchy. The labelling of position by uniform is still common in many institutions: the "attending" physician (clinical instructor or the private physician who admitted the patient) wears a long white coat over his street clothes; the housestaff (residents and interns) wear white jackets and pants or skirts, and formerly often wore white shirts and shoes as well; the medical students wear white jackets over street clothes. In some institutions, the dress differences between medical students and housestaff are breaking down. (Too, not all nurses wear only starched white dresses. I will never forget the first time a nurse wore pants, white to be sure, in a hospital in which I was working in 1970. The place was abuzz about practically nothing else for at least twenty-four hours.) The long white coat is still pretty much the prerogative of the attending physicians however.

Teaching Techniques

Clinical teaching is pretty much by example. You learn what your house staff and attendings have to teach—and what they are interested in. If they "know their stuff" you learn; if they don't, you don't. Although basic content of the clinical clerkships is determined to some degree by the requirements of the several licensing examinations, there is certainly no standardization of clinical teaching between institutions, and sometimes there are problems in this regard within institutions. Lack of standardization can be a special problem when there are major disagreements about what is the correct approach to a particular clinical condition. In an important paper published in the *New England Journal of Medicine,* Dr. Lorrin Koran showed that clinical disagreements often occur in medicine.[15] However, in most instances you learn what your particular instructor believes is correct, sometimes without being told that there even are alternatives.

In Boston, where I went to medical school, virtually all deliveries of babies done at that time were performed using obstetrical forceps—two large metal instruments to be fitted about the baby's head as it appeared in the birth canal, so that the infant could then be pulled quickly through. It occurred to me that women had been delivering babies naturally without forceps for tens of thousands of years, and I wondered why forceps had to be used in normal deliveries. I asked this question of one of the residents under whom I was working and was told simply that "that is the way we do things, that is the best way, and that is really the only way." It was not until I arrived on an obstetrical service in a hospital in New York City during my internship that I discovered that forceps delivery was not "the only way," that most deliveries were aided in that city only by a pair of human hands (gloved), and that (after further inquiry), indeed in *most* of the country, forceps were *not* used in normal deliveries.

Surely it is not incumbent for every clinician to do every procedure the same way, nor for every medical educator to teach either the same thing or the same way. Biomedical knowledge is certain enough only in a minority of instances to be able to demand precise sameness of teaching. However, that last point is exactly the reason why a set of alternatives should be taught. At present, certainty is often taught: "this is the way to do it;" however, uncertainty is often the reality: "there are least two schools of thought on this question." This is one of the major problems arising from having clinical teaching done (only) by example, for the most part by clinicians and/or clinical researchers who also happen to be given teaching responsibilities. Clinical teaching is no more a specialty/profession than is basic science teaching. The person renowned as a "great clinical teacher" these days is more often than not someone who has a great personality, who can thus relate well to both patients and students, and who "knows his stuff," that is who has a prodigious memory. The "pearls of clinical wisdom" roll off his tongue like fine spray does off a waxed boat deck. Only rarely is this person trained to teach students how to think, how to analyze and solve problems, how to evaluate two different approaches to a clinical situation. He knows one approach. It's the one lodged in his memory. That's the one he teaches.

An editorial in the British medical journal the *Lancet,* discussing a British conference on medical education, summarized the present status of medical school teaching in terms that apply equally well in most cases to American medical schools:

> Teachers have little expertise in educational methods. No pressure is placed on them to acquire it and there are few incentives offered to those who wish to improve their teaching. It is assumed that enthusiasm, experience, or knowledge of a subject can compensate for this deficiency. But this is not the case. The best teachers are those who help students to learn effectively; they are not necessarily the most popular individuals or the best lecturers. There is much more to the promotion of learning than the transfer of information . . . At present curricula are designed, time allocated, teaching methods chosen, and examinations prepared without anyone having a clear idea what students should be able to do at the end of the course. Some may believe that such a laissez-faire attitude is a desirable characteristic of university education but it seems a curious way to handle anything as important and expensive as the training of doctors.[16]

Teaching by Specialty

Dr. Morton Creditor, Associate Dean at the University of Illinois College of Medicine at Urbana-Champaign, has pointed out that at most institutions, clinical teaching is done by specialty:

> The medical student [is in turn] taught to think and do like an internist, a surgeon, a phychiatrist, an orthopedist, a pediatrician, etc. It [is] assumed that the student [will] synthesize all of this into being a 'Doctor', but that basic, undifferentiated role model [does] not exist in the high status positions of the medical school if it exist[s] at all. Small wonder that the majority of medical students gravitate toward specialty training and that even those who [go] into the 'primary specialties' such as internal medicine subspecialize at increasing rates.[17]

As Creditor notes elsewhere in his paper, general "physicianship" is nowhere taught in most medical schools. There is no course in "how to be a doctor," although there are many in "how to be an internist," "how to be a surgeon," etc. Is it any wonder that we have a shortage of physicians who are trained to do primary care, which requires a great deal of general physicianship accompanied by enough sense about the problems specialists are trained to deal with to know when to call one in, while we have a plethora of specialists? In some schools, some departments go after clinical teaching time just in order to "expose the students" to their specialty—so that the departments may be able to recruit some of the students to fill the slots in the department's graduate training programs. Of course, clinical departments are just as likely as basic science departments to teach "knowledge" as opposed to methods of information analysis and patient management, otherwise known as problem-solving or the scientific method. Of course, most clinicians and most medical basic scientists come out of the same educational system, and are influenced by the same value sets: research emphasis, rare-disease orientation, absence of a real teaching tradition, and so on. There is little reason to expect them to act differently, since there is no profession of medical educator and obviously no training programs or behavioral criteria for them.

The Place of Memory in Medicine and Medical Education

The management of patient information is the core of medical practice, whether it is episodic or continuous. The mode of information storage and retrieval has a tremendous influence on the mode of medical practice. Dr. Lawrence Weed of the University of Vermont is the developer of a logical system of recording and using patient information called the Problem-Oriented Medical Record, (POMR). Dr. Weed's system, in use in an increasing number of institutions and individual practices, is based on a logical, systematized approach to gathering and recording patient information, to clearly identifying patient problems, to describing plans to deal with identified problems, and to following up the implementation of the plans. It is based upon three principles for good medical care:

1. A system or structure with rules;
2. An audit of performance within the rules and correction of the deficiencies; and
3. An audit of the system itself by examining outcomes, and a change in the system when necessary.[18]

The POMR stands in stark contrast to the information recording system used by the majority of physicians today. Although each physician develops his or her own pattern and tends to be fairly consistent in it, the fact that each has his or her own pattern makes communication between health care providers through records difficult, and in any case, since there are no rules, physicians can and do vary over time within their own system. There is no requirement to list patient problems, only "impressions" and "diagnoses." Nor is there a requirement to clearly state plans of care, and then follow them up. Finally, the present system, as one would expect knowing the system of medical training, is heavily dependent for its implementation upon the individual physician's memory and the body of knowledge in his or her head for its implementation. I have discussed the problems of memory-basing earlier, but Weed puts it simply:

[The] Old Premise [of Medical Education] is: A core of knowledge should be taught. [The] New Premise [of Medical Education] is: A core of behavior should be elicited. . . .

Regardless of what we might say about our philosophy of education, our examination structure gives us away. We examine students and practicing physicians for what they know in terms of medical facts. Sometimes in these examinations we ask them to reason logically with what they know, but nevertheless they are expected to carry a core of knowledge with them.

What has this led to? First, it has probably catalyzed specialization, since if one is going to be examined on what one knows one must narrow the field down in order to pass examinations in a world of such rapidly expanding knowledge. At the time this process is going on, the patient as an organism cannot of course specialize, and the problem of coordinated care is exacerbated. The mere institution of family practice programs may not help the situation if the basic premise is unchanged, since it does not recognize the forces that led to the loss of family practitioners in the first place.

Second, the 'memory,' 'core-of-knowledge' approach led to a mentality in medicine that not only thought it could memorize information it would need for practice, but that it could carry in the mind much information about the patients themselves. . . .

A core-of-knowledge approach allowed us to think that the student's mind was so good that we could give him two years of answers in the so-called basic science years before we told him the questions. . . . Many of our difficulties have their roots in our premises about the role of the human memory and the teaching of the core of knowledge.

Our new premise should be to elicit a core of behavior rather than a core of knowledge, and never examine for or actively memorize knowledge. We should recognize the fact that memory is usage—not IQ, not interest, but usage . . .

[The] core of behavior [to be elicited is]: thoroughness, reliability, a sound analytic sense, and efficiency.[19]

The first step to physician liberation is relieving physicians of as much unnecessary memory work as possible. Computers have much better straight memories than we do. Once computer medical memory systems are perfected, physicians will be freed in their training and their work to do what computers cannot do: clinically apply the scientific method, relate to patients as people, coordinate and integrate care, carry out applied research, and educate patients and staff.

Evaluation of Students

Grading systems have been a matter of great controversy in American medical schools over the past decade or so, and have been the target of many a student revolt. About one-quarter of the schools use the traditional letter/number system. About one-half use a modification of it called "honors/pass/fail," which is really an "A/C/F" system. The remainder use pass/fail, a system in which you either make it or you don't, in theory reducing competition among students.[20] Since many institutions using pass/fail accompany it by more extensive written descriptive evaluations of the students' work, however, it probably does not accomplish that last objective. Most students who support the "pass/fail" system claim that they do so in order to reduce competition. I think that deep down most students who support "pass/fail" do so because such a system usually makes it easier to "get by" in medical school.

Of course, whatever grading system is used, presently it is evaluating test performance, and, as I have noted more than once, tests usually measure knowledge, not ability to perform. A review of the literature by John R. Wingard and John W. Williamson, M.D. has shown little if any relationship between medical school grades and future performance as a physician.[21] The evidence I cited in Chapter 6 shows clearly that there is little relationship between licensure and quality work since studies show that 20 to 40 percent of physicians' work is of less than good quality. Therefore, it can probably also be assumed that the qualifying examinations for licensure, those of the National Board of Medical Examiners and the Federation of State Licensing Boards, are of little value in measuring or predicting performance. Actually, this situation should not be surprising. Medical school examinations by and large measure memory; good medical practice principally requires an ability to *do* tasks well. Again, Weed puts it succinctly:

> Educators took the body of medical knowledge and tried with various teaching techniques, in a modern setting of objectives and examinations, to put that knowledge into the heads of potential physicians, nurses, and other medical personnel. In many instances they assumed it would be used safely in the care of the patient. Medical faculties specialized to an enormous degree to make sure as much information as possible was covered, even though the single student mind could easily suffer from a sensory overload under such circumstances. We fell into the trap of thinking that giving an examination for knowledge at one point in time would ensure performance at that time and for years to come. Even worse, we believed that such transmission of a core of knowledge was necessary and fundamental to good performance.[22]

Weed points out that in the present medical education system, "time and number of courses covered [are] the constant, and achievement the variable . . ." This accounts for the existence of the grading system. (By the way, is it really all right with you if your doctor is correct only 75 percent of the time, especially if one of his classmates who took the same courses is right 95 percent of the time, and in neither case is there a system for routinely catching, *and correcting,* the errors?) Weed counterposes to this: "Achievement should be the constant, and time and number of tasks the variable in medical education and medical practice." In dealing with human lives, there should be absolute standards of performance which everyone professing to do so must achieve. Thus, Weed says, "A person's performance should be audited at random throughout his career, and, according to rules for medical practice, clearly defined and used from the very beginning of medical education." In consequence, "we must abolish the national board examinations as we now know them, and look in an unannounced random manner at how people perform in the real world *according to a core of behavior* (emphasis added)." Weed says, "credentials should be based on performance, randomly audited over a lifetime . . . Nothing short of observing work being done in the actual environment in which a person is expected to function can predict future performance."[23]

From the Particular to the General

One of the most serious faults of American medical school curriculae is that in addition to stressing "knowledge" acquisition (really memory) instead of performance ability, by and large they teach their "knowledge" by beginning with the particular and proceeding toward the general, in relationship to our biomedical understanding of health and disease in man. The latter can be looked at in figurative terms as an equilateral triangle. At the base is knowledge about man in his environment and the distribution of health and disease in populations. This is the purview of the sciences of epidemiology and human ecology. In looking at health and disease, one can, and does, also look at individuals, organ systems, organs, tissues, cells, and sub-cellular structures, and the effects of various stimuli on them. These areas are the purview of the sciences of anatomy, physiology, biochemistry, pathology, and so on. Following this progression, still in the figurative sense, one is moving from the base toward the opposite tip of the triangle, as the focus of study becomes finer and finer. Making the assumption that the purpose of accumulating biomedical knowledge and understanding is to maintain health and prevent disease in man, the base of the triangle can be characterized as the general level, while the point can be characterized as the particular level. To look at in another way, diseases occur biologically within cells—but they affect whole people, and beyond them, populations.

Continuing the figurative analogy, in American medical education, the triangle is standing (teetering?) on its point. We begin our education with the particular and proceed towards the general. In many schools, the morning of the first day is spent beginning to dissect a cadaver. In my school presently, the first class session the students ever have is in microanatomy, the physical analysis of cellular and subcellular structures. After studying cells, tissues, organs, and organ systems for two years or so, medical students finally get to the point where they are asked to look at whole people. This is about as far as most medical students get in proceeding towards the general, except for very brief exposures to epidemiology, usually in an isolated course rated highly by neither the students nor the faculty, and usually poorly attended. Training physicians in this way is analogous to training American historians by beginning with a course on the California Compromise of 1850, rather than with a survey course on the history of Western, if not World, civilization.

After their course in physical diagnosis (in which they do look at whole people) students then generally proceed through clinical clerkships by specialty, and the patients begin undergoing subdivision again. Most physicians, as their education continues, learn more and more about smaller and smaller sub-divisions of the human body. The population, the general level, is hardly ever considered again, much less made a matter for major concern. It is, of course, the disease/cure orientation of modern Western medicine which makes this approach possible. Curing is applied to individuals, not populations. Therefore, disease is taught in individuals, not populations. On the other hand, history has shown that the most effective preventive measures are those applied to populations, and that population health levels have been raised, for the most part, by prevention, not treatment.

A health-oriented medicine would be based on prevention, not treatment. Logically, then, health-oriented physician education would begin with the general and proceed to the particular, the opposite of what we do now. The triangle would be turned from its present tip-balancing position and placed firmly, securely, and comfortably on its base. By putting the triangle on its base, and beginning with the general, the present Disease-Oriented Physician Education system, DOPE, would be replaced by Health-Oriented Physician Education, HOPE. But more of that later, especially in Chapter 13.

Nature-Nurture

If medical schools are training the wrong kinds of doctors with the wrong kinds of attitudes, which the evidence cited in Chapters 3 and 6 indicates is the case, is it due more to what happens to the students while they are in school, or to the type of person selected? Faculties having trouble with their teaching program like to blame the problem on the Admissions Committee: "Boy, are these students terrible. Never study. Never come to class. Flunk the exams. What can we possibly do with this bunch of arrogant ingrates?" In at least some cases, to me this smacks of "blaming the victim."

The way it is done in many schools, medical education is a grinding, dehumanizing, depressing experience. In 1977, I attended my 15th medical school class reunion. I had really disliked medical school, until I reached the clinical years. Naturally, assuming that I was odd man out and attending school during an era when one generally kept one's feelings to oneself, as a student I confided in no one. Imagine my shock and surprise at my 15th when I found that a large proportion of my classmates, now almost all successful in one medical career or another, had felt exactly the same way I did about medical school!

In 1974, Dr. Agnes Rezler of the University of Illinois College of Medicine in Chicago published "Attitude Changes During Medical School: A Review of the Literature." She concluded that: "The findings suggest that the medical school environment fosters cynicism in medical students and that attitude changes induced by participation in special programs are temporary at best unless supported and reinforced by the total medical school environment."[24]

Most medical students come to medical school intending to be practicing physicians. However, the curriculum for the bulk of the first two years ties them to books and labs with little obvious clinical relevance. They are taught in a mode which stresses memorization rather than interpersonal relationships. In light of their expectations on entering medical school, such an approach is bound to make them angry, cynical, depressed. In the clinical years, the bulk of the teaching is highly individualized and randomly sorted for quality. Absolute standards of behavior are not set. Role-modelling by attendings, residents, and interns is a very important determinant of student behavior. Follow the leader is an important principle of medical education, particularly in the clinical years. If the attending you get at a critical point in your career development is a caring person, and is also "successful," you may well become a caring doctor, if you also have what it takes within you. However, a person with caring tendencies who is subjected to arrogant, disease-oriented, medically-mystiqued physicians, who are also "successful," can easily be diverted into that pattern of work. I've seen it happen, only too often.

Obviously, *both* nature and nurture are important in determining the outcome of the medical education process, as they are in all human developmental situations. However, my bias, based on experience and the literature leads me to believe that nurture outweighs nature in influence by about a two-to-one margin.

The Costs of Medical Education

Schools of medicine are expensive places. Drs. John Hogness and Gwynn Akin have pointed out that:

> In 1972, for example, schools of medicine alone accounted for 10 percent of the total expenditures of higher education and had about 10 percent of all employees, although these schools enrolled only about 0.5 percent of all students.[25]

According to the AMA, in 1974–75 the total cost of operating the then 107 fully accredited schools of medicine was slightly over $3 billion. Of this total, almost 40 percent came from the federal government, with the two largest items being contracts and grants for research (20 percent) and contracts and grants for teaching and training (10 percent). An additional 20 percent came from state governments, the bulk of it in the form of direct appropriations to operate the state-owned schools.[26] Thus, nearly 60 percent, $1.8

billion, of all financial support for medical schools is from governmental sources, i.e., the taxpayer.

Third-Party Payments

Governmental funding under Medicare/Medicaid for patient care in teaching hospitals, during which some educational functions are carried out, is *not* included in these calculations, and that category of funding is becoming increasingly important for medical faculty support. The figures discussed in the text are for direct teaching and research costs only. In fact, whenever teaching functions are carried out using patients for whom part or all of the costs of care are paid for by a third party, be it the government or an insurance company, the care becomes less "efficient" in terms of what is happening to that particular patient. Thus, particularly in teaching hospitals, but also in certain kinds of organized ambulatory services, part of the income to the institution from third-party payors goes to cover educational costs, not only for medical students, but for other health sciences students as well.

The amount of patient-care payments supporting medical education and the relative distribution between public and private sources for third-party payments are not known. These matters are subject to a great deal of controversy, however. The nub of the argument is whether or not "service" payments should go in part for the costs of education. If one compartmentalizes "teaching," "service," and "research," in one's mind, then clearly educational costs should be kept separately identifiable and paid for from a separate source. If, however, one sees teaching, service, and research as a continuum which, *when properly designed* (as is now *not* the case), will provide better care for individual patients and groups of patients, then one would take a different tack. In most institutions, part of every third-party payment is earmarked to pay capital construction costs, past, future, or both. If the educational process is seen as developing human capital, then the rationale for allowing third-party payments to cover educational costs, in part at least, is clear.

Distribution of Costs

In 1974, the Institute of Medicine of the National Academy of Sciences issued a major study entitled *Costs of Education in the Health Professions.*[27] The IOM committee which supervised the study was chaired by Dr. Julius Richmond, who later became Assistant Secretary for Health in the first Carter Administration. The Study Director was Ruth Hanft, a principal advisor to Dr. Richmond. The findings are too voluminous to completely summarize here, and I refer interested readers directly to the Report. In considering the particular question of what comprises medical educational cost, the committee concluded that "the costs of education are defined to consist of instruction costs plus those portions of a school's patient care and research programs that are considered essential to education."[28]

The study was carried out principally in 1972–73. For medicine, a carefully selected representative sample of fourteen schools was studied. Annual education costs per student ranged from $6,-900 to $18,650, with an average of $12,650. This means that as of that year, it cost about $50,000 to train one physician in a four-year program. Of the average $12,650 in annual education costs, $7650 was for instruction, $3250 was for education-related research, and $1,750 was for education-related patient care.[29] The 170 percent variation between the lowest- and highest-cost school is interesting to note. Whether there is any variation in the quality of the product by cost of education, and what the extent of the variation is should it exist, is not known. It should be remembered that costs are even higher now.

Average costs were about 25 percent higher in private as compared with public schools. Half the difference is due to additional research and patient care costs related to instruction; the other half to direct instructional costs. Faculty income comprises 43 percent of all instructional costs. Hospital house staff are significant contributors to the educational process: they spend about 10 percent of their time teaching medical students and provide 40 percent of all medical student contact with teachers.[30] House staff are, of course, the least experienced teachers, not trained to teach, not paid to teach, not hired to teach, and have as their major responsibility patient care, at the same they are supposed to be learning themselves.

Volunteer faculty are a major factor in medical school teaching. The complexity of figuring out exactly what their contributions are in terms of time, and then costing out those contributions lead the committee to leave their contributions out of the cost analysis. Those contributons do have some real cost, however, which would have to be added to the already existing high figure.

Although the overall faculty-student ratio in medical schools as determined from AMA data cited early in this chapter is very high, 1 to 1.4, the true faculty-student ratio in terms of full-time equivalent faculty time spent in medical student instruction is actually only 1 to 8, with a range of from 1 to 6, to 1 to 13.[31] This relationship (over-all faculty-student ratio of 1-1.4, teaching faculty-student ratio 1 to 8) confirms the study committee's figures, derived from a direct analysis of faculty worktime, that only "18 percent of . . . total faculty resources [are spent on] instruction of medical students. The allocations of faculty resources to research, patient care, and the instruction of other [kinds of health sciences] students are larger—28 percent, 26 percent, and 28 percent, respectively."[32] This fact, combined with the level of medical faculty salaries, which is determined in large measure by the private, fee-for-service marketplace, is one major reason why medical education costs are so high: most medical school faculty members spend relatively little of their time teaching.

Organization, Regulation, and Quality Control in Medical Education

The Association of American Medical Colleges

Structure

The Association of American Medical Colleges (AAMC) is the major organizational representative for medical schools in the United States. Interestingly, the AAMC has both organizational and individual members, but only the former participate in its governance. The principal benefit for the latter, besides a "feeling of belonging," is a subscription to the AAMC's excellent *Journal of Medical Education.*

Until the late 1960s, the AAMC was popularly known as a "Deans' Club." This is not to say that the organization had not had political power before that time. It had of course been an important factor in achieving the "Flexnerian" reforms, in getting the state boards out of the business of regulating medical schools in the 1920s, in putting accreditation on a firm basis in the 1930s and 1940s, and in struggling for and eventually achieving direct federal aid to medical education in the 1945–65 period. Nevertheless, it was not until the research boom era commenced in the fifties that medical schools began developing administrative structures that were at all complex. Thus a relatively small organization, with a small staff and a low profile, whose Annual Meeting generally consisted of a deans' dinner followed by a few brief reports of business and perhaps one inspirational speech, met the schools' needs. However, as the medical education system grew in complexity, as federal and state government funding became a larger and larger factor in financing operations, as the volume of legislation affecting the health care delivery system grew, the need for reorganization became apparent.

In 1964 the AAMC established a committee headed by Dr. Lowell T. Coggeshall, then Vice-President of the University of Chicago, to review the state of American medical education and the work of the AAMC. The committee's report, entitled *Planning for Medical Progress through Education,* appeared in 1965 and was published by the AAMC itself.[33] It is an important report and is well worth reading. It contained two groups of recommendations, dealing first with the development of American medical education and then with the development of the AAMC. The latter recommendations lead directly to a major reorganization of the Association and its move from relative isolation in Evanston, Illinois, to the national political limelight in Washington, D.C.

A full-time presidency was created, the holder of the post being both the chief executive officer and the chief political spokesman. (Formerly there had been an executive director for administrative matters, and a president, usually a dean of a medical school, elected for a one-year term and serving part-time.) Political power within the Association was divided among a Council of Deans, a Council of Teaching Hospitals, and a Council of Academic Societies, the latter being scientific organizations representing various medical specialty interests. Despite the Coggeshall Committee's recommendation, no provision was made for direct faculty participation in the governance structure, except as faculty members happen to be members of medical specialty societies. The three Councils, joined on a token basis in the early 1970s by a body called the Organization of Student Representatives, meet once a year in the AAMC Assembly, formally the organization's legislative body. The principal day-to-day policy-making group is the Executive Council, composed of elected representatives from the three Councils and the OSR. There are a chairman and vice-chairman annually elected by the Assembly. They, the permanent president, and the executive council, together really run the organization.

Political Posture

On major national medical-political issues the AAMC is fairly conservative. This is to be expected. After all, the AAMC represents a group of organizations, the medical schools, which are generally happy with the way things are going in what they are doing, except that they would just like more money, with as few strings attached as possible, please. To put it another way, pressure for change in medical education is, with few exceptions, not coming from within the system itself, but from the outside. This situation stands in marked contrast with that obtaining at the turn of the century when the AAMC itself was a leading force for reform. The major thrusts from the outside in the present era are asking for major change. The medical schools generally want to preserve the status quo, at least in terms of what they are required to do programmatically. Certain representatives of certain schools would actually like to turn back the clock to an era when there were virtually no controls on research policy, no pressure for training primary care practitioners, no stress on the provision of some direct health care services to persons living in the medical schools' communities. The AAMC represents the schools in the political arena, thus it is not to be unexpected that their positions are fairly conservative, although usually reasonably so. The unthinking

"No," so commonly heard from some other medical organizations, is rare in coming from the AAMC, although it does come on occasion.

On the other hand, the AAMC has taken progressive positions on certain political questions such as increasing minority-group member and female enrollments. Furthermore, the AAMC has a large professional and technical staff of its own engaged in research and development in medical education. There is a great deal of research on many aspects of the medical education process on-going, providing large amounts of useful information, in both the regular "Datagrams" and periodic publications. Some of the work on curriculum development and the development of professonal skills in medical student teaching, for example, is very forward-looking. On numbers of issues, ranging from biomedical research policy to what should be taught in medical schools, many of the staff are privately far ahead of the Association's own elected political leadership which makes the Association's public policy.

Relationships with the AMA

To my knowledge, the history of the AAMC's relationship over the years with the American Medical Association has not been studied in any detail. It appears to me to be generally describable by the word "comfortable." The only major conflict has been over the matter of direct federal aid to medical education, which began after World War II. It was resolved in 1968, when the AMA formally endorsed the concept. There have been some other areas of relatively minor disagreement.

For example, the AAMC believes the hospital housestaff should be classified as students and should not be allowed to organize to bargain collectively with their employers over terms and conditions of employment. The AMA supports the concept of physicians organizing and bargaining collectively, when necessary.

On the other hand, there are major areas of policy agreement, or at least noninterference, on certain very important issues. Both organizations strongly support the concept of voluntary accreditation of medical schools, which one would expect since they do it jointly (see the next section).

The AAMC has until this writing stayed out of controversies

over issues which are very important to the AMA, such as the status of private entrepreneurial fee-for-service medical practice, and national health insurance. On the latter issue, one which certainly affects medical schools, the AAMC has had several working committees, but by mid–1978 had made no definite program proposals, even though the interests of the private practitioners and the medical schools would appear to diverge sharply on many of the major policy issues. However, both organizations strongly, on occasion fiercely, fight "government interference," especially at the federal level, in the "practice of medicine" (AMA) and the medical education system (AAMC). In terms of general political effectiveness, especially at the federal level, it is now generally considered that the AMA has shot its bolt with its correctly earned reputation for constant negativism. The AAMC generally has a good reputation in Congress, although one hears talk that its status is slipping somewhat over its reluctance to consider more than token changes in the medical education system.

Regulation

Government Role

Medical schools are not licensed by any government jurisdiction. They are chartered by state governments to do business as nonprofit corporations. The only limits placed on their operations by such charters are the same as those placed on any other nonprofit corporations. These limits thus do not extend to such activities as curriculum design, admissions policies, degree requirements, and the like. Indirect control of the latter by state medical licensing boards was removed by the agreement between the AAMC and the Federation of State Medical Boards back in the 1920s.

This is not to say that government is not a major factor in medical school operations. Footing 60 percent of the bill, one would expect it to be. However, there is no consistent pattern or system for regulation, related to clearly defined goals and objectives. The influence is rather through conditions attached to the receipt of funds. Thus, it is rather uneven, depending upon particular programs funded. The federal government, as we have seen in previous chapters, has attached certain conditions to the receipt of both research and operational monies. Some are process conditions like procedures for protecting the interests of human subjects in research, and for providing equal opportunity for employment and medical school admission. Others are outcome conditions: beginning a new school, increasing class-size, producing more family practitioners, producing more primary care physicians. Usually these conditions are not of the "you must do it" type, but rather of the "if you do, you get the money" type.

Some state governments have also established programmatic requirements for schools which they own or support. (State-supported schools are not always within the state's boundaries. New York State subsidizes state residents attending a medical school in Tel Aviv, Israel.) State governments have been especially concerned with state-residents-only admissions policies, increasing class size, the creation of Family Medicine departments, and in some states, the establishment of new medical schools.

Governments have thus been reluctant to get into the regulation of day-to-day medical school operations or to become involved in setting over-all goals and objectives for the system. Those activities have been left to the accreditation process.

Accreditation

Accreditation is a voluntary general approach to quality for institutions which I discussed in Chapter 6. For the medical schools, since 1942 it has been carried out by a body called the Liaison Committee on Medical Education (LCME) which has equal representation from the AAMC and the AMA. The LCME is recognized as the official medical school accreditation body by the Office of Education, USDHEW, and the voluntary agency which itself accredits accrediting agencies, the Council on Postsecondary Accreditation. Furthermore, a major state medical board licensure requirement is graduation from an accredited medical school (except in the case of foreign medical graduates). These various recognitions are the sources of power of the LCME. Non-accredited schools cannot receive federal funds, and their graduates cannot be licensed. Thus the LCME is in effect delegated quasi-governmental powers while at the same time governments waive their power to review medical school operations, except in the specific instances described above. Thus there is little public accountability in the medical education system, despite the fact it receives over half its money from governmental sources. In 1976–77, the Federal Trade Commission was challenging the authority of the LCME, claiming that the AMA, if not the AAMC, was engaged in a conspiracy in the restraint of trade. This case, if the FTC pursues it, will probably spend many years in the courts before it is eventually settled.

Having the tremendous authority that it does over a system as complex as the American medical education system, one might expect that its qualifying rules and regulations would be quite detailed and explicit, as, for example are the accreditation standards of the Joint Commission on the Accreditation of Hospitals. However, they are in fact not very detailed at all. The current basic accreditation document, "Functions and Structure of a Medical School," which appeared in 1973, is only about twenty-five hundred words in length. A sort of commentary on the basic accreditation document, entitled "Guidelines to 'Functions and Structure of a Medical School,' " and about twice as long, was published by the LCME in 1976.

"Functions and Structure of a Medical School" is characterized by nothing if not vagueness and a penchant for generalization. (So that readers may judge for themselves, "Functions and Structure" is reproduced in its entirety in Appendix II.) For example, a medical school is defined as "an aggregation of resources that have been organized as a definable academic unit to provide the full spectrum of education in the art and science of medicine in not less than thirty-two months, culminating with the award of the M.D. degree." For the "Educational Program," the document stipulates that: "Each student should acquire a foundation of knowledge in the basic sciences that will permit the pursuit of any of the several careers that medicine offers. The student should be *comfortably familiar* with the methods and skills utilized in the practice of clinical medicine (my emphasis)." Under "Faculty," it is stated that: "The faculty must consist of a sufficient number of identifiable representatives from the biological, behavioral, and clinical sciences to implement the objectives *that each medical school adopts for itself* (my emphasis)."[33] And so on.

The requirements are thus not at all detailed, and are certainly not couched in terms of outcome objectives related in any way to societal needs. The accreditation review process involves periodic visits for several days to the medical schools by teams selected by the LCME. Accreditation visitors are usually senior faculty and administrative personnel from other medical schools, plus AMA and/or AAMC staff, working for the LCME. In addition to the visit, they review a great deal of documentary material the schools are required to prepare. With the generality of the standards, which are structural for the most part in any case, the intrinsic criteria of the team members, (*I* think this is good, *I* think this is bad), must be very important in the accreditation process. Although these days developing medical schools sometimes have accreditation problems, existing ones hardly ever do.

One might think that the vagueness in the accreditation guidelines would produce great diversity among medical schools. However, with a few notable exceptions, medical schools in this country are remarkably similar despite paper differences among them particularly in the arrangement of the curriculum. They are remarkably similar because most of them share a common set of goals and objectives, still primarily defined by the original Hopkinsonian (not "Flexnerian") model: basically inner-directed and inward-turning, founded on the medical mystique, hospital rather than community-oriented, and stressing "knowledge" rather than performance. (See also Chapter 8.) These goals and objectives are not spelled out in the accreditation document, and can continue to exist virtually unchanged precisely because they are not so spelled out. The Hopkinsonian model exists in the heads of most medical school faculty members and administrators, either consciously or unconsciously, again not because it is spelled out anywhere, but because it is the model by which *they* were trained. It is precisely because the goals and objectives of the medical education system are *not* spelled out, but exist only in the minds of those doing the educating, and are therefore not subject to rational review and change, that they have remained as they have for so many years.

The Quality of Medical Education

It is customary for observers of the American medical education system to say, as did the Coggeshall Committee, that in our country are found "a quality of medical education and patient care as good as or better than that found in any other nation."[34] What does this really mean? Even if true, does the comparative standard have any value here? Supposing there were a world-wide food shortage, and while the people in all other countries had 800 calories or less average food intake per day, our people had 900. What that means is that our people would be starving, but not quite so badly as everyone else is. Nevertheless, in that circumstance, our diet could be considered "the best in the world."

If the comparative standard is not too useful in evaluating medical education, perhaps the Coggeshall Committee's conclusions could be arrived at using domestic standards only. In Chapter 6, we saw that there were three types of evaluative techniques: structure, process, and outcome, and we defined them. By reading the medical school accreditation document (see Appendix II), you can see clearly that it relies on structural criteria, and pretty vague and general ones at that. Furthermore, evaluation for accreditation relies on intrinsic application of the standards, a method which can result in a high degree of variability, rather than extrinsic application using a predetermined, written down, thoroughly agreed-to specific criteria.* Then, referring back to the evidence cited in Chapter 6, we find that the structural technique is now considered by most experts to have little validity in judging quality. The most that can be said is that good structure is probably necessary, but definitely not sufficient to produce good quality. Therefore, just because all of the fully established medical schools in this country are accredited means little in determining their quality, considering only the limitations of the structural technique and forgetting those of peer review.

If we want to validly judge the quality of our medical education

*Recall that intrinsic criteria of "goodness" are those existing in the head of the observer, who is chosen for the evaluation job because he or she is considered "good," while extrinsic criteria are spelled out clearly in advance and the observer simply has to apply them.

system, we must rather evaluate its product and outcomes in terms of how they meet the needs of the people for health care. It is in this regard that the system runs into difficulties, as we shall see in the next chapter.

The medical schools have had a great deal of freedom of action over the years, and they have for the most part chosen the paths they have followed. I believe that the evidence I have presented so far in this book, summarized in the next chapter, demonstrates that, in terms of the public's needs for health and health care, the medical schools, largely self-regulated, have not done the best job they could have. They have used their freedom neither to produce diversity nor to produce excellence in meeting the health and health care needs of the people. Aside from its consequences for the people, this behavior potentially has serious consequences for the schools.

In 1910, Flexner thought the government should regulate the medical schools if they did not meet social needs.[35] The schools cast off that burden in the 1920s. But in 1932, the *Final Report* of the AAMC's own Commission on Medical Education was saying that:

> The greatest health problem of the country is that of making modern medical services available to the entire population. . . . The gap between what is known and what is applied has always existed and will continue as additions are made to current knowledge. The extent of that gap, however, can be materially reduced through education of the public, sound regional planning, and the training of physicians and other workers in the broader aspects of the problems involved.

However, the Commission felt that outside regulation was not the way to achieve these goals:

> The Commission has believed from the beginning that an emphasis on educational principles in medical training and licensure can be secured only by modifying the point of view and broadening the interests of those responsible for medical education and licensure, not by recommendations, statistics, new regulations, further legislation or manipulation of the curriculum.[36]

Over thirty years of voluntary action later, another committee sponsored by the AAMC (Coggeshall) could say:

> Perhaps the most emphatic implication of emerging [health care] trends is the need for those responsible for education in the health field to give increasing attention to meeting the requirements of the nation, state, and community for health care and personnel. . . . Those responsible for medical education—faculty members, deans, university officials, trustees, and legislators—will, in decades ahead, need to devote careful attention to appraising the needs of society for health care and health personnel and to developing and implementing plans to meet those needs. Failure to do so will damage the standing of the profession and educational institutions and will invite—even make necessary—less desirable approaches to meeting the health care needs of a growing America. If those responsible for medical education fail to assume and act on a responsibility that is now clearly theirs, it will be assumed by others. The reemergence of medical schools of marginal quality outside the jurisdiction of the university is a clear likelihood. The intervention of government to see that emerging needs are met and to provide the means of meeting them is an even greater likelihood.[37]

Since 1965, government funding has increased and so has government intervention. However, government still has not "taken over," and it is unlikely to do so in the near future at least. However, if (should I say "when"?) that event does occur, with its many desirable, and undesirable, consequences, the medical schools will have only themselves to blame.

SECTION *IV*

Problems and Solutions

12

The Relationship Between the Medical Education System and the Health Care Delivery System

Please do not place the onus of all the faults of our health care system on the medical schools. These institutions have given the country the best educated physicians in the world. These physicians, along with many other health professionals, have provided our people with excellent health care. For nearly thirty years public policy has demanded that these institutions provide an improved scientific base for medicine and that they translate this improved science into action at the bedside. It is fair to say that schools have responded.

—*Robert G. Petersdorf, M.D., President, American College of Physicians*

> *Much of the credit for the new Health Manpower Bill, from the removal by Congress of regulatory controls on the distribution of health professionals to the acceptance of a voluntary approach and the signature of the President, was recently given to the AMA by the Washington based National Journal. . . . Your AMA's effort to resist use of the bill as a vehicle for government dictation of curriculum, regional allocation, federal service, and licensure of physicians was a significant achievement.*
>
> —*Richard E. Palmer, M.D.,*
> *President,*
> *American Medical Association*

> *The simple truth is that if the Association of American Medical Colleges and the American Medical Association had taken the steps necessary to train a proper balance of physicians and to make an active effort to see that the underserved areas of this nation had doctors there would not now be the support in the Congress for direct intervention to achieve these goals.*
>
> —*Senator Edward M. Kennedy*

After reviewing the relationships between health, disease, and health care, and describing the problems of the health care delivery system in the United States as I see them in Section I, I went on to describe the major features of that system in Section II. One of the major conclusions that can be drawn upon analysis of the U.S. health care delivery system is that the physician plays a central, controlling role in its functioning. Historically, the licensing laws, giving physicians virtually exclusive control over diagnosing, prescribing drugs, and surgically operating, have been a very important factor in creating that role. Since it is the medical schools which select and train the doctors, it is obvious that the medical schools have a critically important relationship to the health care delivery system.

The history of medical education in our country was outlined in Chapters 7 through 10; its contemporary profile was described in the last chapter. We have seen that, in general, the role and functioning of our medical schools has not been defined in terms of social responsibility, as Flexner concluded they should be. Instead, most American medical schools have tended to be inner-directed, setting policies to meet the perceived needs of the active medical practitioners and/or the schools' own faculties and administrations. Having this understanding of the history, role, and functioning of the medical education system, we can now proceed to analyze the relationship between that system and the principal problems of the health care delivery system, as I described them in Chapter 3.

Problems in the Health Care Delivery System and their Relationship to the Medical Education System

By now two points should be abundantly clear: (1) Historically it is preventive services, principally of the primary-community type, which have been mainly responsible for the improved health levels observed in Western countries over the past three centuries; and (2) We have a health, perhaps we should qualify the term, "health," care delivery system which is oriented towards disease and cure, rather than health and prevention. For this situation the medical schools, the creators of the doctors, must bear a major responsibility. What is fascinating is that they have maintained their disease-oriented posture in the face of strong recommendations to change, over the years, not only from outside social critics, but from the likes of Abraham Flexner, their own Commission on Medical Education (1932), and their own Coggeshall Committee (1965).

Separation of Services for Acute and Chronic Care

There are economic, political, and social reasons for this situation, but the medical schools must bear some responsibility for it as well. The bulk of medical school teaching is done in acute care hospitals, on patients who are relatively seriously ill. Furthermore, most medical students are infected early on with a serious, usually chronic disease called the "Interesting Case Syndrome," to which I have previously referred. This disease induces the sufferer to think that the common medical and health problems that most people have most of the time are "uninteresting," while the more rare and unusual the medical condition is, the more interesting it is. I cited earlier the case of the Professor of Pharmacology who felt that medical students "couldn't learn anything" in an ambulatory care service. Many patients who come to hospital ambulatory care services have, in fact, chronic diseases or symptoms (including psychosocial problems) not requiring hospitalization. Few medical schools require their students to spend very much time in ambulatory care, particularly general ambulatory care, although this situation is changing.

In many teaching hospitals, a certain attitude towards the elderly sick is not so much taught, as it is inculcated or socialized. One often hears the term "crock" used to refer to the elderly person suffering, perhaps, from senile dementia, generalized arteriosclerosis, or the aftermath of a stroke, with consequent loss of memory, intellectual ability, and control over bodily functions. Very often this patient is poor and has little or no family left to take care of him or her. Or consider the situation in a teaching Veterans' Administration Hospital in which, I am told, aging, alone men, often alcoholics, are commonly referred to by housestaff as "WPOS" (Worthless Piece of S——t). But I wonder if these attitudes are really so surprising when such sci/med establishment leaders as the Dean of the Yale School of Medicine, Robert Berliner, M.D., a former Director of the National Institutes of Health, can say the following, in response to suggestions by Dr. Robert Butler, Director of the National Institute on Ageing that medical students should have a course in geriatrics and that some of their clinical training time should be spent in nursing homes:

There are a lot of problems in society that are reflected in medicine. I don't think giving a course in geriatrics is going to help. As to rotating students through nursing homes, how many nursing homes have you been to? They're pretty dismal places.[1]

Rising Cost

Once again, one can hardly blame medical schools entirely for this most serious problem. However, they have contributed to it, and in analyzing that contribution one begins to see how many of the problems on the list from Chapter 3 are interrelated. As we saw in Sections I and II of this book, physician dependency on the hospital, specialization, excess hospitalization, and excess surgery are major factors in cost escalation. Doctors are taught in medical school to be hospital-dependent. As I have pointed out several times, doctors are the most important determinants of the utilization of medical services, particularly the expensive ones, and are influential in the creation of medical care capital equipment and facilities. Yet few medical students are taught much about health economics in a formal way. In their informal education, they are much more likely to learn about tax-shelters than about skewed demand curves.

Cost consciousness and control and cost/benefit analysis are part of the clinical teaching program in few institutions. Although 80 percent of active clinical practitioners are in private office practice, few programs teach students or housestaff anything about office management, personnel practices, record-keeping, and so on. The medical education system could hardly control rising costs by itself, but it could be a powerful positive influence in the situation.

Financial Barriers to Care

The medical schools are also not a major cause of this problem, but could help to alleviate it, first of all by recognizing its existence. In most medical schools, little is taught specifically on the problems of the health care delivery system. The medical schools generally have been nowhere to be seen in the struggles to lower and eliminate the existing financial barriers to care. To the extent that the fee-for-service private entrepreneurial practice system is itself a barrier to care, the medical schools, heavily dependent as they are for clinical teaching on faculty who are at least part-time in private practice, have absented themselves from that controversy. Furthermore, even though the other major concerned national organizations have produced legislative proposals for a national health insurance plan, even including the American Medical Association, as I pointed out in the last chapter, the Association of American Medical Colleges has yet to do so.

Geographic Maldistribution of Physicians

This is not a problem which the medical schools have created, except perhaps by their admissions policies which until recently excluded most persons who were not white, male, and upper or upper-middle class. However, it is a problem about which the schools have done little or nothing, despite its frequent citation in reports as a serious one, beginning once again with Flexner. Nor for the most part do the schools seem to think that it is a problem for which they have any responsibility. The exceptions to this rule are primarily state-owned institutions whose legislatures have set requirements for dealing with rural health-manpower shortages, such as the University of Illinois. For example, in 1975 the faculty of the Harvard Medical School said among other things, in adopting a set of overall admissions policies:

> The Admissions Committee should not attempt to select students according to predicted future needs of society nor should it set quotas or goals in terms of students professing an interest in a particular career or field of medicine.

As I pointed out in the previous chapter, in 1976, when the current law supporting health manpower education was being debated in the Congress, the AAMC fought hard, and successfully, to eliminate from the legislation the following originally proposed requirements on schools receiving federal support:

1. Some clinical experiences in ambulatory care must be provided at "remote sites" away from the medical school for all students, on the theory that exposure to rural or central city medical shortage areas might encourage some students to return to them to practice.

2. All medical school graduates must serve two years in an "under-doctored" area, a policy similar to that of countries as different as Mexico and the Soviet Union. This proposal of Senator Kennedy's got absolutely nowhere.
3. The schools must require that a certain percentage of their students apply for National Health Service Corps (NHSC) scholarships. The NHSC is a federal service which supplies young physicians on a contract-salary basis to medically underserved areas for two-year terms. An NHSC scholarship provides financial support for a student in medical school on a year-for-year pay-back basis.

All of these programs would have helped relieve geographic maldistribution. The AAMC was very proud of its "victory."

Overspecialization and Specialty Maldistribution

The medical schools have contributed to these problems by sins of commission as well as omission. Virtually every major report on the health care delivery system since the AAMC's own *Final Report of the Commission on Medical Education* in 1932 when only 25 percent of doctors were specialists, through the Carnegie Commission Report in 1970 when only 25 percent of doctors were not specialists, down to the present time, has referred to overspecialization and specialty maldistribution as two of the most serious problems facing the health care delivery system. Now it is perfectly true that biomedical knowledge has been expanding at a phenomenal rate, and that no one individual has been able to comprehend its totality for many decades. It is also true that developments in surgical technique have long since passed the point where in most cases one individual can be considered competent to operate in more than one area of the body. But it is also true that for several decades the medical education system has been turning out more specialists in toto than the population needs, especially in surgery, and it has done nothing about the situation.

You will recall from the previous chapter that Dr. Morton Creditor has pointed out that we do not teach "physicianship" in medical school, but rather than we teach by specialty: clinical clerkship follows clinical clerkship in internal medicine, surgery, pediatrics, psychiatry, and so on. Elective experiences are usually in specialties as well. The response of the general practitioners to the onward march of specialism was not to reveal its fatal flaws as a philosophy of medicine but to try to create yet another specialty: "family practice."

The major teaching hospitals have never come together to try to figure out how many of this or that type of specialist would be needed by the country and then control residency-training positions accordingly. For the most part, residency positions are created primarily to meet hospital service and research needs. Certainly the American Medical Association, which approves hospital residency positions, has never taken national needs into account in its decision-making process. The AMA formally considers only the educational quality of the proposed program. Again in the development of the current health manpower law, the AAMC fought hard and successfully to eliminate any provisions for planning the specialty distribution of residency positions according to national needs.[2] In a discussion of over specialization in the AAMC's Council of Academic Societies at the 1976 Annual Meeting, one of its most respected members argued quite strongly that it was obvious that the only way to solve the twin problems, while preserving "academic integrity," was the voluntary approach. Yet, as I point out in Chapter 9, the voluntary approach to these problems was urged upon its members by the AAMC Commission in 1932. The results have been terrible. For how long do we stick with it?

Deficiencies in Quality and Quality Control

In the quote at the beginning of this chapter, Dr. Petersdorf of the American College of Physicians talks about the "excellent health care" provided to our people by our "physicians, along with many other health professionals." Richard Palmer, M.D., AMA president for 1976–77, said on National Public Radio that: "The pluralistic American health care system presently provides Americans with the best quality health care in the world."[3] (He added that it was private medicine that was doing a great job and that it should be expanded.) The evidence cited in Chapter 6 contradicts these statements. If the medical schools cannot be held responsible for the less-than-optimum performance of a significant minority of their graduates, I'm not sure what they can be held responsible for.

The medical schools strongly support a licensing system whose qualifying examinations measure "knowledge" (read memory), not ability to perform. They have not been in the forefront of the struggle to establish periodic relicensure for physicians. Few medical schools teach their students about the various mechanisms and systems available for objectively auditing and improving the quality of medical care, involving both peer and non-peer review. Rather, in most institutions, what quality control mechanisms exist are those built into the heads of the chiefs of service, other than mechanisms dealing with exceptional circumstances: deaths, surgical operations. Referring back to Chapter 6, this approach represents the use of implicit, rather than explicit, criteria. This is changing now to a certain extent as the JCAH enforces its requirement for the PEP or its equivalent, but there is no information concerning the effect of this change on medical education. It could, of course, be used in the most creative way, involving the students in the auditing and continuing education processes.

The customary approach to quality control ("good" is what is in the chief's head), is totally consistent with the "doctor knows best," and "it's wrong not to know, worse to admit a mistake," attitudes which are built into most students in most schools from the beginning. I once had a student whom I was instructing in history-taking and physical diagnosis leave my group for another teacher because I didn't "know" enough. That is, my memory was not good enough to enable me to answer every question of fact the student asked me. It is my custom, when a student asks me a question the answer to which I do not know, to say first "I don't know," and then to suggest either where they might look up the answer, or which other instructor we might consult together to find out the information. The sooner we institute thoroughgoing systems for catching our errors and correcting them, like the one Dr. Weed has designed for example, the better off we, and our patients, will be. One might say, somewhat uncharitably perhaps: "To err is human; to not admit it, physician-like."

Another aspect of medical school laxity in quality of care measurement and control is the faint, sometimes nonexistent emphasis given to medical ethics and legal medicine. In many schools, students are pretty much left to their own devices to pick up what they can on ward rounds, in the surgical lockerroom, and what have you. The information may be good, bad, or indifferent. The problem is that students are not often taught that there are systematic ways of approaching ethical questions (even if in some situations there is no one "right" answer and one must follow one's own beliefs), that there is a large body of legislation and case law at the federal, state, and local levels dealing with health and medicine, and that there is more to the "malpractice crisis" than rising physician insurance premiums. The major problem is that as with objective quality measurement and control, medical ethics and legal medicine are not built into the educational process in most schools, but are "add-ons" and/or electives, if they are present at all.

Lack of Planning

The medical schools cannot be faulted here directly. Lack of planning is a general health care delivery system problem, and beyond that a general problem in our socio-economic system. In health care, it is importantly related to the private entrepreneurial nature of the bulk of medical practice. Nevertheless, the schools can be faulted indirectly—again for what they don't teach, rather than what they do teach. Health and health care planning is a field with a body of knowledge and techniques. Properly done, it can be effective. Few medical schools spend much time teaching their students anything about health and health care planning, on either the macro (system) or the micro (personal practice) levels. As I pointed out in Chapter 3, since physicians are the major decision-makers in the health care delivery system, nothing much will happen of major significance in planning until the physicians are "trained and brought into the planning system on the one hand, and until a sensible series of controls over their work is created on the other hand." The medical schools have a major responsiblity in this endeavour.

Provider-Patient Communication

As I pointed out in Chapter 3, the physician-patient communication gap is one of the most serious problems we face. From the patients' point of view, it appears to be vying with rising costs as the most serious one. (My own list puts lack of attention to prevention first, the communication gap second, and rising costs third.) How often does one hear the complaint, "My doctor won't talk to me"? As I concluded in Chapter 3, the principal causes of the physician-patient communication gap are the Medical Mystique and physician elitism. The medical schools can be held directly responsible for the creation and maintenance of these two characteristics of doctors. It is the medical schools which teach "doctor knows best," that most patients cannot understand very well, that Greek and Latin words should be used where Anglo-Saxon ones would do very well, that doctors are superior beings (not just leaders) in the health manpower hierarchy, that there is little that doctors can learn either from patients or other health workers, and so on.

It is also what medical schools do *not* teach that is important. Little if any time is devoted to training in health education for individual patients. Little attention is paid to the techniques of how to explain to patients what their illness is and how the therapeutic program should work. There seems to be more literature about patient "noncompliance" (blaming the victim), than there is about how doctors can better explain things to patients. There is little if any exposure to public health education, working either with groups of one's own patients, or with community agencies. These kinds of activities are not important in physician-centered medical practice. They are very important if diseases are to be prevented and the population's health improved. They're not dealt with very much in most medical schools.

Professional Irrelevance

This related back to the separation of services for acute and chronic care and that dangerous, widely prevalent malady of physicians, The Interesting Case Syndrome. Once again, this is a medical school responsibility. Not only do medical schools foster this sickness, but they appear to want to actively infect their students with it. Listen to Sherman Melinkoff, M.D., a medical school dean and prominent leader of the AAMC, writing for a medical audience:

> What makes medicine attractive to bright men? Many diverse features too numerous to list, no doubt, but surely among them are the opportunities for discovery. If any reader is in doubt here, let him contrast his own feelings toward 'routine physical examinations' he may have performed and toward the challenge of trying anxiously to find the obscure cause of a fever or of a severe abdominal pain. . . . There are certain minds, good and useful ones, that thrive on routine tasks or in a degree of team effort in which someone else is always the quarterback. It is doubtful, however, if those men will make the best clinicians.[4]

Pity the poor patient with a common problem. That just happens to be most people, as shown by the data in Chapter 2 and the discussion of the problem of professional irrelevance in Chapter 3. Russell Baker of the *New York Times* has put it very well, in a reproduced set of letters to that well-known medical columnist, Dr. Omniscient:

> Dear Dr. Omniscient: I see where Ramses II, the well-known mummy, has had his fungus infection cured by doctors in Paris and has been sent back to Egypt with a clean bill of health. What kind of a society is this that can cure fungus in a 3,000-year-old mummy but can't even cure the common cold? (signed) Disgusted.
>
> Dear Disgusted: The answer to your question is quite simple. The mummy didn't have the common cold. It had fungus. If it had been suffering from a cold, how do you know society couldn't have cured it? Vintage mummies may not be as resistant to cures as you are."[5]

In Summary

It should now be obvious that the medical education system is a major factor in and cause of many of the observed problems of the health care delivery system. The two systems are closely intertwined, as much as the medical education establishment would like us to think otherwise. The fact is that the taxpayers of this country are spending large sums of money to support a medical education system which is hardly publicly accountable and which is not creating a product that is particularly relevant to the needs of the majority of the people.

Lest you think that I put all of the responsibility for the state of our health care delivery system on the medical education system, I should point out that I do recognize that there are severe problems of inequitable financing and malorganization which can hardly be blamed on the schools: there is the widely prevalent cost-plus reimbursement system for hospitals; then there is fee-for-service private entrepreneurial medical practice. This is also a major cause of our health care delivery system difficulties. I will discuss it briefly in the next section. The medical schools, of course, cannot be held responsible for its existence, but they haven't done anything to remove it either. Although the medical schools do not bear all of the responsibility for our health care delivery problems, they are a significant contributor. If solutions are to be found to health care delivery system problems, changes will have to be made in the medical education system.

Fee-for-Service Private Practice

What It Is

About 80 percent of all American physicians in active practice other than house staff in training are in private entrepreneurial fee-for-service practice, either singly or in groups. In this system, physicians are independent small businessmen contracting with persons ("patients") to provide services. The contracts are usually verbal rather than written and most often do not spell out what services are to be provided, except in the most general terms.

Too, the price is not necessarily given in advance. In fact, many physicians resist discussing fees. Physicians receive a fee for each service, that is they are paid on a piecework basis. In some specialties, particularly surgery and obstetrics, there is one flat rate for the whole set of care: preoperative, the operation, and postoperative.

Fee-for-service private practice is entrepreneurial because income is related directly to the amount of work done, that is, assuming fairly constant rate schedules. The physician must organize, manage, and assume the risks of his practice (business). The more services he provides (sells), the more money he makes. Unlike most small businessmen, physicians don't advertise overtly. Since their numbers are fairly limited, since there are myriad specialties thus creating much smaller effective numbers of physicians in each area of need, and since the provider is an important determinant of demand, physicians don't have to advertise in the way most other entrepreneurs do. That is one reason why the AMA can take such a strong stand against doctors advertising. But that does not mean that doctors do not engage in making their existence known in other ways. There is intra-professional solicitation of various sorts. There may be fee-splitting. There can be subtle encouragement of patients to "tell their friends."

The Contradictions of Private Practice

There are three major social contradictions involving fee-for-service private practice. First, in the fee-for-service system, doctors do well by treating diseases in individual patients. The more diseased persons they treat, the greater their income. Not very much income is derived from keeping or trying to keep people well. However, we have seen that historically the most successful measures for improving health levels have been those applied to the population as a whole: improved nutrition, pure water supply, sanitary sewage and solid waste disposal and so on. In relation to health then, the contradiction is clear: health is most affected by preventive measures of a social nature, while doctors spend most of their time treating disease on an individual basis. Second, health care services are increasingly being financed on a social basis, through general or special taxation and through employer/employee payments for health insurance paid for by society as a whole through higher prices for goods and services. There is a clear contradiction here too: while the financing is social, the payment to the doctors is by individual fees. Finally, in our era, many health services are provided by groups of people most of whom are employed socially. Yet the physician, the principal decision-maker and occasional team leader, is employed individually and separately.

All contradictions are eventually resolved and these will be too. The first is actually the most important one in relation to the peoples' health. However, in our present cost-conscious era it is likely that the second one will be dealt with first. The resolution will not involve returning to a system of individual responsibility for payment.

Fee-for-Service Private Practice and Problems in the Health Care Delivery System

There is not space in this book to do a complete analysis of the relationship between the private entrepreneurial fee-for-service medical practice system and the problems of the health care delivery system. That is a subject which really requires a book of its own. However, we can briefly consider some of the negative influences which fee-for-service private practice has on the health care delivery system.

Neglecting Prevention

Fee-for-service private practice (FFSPP, or PP for short) is based on the treatment of sick people. Under PP doctors do *not* get paid when they keep people well. There is thus no financial motivation behind health promotion and disease prevention. One of our great leaders in public health, Prof. C.-E.A. Winslow put the position well in a 1944 editorial in the American Journal of Public Health:

> So long as the doctor is paid on a fee-for-service basis, his income and his opportunity for service must depend on the treatment of disease, since he will be called in only when something hurts. . . . Only when the doctor is habitually employed on a prepayment basis for health service will preventive and constructive medicine really become vitally significant.[6]

Overspecialization

The way PP has evolved, specialists get paid more for providing services than do generalists, even when the service provided is exactly the same. The supply of physicians in each specialty (except general surgery and a few surgical subspecialties) is fairly thin, driving prices up even in a provider-generated demand system. Since under PP specialists make more money, PP obviously encourages specialization.

Geographic Maldistribution

Under the PP approach, each doctor has the right to choose where he or she wants to practice. At least one study has shown that the most influential factor affecting the geographic movement of physicians has been the geographic change in the distribution of per capita income.[7] To put it crudely, under PP, doctors follow dollars. Is it any wonder that rural areas and central cities are under-doctored?

Overhospitalization and Excess Surgery

Paying a higher proportion of the costs of hospitalization including doctors' hospital fees than of any other kind of service, the health insurance system in this country encourages hospitalization. The PP system, which has steadfastly resisted the broad development of insurance for other kinds of health services, is largely responsible for this situation. Furthermore, the existence of a payment mechanism for some physician services but not others under PP encourages the use of covered services. This is certainly a factor in the excess surgery situation.

Suppression, then Inhibition of the Growth of Prepaid Group Practice

Prepaid group practice (PPGP) offers many advantages to patients: ready accessibility of care, low or nonexistent financial barriers, good availability of specialty consultation services, a full range of supporting services. PPGP offers hospitalization and surgery rates well below the national averages, with no apparent decrement in quality. PPGP can offer a full range of personal preventive services.

PP actively fought the establishment of PPGPs until the late sixties at both the national and local levels. Since President Nixon embraced the PPGP concept in 1971, renaming it "Health Maintenance Organization," the AMA has been cautiously supportive at the national level, especially since the HMO approach also embraces prepayment coupled with solo office practice, and profit-making group practice. However, PP in various local areas continues to oppose the establishment of PPGPs. Doctors are not at all shy in complaining about "unfair competition." If there were no private practice, doctors wouldn't have to worry about "unfair competition." Another aspect of the difficulties presented to PPGP by PP is the high physician incomes PP makes possible. PPGPs have to compete with those high incomes in recruiting medical staff. PPGPs can thus be forced into uneconomic budgets and high medical staff turnover, as medical staff members other than those dedicated to the concept move on to financially greener pastures. This really is "unfair competition."

Nonexistence of National Health Insurance

Since 1920, when the private practitioners took over the AMA leadership from the academic establishment, the AMA has been opposed to NHI. The campaign has been conducted at times with vigor, at times with vitriol, almost always with stubborn negativism. In the mid-seventies the AMA leadership is promoting an NHI proposal which would sanctify fee-for-service private practice, prohibit the use of fee schedules, place what limited controls over the actions of doctors they would countenance in the hands of the state governments only, and put the private insurance industry in control of the financing system. Even with this proposal (hardly "national" health insurance since it would be run by the states), which would aid rather than hinder private entrepreneurship in medicine, is not fully backed by the PP system. The AMA leadership is engaged in a constant battle on its right flank against a strong minority who want to take a "no change at any cost" position. However, whether right or far right, the institution which all factions in the AMA are out to defend is PP.

Deficits in the Quality of Care

One of the essences of private entrepreneurship is independence of action. Thus PP has had little interest in promoting quality control mechanisms other than medical licensing which does much more to limit medical competition than it does to control medical quality. PP likes to limit the scope of hospital medical staff review committees. It certainly doesn't want anyone poking around private offices investigating quality. It has not strongly supported periodic relicensure. In parts of the country, PP has strongly resisted the development of the federally-mandated Professional Standards Review Organizations (see Chapter 6). PP strongly opposed passage of the original law. PP maintains the view that the medical license is a property right. The PP views any attempt to treat the medical license as the privilege it really is as "government interference in the practice of medicine."

Biomedical Research Emphasis of the Medical Education System

All through this book I have referred to the baleful influence of the biomedical research emphasis in the medical education system on the medical education process. In Chapter 10 I showed that biomedical research is not a "natural" component of medical education, at least the extent to which it is carried out in the American medical education system. By indirection it was PP, you will recall, that created the federally-supported biomedical research establishment in the medical schools, by its determined opposition to direct federal aid to medical education in the years immediately following World War II.

The Two-Class System of Medical Care

In a society in which some people are too poor to afford the fees of the PP system while others can afford them, if care is to be provided at all for those who cannot afford private care, it must be provided by some other system. Ergo we have a two-class system: PP and "other." What creates the two-class system then is primarily the payment mechanism. Of course even with social financing and universal financial entitlement to health care, there would still be a two-class system in terms of facilities and manpower supply, and social attitudes of the providers. But without PP the differences would be greatly diminished.

Distortion of the Motivation for Working

To me one of the greatest evils of the PP system is the way it distorts the motivations of physicians to work. Its defenders say that PP ensures good quality (contrary to the evidence of course), that it makes doctors "work hard" and that it cements the doctor-patient relationship. I have been told that without the fee incentive doctors will not get up in the middle of the night, will not work weekends, will reduce the volume of care provided (that might not be so bad), will not do the best job possible, and so on. These arguments are all based on the concept that what the doctor does, he does for money. It is interesting, of course, to hear these kinds of arguments coming from defenders, not critics of the profession.

To me such arguments demean the profession, my profession, as well as fly in the face of facts. There are many salaried physicians who work as hard as they can and do the best job they can. There are many other professions in which people strive to do the best job they can while getting paid on a salary: teaching, engineering, airline piloting, fire-fighting. They do the best job they can because society expects that of them and they expect it of themselves. In the world of business, many hard-working corporate executives are paid by salary. For too many doctors, although certainly not all, PP takes away the human motivation for working and substitutes the monetary one. As we have seen, that situation produces neither good health nor good medical care.

The Road to Change in Fee-for-Service Private Practice

PP is always engaged in guarding its turf, and it regards any federal involvement in anything relating to medical practice as a potential invasion of that turf. In recent years ground has been given, to be sure, but only most grudgingly, after enormous resistance. In fact, so effective has the opposition really been, that despite seeming "losses" over Medicare/Medicaid, various health care planning measures, HMOs, PSROs, and direct federal aid to medical education, PP seems to be in better shape then ever.

The only way to eliminate private entrepreneurial fee-for-service medical practice in this country is to attack it frontally. Indirection will not do. One must be politically realistic, however. PP will not be legislated out of existence overnight. It seems to me that one politically feasible way to do it, in the context of national health insurance, would be a grandfather clause—grandfathering PP *out* rather than *in.* The law would simply provide that no physicians licensed after some certain date subsequent to the enactment of NHI could be paid on a fee-for-service basis by NHI. All physicians presently in practice, and perhaps including those already in training with whom some kind of social contract could be said to exist, could be paid on a fee-for-service basis, if they so chose. However, the die would be cast, and the road would be open to placing the organization of the profession on a social basis, to match the social basis of its principal task, improving the health of the people.

Proposed Solutions to the Problems of the Health Care Delivery System

Major Inputs and the Need for Change

The major inputs to the health care delivery system are financing, facilities, organizational structure, and manpower. For there to be a change in the quantity or quality of the system's output, there must be change(s) in the quantity or quality of one or more of the inputs. Now there are those, usually representatives of organized medicine or their spokesmen, who say that no change is required. AMA representatives and Harry Schwartz are examples of this point of view (see Chapter 3). As I have shown throughout this book, with data, with history, and with quoted statements from persons representing many different viewpoints, the preponderance of opinion in this country outside of the medical profession is that the product is not satisfactory and that change is needed. Two debates, then, rage simultaneously: whether or not change is needed at all, and granting that change is necessary, what kind of change should it be. I will not comment extensively on the first debate. By this time it is obvious where my sympathies lie. About the second debate some comments should be made.

Financing, Facilities, and Organizational Structure

Most of the major proposals for change now on the table concern financing, facilities, and/or organizational structure. Some people stress the need for national health insurance or a national health service, some financing system in any case providing universal financial entitlement to care with no or low financial barriers to care. In this view, the main problem or at least the first problem of the health care delivery system is uneven and unequal access to care. Another position states that the major problem lies with the facilities. There are too many hospitals and not nearly enough ambulatory care services. What we really need, so this argument goes, is to reduce our hospital bed supply, while vastly expanding hospital ambulatory care and health maintenance organization-type services.

A third position holds that the real problem is to be found in the system's organizational structure, or lack thereof. I do not agree with those who hold that we have a "non-system." We have a system all right, with loci of power and centers of control. It is just that they are multiple, the table of organization is extremely complex, and the most powerful effective controllers of the system, the doctors, don't always show up in clearly labelled boxes on a chart. But at any rate, some persons think that the solution lies in creating a neat, clear table of organization with solid lines running between the boxes according to one preference or another. One opinion would turn the whole thing over to the federal government. A second would put primary authority in the hands of the state and local health departments. A third would give it to local voluntary hospital boards of trustees. A fourth, under some kind of national health service, would place in charge new local voluntary agencies and call that arrangement "community control."

Manpower and the Road to Change

Changes in financing, facilities, and organizational structure of some sort are all *necessary* if the output of the health care delivery system is to be changed. However, change in one, two, or even all three of these inputs is not *sufficient* to produce significant change in output. Health services are delivered by people, not by money, buildings, or organizational charts. If the manpower isn't changed, the product won't change that much, even if it is easier for everyone to buy.

What has happened in Great Britain in the thirty years of the National Health Service (NHS) illustrates this point well. The NHS provides universal entitlement to health care with few financial barriers to care. Since the late sixties there has been some movement away from dependence on hospitals as the major facility class to the development of group medical practice centers. The whole organizational structure has changed, twice, since the inauguration of the NHS in 1948, once in that year and then again in 1974. In both structures, the ultimate control is central in a ministry of health, the lines are solid, and the boxes are clear. However, medical practice, what goes on between doctor and patient, what the doctor does with his time, how the doctor views his role, has changed little since 1948. This in fact is not surprising since it happens that despite major changes in financing and organization, medical education, the creator of the doctors, has changed hardly at all in Great Britain in the last thirty years.

Regardless of the financing mechanisms, the facilities, and the organizational structure, if you don't change the people who are doing the job, you haven't done much at all. This is not to say that change in manpower is sufficient by itself either. You could have the most prevention-oriented communication-conscious doctors in the world and if people could not pay for their services, no improvement would occur. However in my view we should probably begin with changing the manpower, or at least we should not fool ourselves into thinking that there will be major changes in health care delivery system outcomes without changes in manpower.

Changes—Health Manpower

Supporters of the view that changes in the quantity and quality of health manpower are necessary if significant changes in outcomes of the health care delivery system are to be achieved take several different tacks. They all recognize the centrality of the physician in the present system, the problems the physician, as he is presently trained and works, creates in the system, and the necessity of doing something to alter the present situation. But after that, the several schools of thought part company. One approach is to let the physician go on working pretty much as he or she does now, and by implication leave medical education alone, while filling the service gaps created by the work patterns of the contemporary physician with other kinds of health workers. This approach would generally let the doctors carry on business-as-usual, giving up as an impossibly difficult task any attempts to change either existing doctors or the medical education system.

A variation on this theme is that doctors, if not all health workers, are bad for you, and never have been nor ever could be good for you. They are best ignored entirely, and you will be much better off if you just take care of yourself. The do-it-yourself school has attracted many adherents in home-building, auto mechanics, and boat maintenance. Why not in health services?

Ignore the Doctor: Change Something, Anything, Else

An interesting view is one which recognizes the centrality of the physician in the health care delivery system and also recognizes that the system has certain, perhaps serious problems, but says that the doctors are doing a great job, and that change should affect anything *but* the physicians. This is generally the approach of the sci/med establishment. For example, listen again to Dr. Robert Berliner, Dean of the Yale School of Medicine:

> The traditional role of the physician is as the provider of medical care, not as the provider of health care. "Aha!" the critics say. "That is exactly the trouble with medicine; it's not interested in keeping people well—only in trying to cure them when they get sick!" However, the fact is that medicine can do relatively little to keep people healthy. As has [been] pointed out, much ill-health derives from economic and social factors far beyond the competence of the physician to remedy. . . .
>
> The appropriate principal role for the physician is, in my opinion, the traditional one: namely, to try to effect the restoration to health of the individual patient. And the appropriate role of medical education is, accordingly, to provide the physician with the background that will maximize his effectiveness in this role.[8]

Or consider the views of Dr. Franz Ingelfinger, the recently retired editor of the sci/med establishment's most prestigious journal, the *New England Journal of Medicine.* He characterized virtually all critical analyses of the United States health care delivery system as "Those Anti-Doctor Books," in an editorial of that title. He suggested to his readers: "Make a synopsis of any one of these anti-doctor books that are being published in such profusion, and you have an outline for nearly any one of them." His "outline," preceding the above statement, is based on his reading of Spencer Klaw's *The Great American Medicine Show.*[9] According to Ingelfinger, Klaw says:

> . . . that medical care is too costly, with inappropriately small returns for money spent, that private insurance is inadequate, with too limited coverage for many, that hospitals are over-utilized and are not motivated to economize, that Medicaid has not relieved either the indignity or the inferiority of care for the poor, that pharmaceutical companies enjoy huge profits by their successful promotion of brand name drugs, and that doctors, while taking advantage of a sellers' market and using an entrepreneurial fee-for-service system to impose excessive charges, practice poor-quality medicine marked by over-prescribing and over-operating, by haste if not incompetence, and by a specialty-oriented focus on the organ rather than the whole person.
>
> So what else is new?[10]

Klaw, of course, was criticizing the whole *system,* but Ingelfinger chose to label it an anti-*doctor* book. Of course, by doing so he serves to confirm the theory of physician dominance. One can then draw the conclusion, although Ingelfinger hardly would, that nothing indeed can be changed without changing the physician. But Ingelfinger doesn't buy that either, as he reveals in a subsequent editorial:

> The physician, of course, should be aware of the multiple influences that bear on health—the economic, marital, political, environmental, and all other factors that determine how a given individual feels. . . . But the doctor's basic responsibility is cure. Yes, CURE. . . . His primary concern, in spite of all the utopian claims to the contrary, is sickness, not overall health.
>
> If the role of the physician here expounded—an exposition sure to evoke protest—were clearly recognized, many current problems would become more manageable. Medical pedagogy, both in and after medical

school, could once again concentrate on scientifically accurate diagnosis and treatment, as could the average physician . . .[11]

Dr. Ingelfinger appears to want it both ways. There are many problems in the health care delivery system, but virtually any critique of any aspect of the system is labelled by him as "anti-*doctor*" (emphasis added). Nevertheless, according to Ingelfinger, doctors and medical education are as they should be now—possibly having been at an ideal place about fifteen years ago. There must be no change in medical education except to go backwards, slightly. Change anything else, he said in his "Anti-Doctor Book" editorial; just leave *us* alone.

Thus we have three variations on the "ignore the doctor" position:

1. Ignore the doctor for he is a lost cause. Train others to meet the needs the doctor cannot meet, and just work around him.
2. Ignore the doctor, and most other health workers. They are harmful to you anyway. Take care of yourself.
3. Ignore the doctor because he is doing a great job, or at least would if he were only left alone. Change anything else you want to, from lifestyle to payment mechanisms. Maybe you will thus alleviate some of the serious problems we admit do exist. But please, leave us alone. We have nothing to do with any of that other stuff anyway.*

It should be obvious by now that I find all of these positions unacceptable. Ignore the doctor and train other health workers? Why then should the taxpayers continue to bear so much of the burden of training the expensive, high-earning private entrepreneurs who are responsible for so much of the high cost of health care? Why then should medical licensure be maintained to protect their monopoly? One answer would be indeed to end medical licensure, as Milton Friedman the University of Chicago economist has proposed for so many years. Ending medical licensure *might* reduce medical dominance. It *might* lower costs through increased competition, or it might in fact raise them since there would be many more private entrepreneurial providers creating demand. After all no less a personage than the Chief Justice of the United States said in the spring of 1977 that one reason for the

*In the principal policy address at the 1977 Annual Meeting of the AAMC, the Alan Gregg Lecture, Dr. D.W. Seldin took precisely this position.

increasing litigiousness of our society is the rapidly increasing number of lawyers. It would *not* produce health-orientation, and a likely result would be a state of chaos.

Ignore the health care delivery system entirely? Many more prestigious authorities than I have dealt most effectively with Professor Ivan Illich, the current popularizer of this harmful view. Ignore the physician, *because he is doing such a great job,* and deal with everything else? I have written this book to expose the fallaciousness of that position. No, indeed it is the physician who must be changed if we are to realize progress in our health care delivery system. Physician change alone is no more sufficient than is change in financing, facilities, or organization alone. But it is certainly necessary, and because of the long lead time required to effect changes in medical education, the process should begin now.

Meeting the Needs of the People: Physicians for the Twenty-first Century

Rational Task Analysis

The set of tasks that must be performed by the health care delivery system is obviously much too large for any one person to carry out. There are in fact several hundred formal job titles and subtitles in the health care field, with responsibilities divided among them. A variety of factors have influenced the way in which the responsibilities have been distributed: historical, political, economic, social. Rationality and logic, however, have played little part in the "divvying up" process. The licensing laws defining the powers and responsibilities of doctors and nurses were for the most part written late in the last century and early in this one. The definitions were based very much on the social role and political power of the medical profession at that time, the social position of women, and the existing state of biomedical knowledge. Times, knowledge, abilities, and social needs have changed a great deal since that day, but the licensing laws have not. What people are actually doing changes too so that educational programs, geared mainly to ensuring passage of licensing laws, may end up either over-training or under-training people in relation to their actual work.

Licensing laws as now written especially for the medical profession, and to a lesser extent for the other licensed health care provider groups, exist very much to meet the needs of the licensed profession, not very much to meet the needs of society. If social needs are to be met, what makes sense is to list all the health care delivery tasks that need to be done and divide them into groups such that one person can reasonably acquire the knowledge and skills needed to carry out each group well. This is called "rational task analysis." Having done this, one can design educational programs to create people who can do the tasks, neither over-training nor under-training them, develop evaluation tools which can measure the effectiveness with which the tasks are carried out, and institute quality control mechanisms to maintain performance at the highest possible level.

Rational task analysis has been undertaken by a number of investigators in recent years, including Dr. Archie Golden and his colleagues at Johns Hopkins[12] and Dr. Robert Kane and his colleagues at the University of Utah. A great deal more has to be done, of course, but it should be understood that as complex a job as it is, it is much easier to do rational task analysis than it is to implement the results of the process.

Goal-Directed Medical School Design

Once one has rationally defined and described a set of tasks for the physician, then one can undertake rational design of a medical school. Dr. Kane and his colleagues put it well in beginning their paper "Toward Defining the End Product of Medical Education":

> Curricula in medical schools across the country have been in a state of constant ferment. In seeking beneficial change, many medical schools have concentrated attention on the sequence of courses. Too often proposals urge a rather arbitrary new structure, such as organ systems or early clinical experience, which represents only a repackaging and renaming of old information. The same lecture or the same ideas may be delivered through a different department or some other individual or perhaps at a different time. Yet changes, to be significant, must not be dictated by fashion, whim, or even desire for improvement; they must be

solidly founded on a clear concept of the desired outcome in terms of the expected behavior of the student after he has successfully completed the medical school curriculum and enters practice.

They conclude by pointing out that:

> One must first define the end product in terms of what [the physician] should be able to do. From this description one can specify levels of competency and hence behavioral objectives. In turn, the means for teaching (or more correctly, learning) these behaviors become the curriculum. Evaluation of the student is based on the degree to which the end product proves effective in practice. It is thus safe to say that this type of curricular building calls for beginning at the end.[13]

Following this sound advice, before proposing reform measures for medical education, one must describe the appropriate role for the physician. To me, the only way to do this is in terms of the needs of the people.

A Health-Oriented Health Care Delivery System

In Chapter 2, I discussed the evidence that demonstrates the importance of preventive measures, particularly community ones, in improving population health levels over time. I also showed that many of our current major killer and non killer diseases could be controlled, if not eliminated, by using known, available preventive measures, even when the disease cause is unknown or uncertain. We presently have a disease-oriented "health care" delivery system which generally waits until disease, illness, or injury strikes and then attempts to cure it. However, if health is our goal, and let someone say it is not, then we must become health-oriented so that the "health care" delivery system can be replaced with the health care delivery system.

The most important task of a health care delivery system is health promotion, teaching, and helping people to live healthy lives in general. Health promotion does not include disease-specific preventive measures. It does comprise proper nutrition, adequate rest, exercise, healthful working environments, environmental pollution control, and the like. The second most important task of a health care delivery system is disease-specific prevention: immunization, cigarette smoking and alcoholic beverage control,

control of disease-specific environmental and industrial toxins, and case-finding and contact investigation. Early detection of existing but clinically unapparent disease, when early detection can prevent or delay death or complications, can be considered prevention as well. The third most important task is treating disease, illness, and injury in individuals. Although apparently of little importance to population health levels, treatment is of vital importance to the sick person. It must be done, must be done well, and at a cost that is affordable to the individual and the society.

Role, Structure, and Function of a True Health Care Delivery System

The Political Process

It is not my intention here to lay out a blueprint for a health care delivery system of the future. That could well be utopian, and certainly would be beyond the scope of this book. I am simply going to state some general principles. In order to deal with many of the current health problems, in order to implement many health promotive and disease preventive measures, the political process will have to be involved. One cannot otherwise deal with problems of food additives, pesticide exposure, cigarette smoking, alcoholic beverage consumption, industrial toxins, and so on. There will certainly be resistance to change, and some affected economic and social interests will howl in pain if their *modae vivendae* are affected, even if the health benefits of change are clearly demonstrated. But of course neither the involvement of the political process in health and vice versa, nor the resistance to change are anything new.[14]

Ibsen's *An Enemy of the People,* written in the late nineteenth century, is a marvelous dramatization of the conflict between the public's health and commercial interests. In the 1850s, a London doctor named John Snow clearly demonstrated that a cholera outbreak was related to water supplied by a private company drawn from the Thames below the London sewage discharge point. Only the government was able to force the company to move its pipe. In the late nineteenth century, private doctors strongly resisted a law requiring them to report cases of tuberculosis, an important element in the control of that particular disease. They called it "government interference in the practice of medicine." (Sound familiar?) The political process eventually brought about compliance. It is the political process which has been responsible for such measures as pure water supply and sanitary sewage disposal, the control of food purity, elimination of child labor, the shortening of the work day, industrial safety and industrial pollution controls to the extent they exist, and so on.

The health care delivery system does not institute such measures. But if it is to be concerned with *health,* neither can it separate itself from the political process that does handle these measures. It cannot attempt to insulate itself from the real world and say, as so many leaders of both the medical education establishment and the private practice sector do: "Oh that's *life style.* We don't have anything to do with *that.* And anyway, it's really uncontrollable. That is the business of the politicians and personal choice. Leave us alone to treat and cure." That is *disease* orientation, not *health* orientation.[15]

Health orientation recognizes the importance of the political process to health. It recognizes that in a democracy, decisions are not made by fiat but as a result of the free interchange of ideas and the balancing of all affected interests. It recognizes that the health care delivery system is the advocate of health, and that it must provide the scientific knowledge and understanding upon which health advances can be made. Under health orientation, the health care delivery system clearly recognizes its responsibility to engage in public debate, to attempt to educate and influence both the public and its government.

In a position paper on "Environmental Quality and Human Health," the American Medical Association itself has said the following:

> The medical profession must develop a broader base of concern to permit a preventive medical approach that will include environmental factors in control of disease. *Traditionally, physicians have been disease-oriented with emphasis on the treatment of illness.* [My italics.] Attention must also be directed to the health consequences of environmental changes so that prevention and protection aspects are not neglected. To continue to expend money and professional effort merely to treat clinical conditions

without concern for their environmental etiology would not solve the basic problems.

In the same paper, under "The Role of Medicine," the AMA said:

> The AMA suggests that all levels of legislative bodies and government agencies should utilize the unique capabilities of members of the medical profession to lend an essential dimension—consideration of human health—in the deliverations and decisions on environmental quality and protection.[16]

Health orientation does not keep the medical professions out of political debates on *health* matters. At present, the profession comes roaring into the political arena primarily when matters of professional economic self-interest are being decided. Despite their frequent plaints and complaints about the "politicization of health," and "government interference in the practice of medicine," over the decades both the AMA and AAMC have shown no reluctance to enter the political arena to get government assistance when they thought they needed it, whether it be for licensing laws or government financial aid to medical education. If only the two associations acted as decisively in supporting governmental regulation of environmental hazards.

The fact of the matter is that the only separation of medicine and politics is an artificial one. It was Rudolf Virchow, the nineteenth century founder of the science of pathology, who said, "Medicine is a social science, and politics is nothing else but medicine on a large scale."[17] Overblown? Perhaps. But in discussing the relationship between health and unsanitary living conditions in Upper Silesia, Virchow was certainly right when he said:

> A new time has come. Radical changes have taken place in the thinking of people. Medicine cannot stand aside. It too must act to bring about much needed reforms in its field.[18]

In our own era, Harvard's Dr. David Rutstein, and colleagues said:

> [I]n every kind of unnecessary disease, disability, and untimely death, the physician has the initial and also some continuing responsibility. He is the only one competent to provide the leadership and the professional guidance to the politician, the administrator, industry, the public, and to

the patient himself. They may not, of course, take the physicians' advice, but that does not relieve him of the responsibility for the input of the scientific facts and the professional knowledge that are directly relevant to the improvement of human health and to the prevention of community decisions that may result in unnecessary disease, disability, or untimely death.[19]

Participation in the political process on behalf of health is one of the most important roles for a health-oriented health care delivery system. That system must be structured so that it can carry out that role most effectively.

Organizational Structure

Policy setting and the establishment of standards should be done centrally. Administration of day-to-day operations should be decentralized to the greatest extent possible. Health services should be regionalized under a system of rational planning. Health services should be distributed on the basis of demonstrated need for care. Complex specialty and referral services should be geographically situated in such a way that maximum economical use is made of them, at the same time that availability is optimized. Responsibility for program planning and evaluation, one of the most important functions of the organizational structure, should be shared between the local, state, and federal levels to ensure as high a degree of local autonomy as possible, within a goal-oriented national planning system.

Quality Assessment and Control

Quality control for services should be carried out locally, but should be monitored centrally to ensure that standards are being met. Process and outcome measures should be used for the most part, with a deemphasis on the reliance on structural standards. Peer review, monitored by outside authorities, should form the basis of the case-specific quality assessment system. The assessment systems for both licensure and relicensure should be converted from memory-basing to competency-basing. The judgment of the efficacy of drugs and procedures should be the responsibility of the quality control system.

Financing and Payment Mechanisms

The balance between expenditures for treatment and expenditures for prevention, now tilted heavily towards the former, must be altered. Our ability to carry out cost-benefit analyses must be greatly improved. There must be universal entitlement to treatment services, with low or no financial barriers to care. The reimbursement system should be altered so as to encourage preventive health care and early diagnosis and treatment in ambulatory settings, discourage hospitalization, and discourage piecework.

Facilities

The hospital, the ultimate physical structure of a disease-oriented system, must be deemphasized. Hospital beds must be closed and/or converted to other uses. The major facility in a health-oriented system would be a health center responsible for the broad range of personal and community preventive measures and health promotion for its community, for health-related political involvement, and for ambulatory treatment services for the sick. This idea is hardly new. Herman Biggs, M.D., a former New York State and New York City Health Commissioner put it into legislative language in New York State in 1920.[20] A few facilities of this type, minus perhaps the overt political function, presently exist in Japan and Sweden. In a health-oriented system, treatment services would be provided by multidisciplinary group practices. Thus the present contradiction between individual medical practice and the social nature of the modern approaches to health maintenance and the control and treatment of many diseases would be resolved.

Health Manpower

It is obvious that a health-oriented health care delivery system requires health-oriented manpower at all levels. Changes in the training and functioning of many categories of health personnel are required. However, in this book, I am concerned with physicians, and so in dealing with health manpower questions, I must limit my remarks. Of course changes in the role, functioning and education of physicians of the type I am recommending have many important and serious implications for the role, functioning, and education of most other health care providers. Space and time require me, however, for the most part to ask the reader to draw his or her own conclusions about those implications from what I have to say about physicians.

Physicians in a Health-Oriented Health Care Delivery System

Leadership

The principal responsibility of the physician in the health-oriented health care delivery system is to provide its leadership. (This of course assumes that physicians will be trained for that function, which they patently are not now. The next and last chapter of this book is concerned with that reformed training.) The system, like any system, will need leadership. The social nature of the health task requires a team to carry it out. History has shown that leaderless teams or those with rotating coaches don't function very well. Perhaps in the future they will be able to function well when people have a different psychology, but for the present era, leaders are necessary. Why then the physicians?

The basis of health service is biomedical science. It is the physician whose education and training are most firmly based in biomedical science. It is presently taught in the wrong way: memorization of "facts" instead of the scientific, problem-solving method; biomedical "knowledge" for its own sake instead of clinical relevance. But training can be changed. Emphasis can be changed so that they are in proper proportion to social needs. The scientist-leader will be necessary. If it is not to be the physician, then a new species will have to be created, one whose training encompasses a great deal of science. To discard what is good in physician training just to get rid of the bad would be of course a prime example of throwing out the baby with the bathwater.

Now there are those among both the strongest critics of medicine and medical education as they are now conducted and their strongest defenders who would agree that in fact nothing should be done about either the doctor or medical education. The former give up physician reform as an impossible task and would state that under health orientation indeed a new leadership profession should be created. The latter (such as Ingelfinger and Berliner) state that everything is fine in medicine and no changes should be made. They are all for health, or so they say, but they ask that someone else do it.

If we were to move to health orientation while leaving medical education and the present medical role alone, however, the following events would have to take place:

1. The physicians would have to give up their dominant position in the health care delivery system. Since that dominance is created in significant measure by the medical license, sooner or later they would be forced to give it up or at least see it markedly modified.
2. The physicians would have to give up their high incomes since they would be limiting themselves to a task of tertiary importance, treatment.
3. Since they would be limiting themselves to treatment, they eventually have to give up their heavy demand on the public purse for the support of:
   a. The training of practitioners.
   b. Researchers who want to do what they want to do when they want to do it.
4. Physicians would have to be prepared to see leadership powers transferred to a new profession concentrating on health promotion and disease prevention, with consequent public financial support for its training.
5. The physician would be confined to the role of clinical technician, within the broad spectrum of health services personnel. "You mean to tell me that you *only* treat?" one might say. "Don't you *know* that it's prevention that's the key?"

Clinical Work

In a health-oriented health care delivery system, physicians would be divested of most responsibility for providing primary care treatment services. Physicians are simply over-trained for that kind of work, and regardless of what medical school curriculum one would envision, it is simply not necessary to spend all the years in training that a physician does in order to do primary care. There are a number of studies now which have demonstrated that in primary care, nurse practitioners and physicians' assistants when appropriately trained can do the job as well or better than physicians.[21] The director of one of the first nurse practitioner programs in the country, operated in combination with the largest family medicine residency in the country, has told me that he sees no difference between what the nurses and the residents are doing in clinical primary care. The role of the physician in primary care, remembering that we are considering the multi-disciplinary group practice model only, will be to lead, supervise, consult, educate, make more complicated clinical decisions, evaluate, plan, and so on. To do this, he or she will have to have some direct training and experience in primary care practice, but will not have to do it every day.

There will be technical specialist physicians to take referrals from the primary care level, and work at the secondary and tertiary care levels. They will be specialists, just as there are specialists now, but there will be some important differences. They too will work in multi-disciplinary group practices, whether health-center or hospital-based. They will not be an elite guard. Their distribution among the specialties and geographically will be controlled by national planning. (This does not have to be done in a terribly coercive way. Doctors can be told where they may *not* go, not where they *must* go. Applicants for residency training can be told what specialties are open, not which one they *must* choose.) But most important, their training will be health-oriented because they will be working in a health-oriented system. In medical school, they will study the processes of prevention and health-promotion as a base for their future clinical work just as medical students now study basic medical science. Basic medical science will continue to be important but it will include health as well as disease, and of course it will be taught differently.

Physicians in the Twenty-first Century

Physicians in the twenty-first century will be problem-solvers, not fact-memorizers. In this regard, they will have learned that the computer is a liberating force, not a constricting influence. They will be health-oriented, not disease-oriented. They will lead the health care delivery system for reasons of social good rather than personal gain. They will understand the relationship between politics and health and will be able to use the political system to promote health. Some will be clinical specialists, others team leaders, still others program administrators. They will know how to communicate with their colleagues as well as with their patients. They will have to spend time in specialty training after basic medical education to be able to fulfill their various roles, just as physicians do now. But that basic medical education will be very different from what we have now, as we shall see in the next and final chapter.

13

Health-Oriented Physician Education

The practice of medicine in its broadest sense includes the whole relationship of the physician with his [or her] patient. It is an art, based to an increasing extent on the medical sciences, but comprising much that still remains outside the realm of any science. The art of medicine and the science of medicine are not antagonistic but supplementary to each other. There is no more contradiction between the science of aeronautics and the art of flying. Good practice presupposes an understanding of the sciences which contribute to the structure of modern medicine, but it is obvious that sound professional training should include a much broader equipment.

The most common criticism made at present by older practitioners is that young graduates have been taught a great deal about the mechanisms of disease, but very little about the practice of medicine—or, to put it more bluntly, they are too 'scientific' and do not know how to take care of patients.

—Francis W. Peabody, M.D.
1927

Much of the public dissatisfaction with health and medical care is due to the premature and inappropriate mobilization of an expensive technology on behalf of ordinary problems. Traditional medical education contributes to the mismatch by producing a physician who substitutes technocracy for science. This is the result of an educational process which is a synthesis of specialties. This problem will not be resolved by creating additional specialists for newly fabricated specialties. What is proposed is a restructuring of basic medical education toward the end of recreating the physician as the core and substance of the health care system.

—*Morton Creditor, M.D.*
1976

The basis of the Health-Oriented Physician Education (HOPE) system is an ideology that states that the primary purpose of a health care delivery system is to protect and improve the health of the people it serves. The concerns of the system itself and of its workers, while important, are secondary to the interests of the people for health. HOPE is focussed on a health-oriented health care delivery system.

The HOPE system is neither a particular curriculum pattern, nor a particular educational administrative structure, nor a particular student admissions policy, nor an ideal set of institutions in particular places in which instruction is to be carried out. Since Flexner, many proposals for medical education reform, or "re-form," have been couched in those terms. They have either not been implemented or have meant little in terms of the outcome of the medical education process. A favorite game in medical schools has been curriculum rearrangement, without change in the basic ideology of medical education. However, as Robert S. Harnack has said: "Changing curriculum in the medical school is like rearranging the lifeboats on the *Titanic.*"[1] In contrast, the HOPE system is a set of educational and pedagogical principles and approaches to learning, work, and life designed to produce a health-oriented physician.

In Sections I and II of this book I showed that presently in our country we do not really have a *health* care delivery system, even though, bowing to convention, I do use the term to describe that industry which applies biomedical knowledge to the care and treatment of human ills. Rather, we have a disease care delivery system. This disease care delivery system is served by a Disease-Oriented Physician Education system, DOPE, described in Section III and Chapter 12. It is difficult to find the true ideology of DOPE stated succinctly anywhere, but the writings of people like Doctors Berliner and Ingelfinger state clearly that its focus is disease and that health, while important, is someone else's, anyone else's, responsibility. Furthermore, the actions of the major professional organizations (the American Medical Association and the Association of American Medical Colleges and a powerful organization I have discussed little in this book, the American Hospital Association), in order to protect the turf and status of the "health" care providers, indicate that they view as an important function of the disease care delivery system the protection and fostering of the interests of those who work in it, particularly those at the higher levels.

The ideology of the disease care delivery system completely ignores the historical fact of the primacy of prevention in improving the health of the people. This historical fact is, of course, a cornerstone of the ideology of HOPE. HOPE is designed to provide physicians for a health-oriented health care delivery system. DOPE provides physicians for, and is a major factor in perpetuating, the disease care delivery system we now have. HOPE recognizes the physicians' fundamental responsibility for the health of the people, and states that the profession stands ready to deal with that responsibility in all of its ramifications: political, economic, and social, as well as scientific and medical.

HOPE and the Role of the Physician

If we are to have a true health care delivery system, HOPE is necessary whether or not physicians relinquish their primary care role. (In the previous chapter, I predicted that they would eventually relinquish that role because it is becoming apparent that high quality primary care can be provided by persons who have quite a bit less training than do physicians.) Flexner established the principle that if medicine is to be scientific, all physicians, regardless of specialty and regardless of research interests or lack thereof, must have a solid educational grounding in biomedical science and the scientific method. Likewise, if we are to have a true *health* care delivery system, all physicians must be health-oriented and must have a solid educational grounding in the science of health promotion and disease prevention.

Both the leadership group and the specialist individual clinicians would be health-oriented. Just as it is silly to say of a surgeon, "Why does he have to know science, he just cuts," so it is silly to say of any physician, "why does he have to know prevention, he just treats." Primary care physicians, if they remain, certainly must be health-oriented. For primary care providers, physician or nonphysician alike, health-oriented education is vital because of the importance of personal preventive services in primary care. If physicians refuse the leadership role in the health-care delivery system I described for them in the last chapter, regardless of whether or not they relinquish the primary care role, they will eventually become nothing more than disease-oriented clinical technicians. History will roll over the profession. Thus continuing DOPE is nothing more than a historical dead end.

The Major Components of HOPE

HOPE has five major components, upon which I shall elaborate in some detail below. First, there is a philosophy: the basis of medical practice which serves the interests of the people for constantly and consistently improving their health is prevention-orientation. Second, there is the active practice of healthy living in the educational process. If the leaders and practitioners of the health care delivery system do not lead healthy lives, how can they possibly influence and teach others to do so? Third, there is an educational process: problem-based learning, the active use of the scientific method. To properly teach people who can correctly apply the scientific method in their every day work, we must teach them to use the scientific method from the very beginning of their education.

Fourth, HOPE has a technique: computer-assistance. HOPE recognizes that in this era of rapidly expanding biomedical understanding, it is only the computer which can free the physician from the tyranny of memory so that he or she can actively and accurately apply the scientific method. Fifth, HOPE has a pedagogy, a profession of teaching. Historically and presently, almost all teachers of physicians have been educational amateurs. There is no profession of medical educator. Medical school teaching is not itself taught. Thus the good teacher and there are some, is more often than not the happy accident of history, personality, and personal inclination. HOPE approaches the subject quite differently.

In describing the HOPE system, I purposely do not go into details of curriculum design, admissions policy, faculty organization, and so forth. On the one hand, I believe that getting that specific would be Utopian. On the other hand, I believe that if the principles of HOPE are adopted there are a variety of specific ways in which they could be implemented, as long as the goals and objectives of health-orientation are kept in mind. Once the ideology is adopted, the logical variations on the theme in practice will become self-evident.

Prevention-Orientation: What It Is

Prevention-oriented medical education has three principal features. First of all, unlike the present particular-to-the-general approach, under prevention-orientation medical education begins with the general and moves toward the particular. Thus instead of beginning with cells and molecular processes, students would begin with society. They would study epidemiology, the science of the distribution of health and disease in populations and the factors affecting them. They would study medical history, and economics, sociology, and political science as they apply to health, disease, and medicine. To create clinical relevance, these subjects would be taught using real cases of both individual patients and populations. All learning would of course be problem-based (see below). Thus before proceeding to study individuals and their many parts and sub-parts, medical students would understand human ecology, that is the science of the relationship between man and his environment, since the latter is the primary (although not the only) determinant of health.

Second, the entire curriculum would be permeated with the concepts of prevention. The introductory curriculum segment on human ecology would not simply be an enlarged course in "Preventive Medicine," still standing apart from the rest of the curriculum as so many of the (small) courses in preventive medicine do now. Rather, as students worked their way through the biomedical, and then the clinical sciences, using always the problem-solving process, prevention would continue to be stressed: How could the family of this child with a serious genetic defect have been counselled before conception and/or the birth of the child? How could this particular case of emphysema in a heavy cigarette smoker have been prevented? How could this premature death from coronary artery disease been dealt with? How could hypertension in a patient who now has a crippling stroke been detected and controlled earlier? How would better access to treatment prevent this patient's appendix from rupturing? And so on.

In each of the examples given above there is obviously what is called "basic science," the biochemistry, physiology, genetics, and pathology of a particular disease process. There is also clinical science: diagnosis and therapeutics. There is also a preventive aspect of each, often involving history, politics, economics, and sociology. Presently, the "basic" and "clinical" sciences, and prevention if taught at all, are compartmentalized and separated. In real life, however, they form a continuum with the border areas between them being quite gray. Prevention-orientation recognizes, illuminates, and makes rational the continuum. In fact, prevention-orientation makes "basic" science real and understandable because it teaches "basic" science in the context of clinical, that is, treatment and preventive, medicine.

As I pointed out in Chapter 2, a great deal is known about community preventive measures which could greatly improve the health of the population: control of cigarette smoking and alcoholic beverage consumption, reduction in environmental carcinogens, improved industrial hygiene, proper nutrition, and so on. Available too are known personal preventive measures which can be applied in a systematic way. For example, Dr. Lester Breslow Dean of the School of Public Health, University of California at Los Angeles, and Professor Anne R. Somers of the New Jersey College of Medicine have described a "Lifetime Health-Monitoring Program" (LHMP) which can be applied by individual clinicians to individual patients.[2] The LHMP organizes known individual preventive and early-detection measures by age group and applies them in a coordinated fashion only rarely undertaken at the present time. In prevention-orientation, clinical teaching of medical students would feature the LHMP or its equivalent as a framework to be modified as new knowledge accumulates.

The third feature of prevention-orientation is a stress on the importance of doctor-patient communication. Studies cited in earlier chapters indicate that communication difficulties, usually phrased as "my doctor won't talk to me," rank with high cost as the two principal concerns people have with the health care delivery system. Prevention-orientation recognizes communicative ability, with individual patients, colleagues, the general public, and the political area, as one of the most important skills a physician can have. Only the Medical Mystique says: "Communication skills are unimportant. I'm a *doctor;* therefore you must listen, and believe."

Under prevention-orientation, medical students will be consciously taught how to communicate effectively with individual patients. This is necessary both for good therapeutics (understanding treatment regimens and so forth), and for good personal preventive medicine. Persuading individuals to stop smoking cigarettes on a one-to-one basis is probably not an effective way to control cigarette smoking in the population, any more than getting people to boil their drinking water is an effective way to deal with polluted water supply. However, each individual who does stop smoking is a person helped to better health, just as is each person who has a broken leg set properly.

For physicians to be useful members of health care teams, they must be consciously trained in effectively communicating with their colleagues, physician and non-physician alike. Sensitivity training, important for all levels of communication, is especially important here. Those physicians who engage in community preventive programs must also be trained in communicating with the public and with the political process. Community prevention will not advance by itself. The process must be led. Physicians can do it, if properly prepared. If they don't, others eventually will.

The Practice of Healthy Living

If a healthy population is the goal of HOPE, then the teachers and practitioners of medicine ought to live healthy lives themselves. "Do as I say, not as I do" really has no place in HOPE. The process of furthering the health of the population ought to begin with the example set by the leaders of the health care delivery system. It would be a good idea for a gymnasium to be at the center of every medical school, so that it could be used by faculty, staff, and students on a regular basis. Cigarette smoking, excessive consumption of alcoholic beverages, and abuse of drugs ought to be discouraged. Those habits should not be prohibited, but it should be made clear to faculty, staff, and students that persons with problems of that sort really should deal with them. Appropriate prevention and treatment programs should be provided. Obesity should be recognized as a problem as well. Proper nutrition in all respects would be encouraged by educational programs and by the institution's own food service.

A full range of psychological counselling services would be available to all as well. Sensitivity training would be an important part of the ongoing experience for faculty, staff, and students. Furthermore, provisions would be made to deal with the internal anxieties created in most people who work with disease: "will I get such and such? do I have it? that's a pretty awful condition." Few medical schools do this now although, in my view, a great deal of the anger expressed by some physicians is nothing more than the physician's response to his or her own anxiety which he does not know how to deal with in any other way. The health care delivery system can hardly expect to produce a healthy population if its own personnel are not healthy themselves.

Problem-Based Learning

Problem-based learning is the application of the scientific method to the educational process. As I have shown, we currently teach "fact" acquisition and memorization. However, as Flexner so correctly and eloquently pointed out, the principal task of the physician is the ability to solve problems, that is to apply the scientific method. As he said:

> The main intellectual tool of the investigator is the working hypothesis . . . Upon this he acts, and the practical outcome of his procedure refutes, confirms, or modifies his theory . . . This is essentially the technique of research: wherein is it irrelevant to bedside practice? (Appendix I.1.)

There is one medical school in North America which has developed problem-based learning in medical education to a high degree, the McMaster University School of Medicine in Hamilton, Ontario, Canada. I don't think that the McMaster approach to problem-based learning represents perfection itself, and I don't believe that any McMaster faculty would claim that it does. Nor has the program, only in operation since the late-sixties, a short time in medical education, been completely evaluated. Nevertheless, in most respects, the McMaster Program represents "state-of-the-art" in problem-based learning for medical education. Thus I will let McMaster faculty describe the program's principles for us.

Drs. Victor Neufeld and Howard S. Barrows of McMaster listed the "general goals of the program, stated in terms of *outcomes for the student*" (emphasis added) in a paper published in the *Journal of Medical Education* in 1974:

> 1. To identify and define health problems and to search for information in order to resolve or manage these problems;
> 2. Given a health problem, to examine the underlying physical or behavioral mechanisms; (A spectrum of phenomena might be included, from molecular events to those involving the patient's family and community.)

3. To recognize, maintain, and develop personal characteristics and attitudes required for professional life;
4. To develop the clinical skills and to learn the methods required to define and manage the health problems of patients, including their physical, emotional, and social aspects;
5. To become a self-directed learner, recognizing personal educational needs, selecting appropriate learning resources, and evaluating progress;
6. To be able to assess critically professional activity related to patient care, health care delivery, and medical research;
7. To be able to function as a productive member of a small group which is engaged in learning, research, or health care; and
8. To be aware of and be able to work in a variety of health care settings.[3]

In the same paper, they go on to describe "biomedical problem-solving," that is the problem-solving technique applied specifically to medical education:

Given a description of a patient or other clinical situation, the tutorial group or individual student should carry out the following sequence of activities: a series of questions, which may be stated in lay terms, will be listed as they arise from the biomedical problem; these questions will be translated into issues in structure, function, behavior, and response to stimuli; acting singly or in a group, students will identify and study in depth educational resources which provide information relevant to issues previously identified; the students will then synthesize this information into a cogent explanation of the clinical situation, either during a group tutorial session or individually; the development of additional questions, suggestions, and hypotheses for further steps in the evaluation and/or management of the clinical situation follows logically from this synthesis, and emphasizes the fact that biomedical problems can be pursued in a number of directions and tend to be open-ended; the tutorial group will complete the process by evaluating individual and group performances, the biomedical problem itself, and the related learning resources.

The assumption of sequential learning [the conventional method of medical education] is challenged by this approach. Sequences are based on arbitrary decisions which are frequently unrelated to real life situations. It is commonly assumed that normal structure and function should be learned prior to the abnormal, and yet only by comparing the abnormal with the normal can the range of normal become clear to the student.

The sequence myth includes the idea that basic science must be learned prior to clinical science. In the McMaster program, basic science and clinical science are interwoven. The central focus is on the series of biomedical problems. When tackling a clinical problem, the student asks questions about basic mechanisms, both physical and behavioral. Over time, the student spirals through the same content area several times in the program, each time at a more sophisticated or broadly applied level.

Also challenged is the assumption that information is required before problem-solving can begin. In general, we tend to forget the fact that students bring a wide variety of expertise to the program; that, to some extent, they can think logically (based on many years of problem-solving experiences in their personal lives and possibly in their schooling); and that, at the very least, they possess an intelligent 'lay public' baseline of information. Thus, with the recognition of an appropriate level of activity, problem-based learning can start at the beginning of the program.

Is problem-solving a legitimate goal in itself, or is it a vehicle to 'get at the content'? The acquiring of problem-solving approach is a stated goal of the school. It is useless to have a stockpile of information without a method of handling it. On the other hand, given a good approach to problem-solving, students will be able to define the information they require to handle encountered problems, not only during their medical school experience but also in medical practice. . . . Rather than knowledge acquisition per se, it is the use of information in the solution of problems that is encouraged.

When problems are used effectively . . . not only are the 'process goals' reinforced but also specific 'content goals' are tackled. The content focus is determined in the selection of the problem and in the specific issues defined while discussing it.

Problem-based learning includes more than simply learning around clinical problems. It represents a fundamental intellectual process which can be applied to physiologic problems in a research laboratory, to a problem of family dysfunction, or to problems of health care in the community.[4]

Key to problem-based learning are the "small group tutorial" and the proper preparation of "learning resources." Students do not tackle problems on their own but in groups, with a faculty tutor. Tasks are divided among the students; responsibilities are shared. The group becomes involved with the learning of each of its individual members. Thus not only is problem-solving taught, but group process, so important to a socially-oriented health care delivery system, is taught as well. The function of the faculty tutor is not to lecture or answer "fact" questions, but to guide the student group in solving the assigned problem, facilitating that process to the greatest degree possible.

The preparation of the "learning resources" is also enormously important. Students are not simply thrown out into the world and told to "go solve the problem." Textbooks are used. There are prepared sets of reprints and articles. There is a great deal of audio and audio-visual material available in the library for student use. The computer is used extensively as a teaching tool. There are "simulated patients" available, actors, usually amateur, who are trained, fairly easily it happens, to reproduce the history, symptoms, and sometimes even the signs*, of a patient with a particular problem. There are faculty experts in various content areas who are available to the students as "resource people," again not so much as "question-answerers" and "knowledge givers" as expert guides to problem solving in specialized areas. Finally, there are sets of cards, called Portable Patient Problem Packs (P_4), containing the elements of real patient cases arranged sequentially, which force the student to justify choices made while working through the history, physical, and laboratory examination of the patient, to assist in the development of clinical assessment skills. A tremendous amount of faculty time and effort must go into developing the learning resources if the problem-based learning system is to be a success.

Dr. Barrows and his associate Robyn Tamblyn have this to say to students about the power of problem-based learning:

> Problem-based learning allows you to identify what knowledge needs to be learned, how it is to be learned, and to what depth. It allows you to synthesize information from a variety of fields and disciplines to gain an understanding of a patient, a patient problem or health problems. It allows for tailor-made instruction adapted to your own needs, background, career goals and style of learning.
>
> Information learned in this manner is better remembered and more readily applied to new problems than information gained from more traditional forms of discipline-oriented teaching.[5]

*A symptom is something reported by a patient: "I have pain in my chest." A sign is something found on physical examination: a doctor detects a reduction in the loudness of sounds made by breathing when he listens with a stethoscope over the painful chest area to the sounds of respiration.

Health-orientation requires the ability to think clearly and use the scientific method in all spheres of medicine, from genetic research to securing legislation for community prevention programs. Problem-based learning is the key.

Computer Assistance

Computer assistance will liberate the physician from the tyranny of memory. Computer assistance will free the physician from the necessity to concentrate on recall, which computers do much better than we do any way, so that he or she can lead, plan, integrate, solve problems, teach, learn, communicate, and coordinate. Computer assistance (see Dr. Weed's statement, Chapter 11) will allow us to have a built-in, ongoing quality measurement system with immediately available feedback loops for quality control and improvement.

In a true *health* care delivery system, then, the computer will have three principal functions. First, it will store and retrieve medical records, in the problem-oriented mode, of course. Second, it will store and keep available for immediate use current and continually updated biomedical knowledge about the broad range of the more common diseases. Third, it will provide the basis for a rational quality control system. In the HOPE system, of course, medical students will be taught how to use the computer in these three functions, and it will also be used directly as a teaching tool in patient and system simulations.

Dr. Weed has presented the basic rationale for computer assistance. He has also shown how computer assistance is integrally linked with problem-based learning. He states two premises concerning "The Resources and Capital Investment of a Medical School," one old and one new:

Old Premise: Faculty, research facilities, specialized extensive clinical facilities, and teaching facilities are the principal resources of a medical school.

New Premise: The principal resource of a medical school is the student's natural capacity to learn on his own and solve problems on his own in an environment that allows and encourages him to do so, and provides essential feedback.

. . . although not always stated explicitly, it is an underlying premise of modern medical schools that they require a huge capital investment, with extensive research laboratories, large numbers of specialized faculty, and multimillion dollar budgets. This, for the most part, grows out of the old premise. When one focuses on knowledge to the exclusion of other things, one is forced to overemphasize educational facilities that produce new knowledge and encourage attempts to transmit memorized knowledge. It is of course appropriate that we have research institutes for the accumulation of new medical information, but if they are properly organized, and if students learn a significant core of behavior, the cost of medical research need not be charged to medical education. . . .

The new premise should be that the greatest resource of the medical school is the student's capacity to solve problems on his own, using every tool, new and old, available to him. The function of the school should be to emphasize and develop that capacity, so that instead of breeding people who need more and more intellectual diaper-changing and postgraduate education, we have individuals with resourceful, independent minds who will naturally turn to books and all other sources of information and skills that abound in our society, independent of the formal development and expenses of a medical school and its faculty.[6]

The McMaster and Weed systems, since they are based on the same philosophy, would seem ideally suited for merger.

The Pedagogy of HOPE

Pedagogy means "the profession or science of teaching."[7] In the HOPE system, such a teaching profession would be created for medicine. As I have pointed out before, medical students are presently taught by people who are, by and large, amateur teachers. Furthermore, the average medical school teacher spends less than one-fifth of his or her time teaching medical students (see in Chapter 11, "The Costs of Medical Education"). Disease orientation and a stress on "fact" acquisition actually do not really require professional teachers. They require, for the most part, only people who are good at telling students what they, the teachers, "know," and then asking the students to remember it.

The current approach is not useful in the HOPE system. Besides being prevention-oriented, HOPE system teachers must be expert in the problem-based learning approach, as well as in the use of the computer in its various applications to medicine. In terms of research, the professional medical educator will study teaching, learning, and knowledge acquisition and transmittal.

It is unclear at this time on what basis the profession of medical educator might be established. It might become a postgraduate field of its own leading to a separate doctorate, the Doctor of Medical Education, or perhaps a Master's degree that physicians can take after earning a doctorate in medicine, much as physicians now earn Masters of Public Health after the M.D. On the other hand, the education for medical school teaching might become part of residency training programs in certain specialties, in centers concentrating on developing academic staff. Or there might be short-term certificate programs and in-service, continuing education programs. Or there may be some combination of two or more of these approaches. Whatever the pathway(s), it (they) must be established if medical education itself is to become an enterprise consciously planned in relation to societal needs. To do that, we cannot continue to have a system which relies on untrained teachers who teach because "it's part of the job," and whose only guide in their work usually is how *they* were taught when *they* were in medical school.

In addition to its educational advantages, the development of a profession of medical educator should reduce the cost of medical education through a more economical use of faculty resources for teaching: one would not expect full-time professional medical educators to spend only 18 percent of their time teaching medical students! The total number of medical faculty probably could be reduced, thus saving money.

Now this is not to say that all part-time or occasional teachers in medical schools would be replaced. Hardly. That would be foolish both educationally and economically. As costly as medical education is, a great deal of teaching, particularly clinical teaching, is done by volunteer faculty, and house staff. It would be very costly to replace them entirely with full-time staff. Also, HOPE is intended to provide more clinical relevance to medical education, not less. For clinical relevance, the active participation of practicing clinicians is needed. However, with professional medical educators on hand, the work of the volunteers, presently largely un-supervised and uninstructed, and of widely varying quality, could be brought under much better direction. The volunteer faculty could be made into effective teachers, and everyone would benefit. The same line of reasoning would in fact apply to the work of any part-time teacher, whether laboratory researcher or paid full-time clinical staff member.

The creation of the profession of full-time medical educator will succeed, of course, only if certain conditions are met:

1. The new profession, however created and certified, must be recognized as being in charge of medical education.
2. The pay and benefits must be comparable with those for other full-time medical school faculty members, whether they be in research or clinical work.
3. Opportunities for advancement and career development must be present, and one must be judged for advancement on one's abilities and work *as a medical educator.*

How Is All of This To Be Accomplished?

Not easily. It is obvious that the level of resistance to change on the part of the sci/med establishment is enormous, as we have seen throughout this book. Presently, change, sometimes representing an advance in meeting the needs of the people and sometimes not, is made grudgingly and usually only in response to an increased outpouring of governmental (taxpayers') dollars. In fact the need for change is simply not recognized by a sci/med establishment which just says, over and over, "American medical education is the best in the world," a patently meaningless statement, as I have previously discussed.

The fact is, as I believe I have shown, the needs of our people for health care are not being adequately met, the medical schools bear a major responsibility for that situation, and they are doing nothing to improve it. That is a most unfortunate state of affairs because it means that change will be made entirely in the political arena and forced on the medical schools from the outside. In a democracy it is entirely appropriate that the political process be involved in change in any one of its major institutions, but the results will be quite different depending whether or not the institution involves itself in the change process, or just sits there saying "No, no, no!"

In 1917, Dr. Alexander Lambert, a leader of the American Medical Association admonished it, in reference to then-pending proposals for national health insurance:

> Blind opposition, indignant repudiation, bitter denunciation of these laws is worse than useless; it leads nowhere and it leaves the profession in a position of helplessness if the rising tide of social development sweeps over them. The profession can, through its influence in the community, prevent for a time these laws being passed and it can, by a refusal to cooperate, still further retard them, but in the end the social forces that demand these laws and demand an improvement in the social existence of a great mass of the people of the nation will indignantly force a recalcitrant profession to accept that which is unjust to it and that which is to its detriment.[8]

Of course one can say that the AMA has managed to hold off national health insurance for over sixty years at great benefit to (the pockets of) its membership, but at the cost of what untold suffering, medical and financial, of many individuals in this country. And will the product, when we finally do get it, be better or worse for both the doctors and the people? Dr. Lambert's thought is still most applicable.

In speaking directly to the medical schools in 1965 on the need for change in medical education, one of their own, Lowell T. Coggeshall, M.D., echoed Dr. Lambert's thoughts:

> If action is not taken by those best equipped to plan and implement changes—the persons now responsible for medical education—action will continue to be sought by the public at large and the initiative for action will be assumed by forces less well equipped. Most likely, public appeals channeled through legislative representatives will result in increasing assumption of responsibility by federal, state, and local governments.[9]

As is evident from previously quoted statements of people like Doctors Berliner, Petersdorf, and Ingelfinger, and from the positions of the AAMC and the Carnegie Council on Policy Studies in Higher Education on various questions of medical education reform, warnings of this type are simply not being heeded. As I have previously noted, the general position of the sci/med establishment is: "Leave us alone. We know what we are doing. But, oh yes, please throw more money at us."

However, that will not continue to happen, at least in the long run. Since history always resolves contradictions, in one way or another, the contradiction between what the medical schools are doing and what the needs of the people are will be resolved. The question concerns the degree of difficulty and pain to be encountered in the resolution.

Political Routes to Change

The first step toward change in medical education involves a major increase in public awareness of just what the problems are and how much the present system is costing the taxpayer. It is my hope that this book will, among other things, contribute to that educational process. There are a variety of measures which could be undertaken to force change in the medical education system if it continues to refuse to modernize itself. I will not at this point consider them in detail, but simply list them:

1. Attach requirements for change to the allotment of money, the present main approach.
2. Supply financial aid to medical schools under a contract mechanism with specific performance requirements.
3. Change state licensing laws for physicians, possibly substituting a single national licensing law, such that medical schools would be forced to change in order to qualify their graduates for licensure. (This approach was favored by Flexner.)
4. Directly license medical schools by state or federal government. (Flexner also looked with favor on this approach, as a last resort.)
5. Provide national health insurance monies, when they come, under a contract mechanism.

Of these, licensure of medical schools, a Flexnerian idea ironically enough, is probably the most efficient. Flexner presented the rationale for it much more eloquently than I can. (See Appendix I: e., f., and g.)

Concluding Thoughts

Now is a time for creativity, experimentation, and careful evaluation. The constant nay-saying and blocking of change on the part of the sci/med establishment must stop, but we must continually remember that we are not here dealing with individual villains. Individuals may be a spokesmen for a system but they are not to blame, as people. We are dealing with severe *system* problems, created by history, and the representatives of the system are created by history too. We must look beyond "good" and "evil" persons and see the history behind them. We must realize that just as history creates contradictions, so it resolves them. It is in the hands of the people to guide history towards the most useful resolution.

Change has occurred before in American medical education; it will occur again. The potential for advancing the health of the people is enormous. I believe I have demonstrated that. We must now take what is best in American medical education, in people, facilities, and programs, and combine them with new ideas and new ways of doing things to meet new conditions. This is a great challenge. I am confident that the American people can meet it.

APPENDIX *I*

The True Flexnerian Program

The following are quotations from the *Flexner Report* with page references in parentheses.

I.a. The overwhelming importance of preventive medicine, sanitation, and public health indicates that in modern life the medical profession is an organ differentiated by society for its own highest purposes, not a business to be exploited by individuals according to their own fancy. There would be no vigorous campaigns led by enlightened practitioners against tuberculosis, malaria, and diphtheria, if the commercial point of view were tolerable in practice. And if not in practice, then not in education. The theory of state regulation covers that point. In the act of granting the right to confer degrees, the state vouches for them; through protective boards it still further seeks to safeguard the people. The public interest is then paramount, and when public interest, professional ideals, and sound educational procedure concur in the recommendation of the same policy, the time is surely ripe for decisive action. (p. 19)

I.b. The practitioner deals with facts of two categories. Chemistry, physics, biology enable him to apprehend one set; he needs a different apperceptive and appreciative apparatus to deal with other, more subtle elements. Specific preparation is in this direction much more difficult; one must rely for the requisite insight and sympathy on a varied and enlarging cultural experience. Such enlargement of the physician's horizon is otherwise important, for scientific progress has greatly modified his ethical responsibility. His relation was formerly to his patient—at most to his patient's family; and it was almost latogether remedial. The patient had something the matter with him; the doctor was called in to cure it. Payment of a fee ended the transaction. But the physician's function is fast becoming social and preventive, rather than individual and curative. Upon him society relies to ascertain, and through measures essentially educational to enforce, the conditions that prevent disease and make positively for physical and moral well-being. It goes without saying that this type of doctor is first of all an educated man. (p. 26)

I.c. To the intelligent and conscientious physician, a typhoid patient is not only a case, but a warning: his office it is equally to heal the sick and to protect the well. The public health laboratory belongs, then, under the wing of the medical school. It is the clearinghouse into which data from an entire state should pour. Tax-supported institutions are most favorably circumstanced in this respect. The material which they readily accumulate is at once a basis for teaching, for investigation, and for practical sanitation. Thus the laboratory sciences all culminate and come together in the hygienic laboratory; out of which emerges the young physician, equipped with sound views as to the nature, causation, spread, prevention, and cure of disease, and with an exalted conception of his own duty to promote social conditions that conduce to physical well-being. (p. 68)

I.d. Inevitably, the way to better medical education lies through fewer medical schools; but legal enactments on the subject of medical education and practice will be required before the medical schools will either give up or relate themselves soundly to the educational resources of their respective states. . . . Whatever the standard fixed, it would thus be intelligently enforced. The school catalogues would then announce that no student can be matriculated whose credentials are not filed [with the state board of medicine] within ten days of the opening of the session, and that no M.D. degree can be conferred until at least four years subsequent to complete satisfaction of the preliminary requirement. These credentials, sent at once to the secretary of the state board, would be by him turned over to the registrar of the state or other university, whose verdict would be final. (pp. 49–50)

I.e. The right of the state to deal with the entire subject [of medical education] in its own interest can assuredly not be gainsaid. The physician is a social instrument. If there were no disease, there would be no doctors. And as disease has consequences that immediately go beyond the individual specifically affected, society is bound to protect itself against unnecessary spread of loss or danger. It matters not that the making of doctors has been to some extent left to private institutions. The state already makes certain regulations; it can by the same right make others. Practically the medical school is a public service corporation. It is chartered by the state; it utilizes public hospitals on the ground of the social nature of its service. The medical school cannot then escape social criticism and regulation. It was left to itself while society knew no better. But civilization consists in the legal registration of gains won by science and experience; and science have together established the terms upon which medicine can be most useful. (p. 154)

I.f. Such control in the social interest inevitably encounters the objection that individualism is thereby impaired. So it is, at that level; so it is intended. The community through such regulation undertakes to abridge the freedom of particular individuals to exploit certain conditions for their personal benefit. But its aim is thereby to secure for all others more freedom at a higher level. Society forbids a company of physicians to pour out upon the community a horde of ill trained physicians. Their liberty is indeed clipped. As a result, however, more competent doctors being trained under the auspices of the state itself, the public health is improved; the physical well-being of the wage-worker is heightened; and a restriction put upon the liberty, so-called, of a dozen doctors increases the effectual liberty of all other citizens. Has democracy, then, really suffered a setback? Reorganization along rational lines involves the strengthening, not the weakening, of democratic principle, because it tends to provide the conditions upon which well-being and effectual liberty depend. (p. 155)

I.g. The state boards are the instruments through which the reconstruction of medical education will be largely effected. To them the graduate in medicine applies for the license to practise. Their power can be both indirectly and directly exerted. They may after examination reject an applicant—an indirect method of discrediting the school which has vouched for him by conferring its M.D. degree . . . A more direct and therefore more salutary method is needed, however, in dealing with schools bad beyond a reasonable doubt. In such instances the board should summarily refuse to entertain the applicant's petition because his medical education rests upon no proper preliminary training or was received under conditions that forbade thorough or conscientious instruction: the full weight of its refusal would fall with crushing effect upon the school which sent him forth. No institution can long survive the day upon which it is thus publicly branded as feeble, unfit, or disreputable. For the purpose, however, of saving the victims whose cruel disappointment will in time destroy these schools, the arm of the state boards should for the present go beyond the rejection of individuals to the actual closing up of notoriously incompetent institutions. The law that protects the public against the unfit doctor should in fairness protect the student against the unfit school. (p. 167)

I.h. If the written examination were relegated to a subordinate position, the weight of the test would fall upon the applicant's ability to do things; schools incapable for whatever reason of training students in the necessary technique would be rapidly exposed through the annual publication of statistics proclaiming their failure. The state board results, now so frequently misleading, would be a trustworthy index which the more intelligent students would carefully scan; and those schools only survive whose records entitle them to live. Of such overwhelming importance, indeed, is the character of the license examination that, if thorough practical examination were instituted, all the other perplexing details we have discussed would become relatively immaterial. (pp. 169–70)

I.i. Despite imperfect and discordant laws and inadequate resources, the state board has abundantly justified itself . . . Reciprocity between states whose laws are measurably concordant and whose ideals are taking similar shape tends to demonstrate the fundamental sameness of the problems requiring solution. Out of these first cooperative efforts, a model law will emerge; federated action may become possible. Perhaps the entire country may some day be covered by a national organization engaged in protecting the public health against the formidable combination made by ignorance, incompetency, commercialism, and disease. (p. 173)

I.j. What the student did not readily apprehend could be drilled into him—towards examination time—by those who had themselves recently passed through the ordeal which he was now approaching; and an efficient apparatus that spared his senses and his intellect as entirely as the drillmaster spared his industry was readily accessible at temptingly low prices in the shape of 'essentials' and 'quiz-compends'. . . . However, the practical outcome of . . . investigation is not communicable by rote; it cannot be reduced to prescriptions for mechanical use by the unenlightened practitioner. Modern medicine cannot be formulated in quiz-compends; those who would employ it must trouble to understand it. Moreover, medicine is developing with beneficent rapidity along these same biological and chemical lines. Is our fresh young graduate of five and twenty to keep abreast of its progress? If so, he must, once more, understand; not otherwise can he adopt the new agents and new methods issuing at intervals from each of a dozen fertile laboratories; for rote has no future: it stops where it is. (pp. 21, 25)

I.k. The reconstruction of our medical education on the basis of two years of required college work is not, however, going to end matters once and for all. It leaves untouched certain outlying problems that will all the more surely come into focus when the professional training of the physician will generally expand, and to support such expansion, he will crave a more liberal and disinterested educational experience. (p. 48)

I.l. The main intellectual tool of the investigator is the working hypothesis, or theory, as it is more commonly called. . . . Upon this he acts, and the practical outcome of his procedure refutes, confirms, or modifies his theory. . . . This is essentially the technique of research: wherein is it irrelevant to bedside practice? The physician, too, is confronted by a definite situation. He must needs seize its details, and only powers of observation trained in actual experimentation will enable him to do so. The patient's history, conditions, symptoms, form his data. Thereupon he, too, frames his working hypothesis, now called a diagnosis. It suggests a line of action . . . The sick man's progress is nature's comment and criticism. The professional competency of the physician is in proportion to his ability to heed the response which nature thus makes to his ministrations. The progress of science and the scientific or intelligent practice of medicine employ, therefore, exactly the same technique. To use it, whether in investigation or in practice, the student must be trained to the positive exercise of his faculties; and if so trained, the medical school begins rather than completes his medical education. It cannot in any event transit to him more than a fraction of the actual treasures of the science; but it can at least put him in the way of steadily increasing his holdings. . . . In the end the scientist alone draws the line accurately between the known, the partly known, and the unknown. The empiricist fares forth with an indiscriminate confidence which sharp lines do not disturb. (pp. 55–56)

I.m. The backbone of the structure [for clinical teaching] is the clinic in internal medicine. . . . To sample a school on its clinical side, one makes in the first place straight for its medical clinic, seeking to learn the number of patients available for teaching, the variety of conditions which they illustrate, and the hospital regulations in so far, at least, as they determine (1) continuity of service on the part of the teachers of medicine, (2) the closeness with which the student may follow the progress of individual patients, and (3) the access of the student to the clinical laboratory. . . . Excellent didactic instruction is no compensation; successful passing of written state board or other examinations is no proof that the school has managed to do without. (pp. 93–94)

I.n. . . . there is little reason to believe that the divided school will ever function as an organic whole, though it may be tolerable as a halfway stage on the road from the proprietary school to the complete university department. "I cannot help wondering," said President Pritchett [of the Carnegie Foundation] "how it would affect the pedagogic and professional ideals of an engineering school if its first two years were given in one place and the last two years in a place two hundred miles away. My impression is that there would be two separate schools with very little more reaction, the one upon the other, than exists between any other two schools so located." Thus far the difficulty seems hardly to have been suspected: the dean of Nebraska at Lincoln is a busy professor who has no real hold on the clinical men at Omaha; the dean of California is superintendent of the hospital in San Francisco, with no real control of what goes on at Berkeley, and surely without any possible control over the second clinical department at Los Angeles; Kansas practically accepts the split by setting up a dean at each of the two ends, though they are only an hour and a half apart; Mississippi, with even better reason, does the same, for the journey from Oxford to Vicksburg, not great when measured in miles, takes the better part of a day if one is lucky enough to make the necessary railroad connections. (p. 73)

I.o. There is room for men of another type—the nonproductive, assimilative teacher of wide learning, continuous receptivity, critical sense, and responsible interest. Not infrequently these men, catholic in their sympathies, scholarly in spirit and method, prove the purveyors and distributors through whom new ideas are harmonized and made current. They preserve balance and make connections. The one person for whom there is no place in the medical school, the university, or the college, is precisely he who has hitherto generally usurped the medical field—the scientifically dead practitioner, whose knowledge has long since come to a standstill and whose lectures, composed when he first took his chair, like pebbles rolling in a brook get smoother and smoother as the stream of time washes over them. (p. 57)

I.p. It follows that in other respects, too, the clinical professors will be on the common university basis: salaried, as other professors are. Of course, their salaries will be inadequate, i.e., less than they can earn outside—all academic salaries paid to the right men are. But there is no inherent reason why a professor of medicine should not make something of the financial sacrifice that the professor of physics makes: both give up something—less and less, let us hope, as time goes on—in order to teach and to investigate. The clinical teacher should indeed not arbitrarily restrict his experience: he may wisely develop—preferably in close connection with the hospital—a consulting practice . . . for at all points only good can come of educational contact with unsolved problems—practical or other. But a consulting practice—developed in a professional or commercial, rather than in a scientific spirit—may prove quite as fatal to scientific interest as general practice. University hospitals, academic salaries, etc., make the conditions in which clinical medicine may be productively cultivated. They do not, however, create ideals; and without ideals, superabundant and highly paid consultations are perhaps as demoralizing as superabundant low-priced "calls." (p. 102)

APPENDIX II

Accreditation of Schools of Medicine: Policy Documents and Guidelines

OFFICIAL POSITION OF
Liaison Committee on Medical Education of the Council on Medical Education, American Medical Association, and the Association of American Medical Colleges

Functions and Structure of a Medical School*

I. Introduction

This is a statement of the Liaison Committee on Medical Education, of the Association of American Medical Colleges, and of the Council on Medical Education of the American Medical Association. It is intended that this material be used to assist in attainment of standards of education that can provide assurance to society and to the medical profession that graduates are competent to meet society's expectations; to students that they will receive a useful and valid educational experience; and to institutions that their efforts and expenditures are suitably allocated.

The concepts expressed here will serve as general but not specific criteria in the medical school accreditation process. However, it is urged

*The basic medical school accreditation document, it is approved by the Assembly of the Association of American Medical Colleges, November 1972, and the House of Delegates of the American Medical Association, June 1973. There are two official commentaries on it, intended to provide medical schools with help in interpreting the rather brief basic document: "Guidelines to 'Functions and Structure of a Medical School'," and "Supplemental Guidelines for Medical Schools with Branches or Multiple Campuses." The three documents are published together as *Accreditation of Schools of Medicine: Policy Documents and Guidelines*, available from either the Council on Medical Education of the American Medical Association, 535 N. Dearborn St., Chicago, Ill., 60610, or the Association of American Medical Colleges, 1 Dupont Circle, N.W., Washington, D.C., 20036.

that this document not be interpreted as an obstacle to soundly conceived experimentation in medical education.

II. Definition and Mission

A medical school is an aggregation of resources that have been organized as a definable academic unit to provide the full spectrum of education in the art and science of medicine in not less than 32 months, culminating with the award of the M.D. degree. The educational program must be sponsored by an academic institution that is appropriately charged within the public trust to offer the M.D. degree.

As an institution of higher education, a medical school has four inherent responsibilities which embody the concept of a continuum of education throughout professional life. These are:

A. The principal responsibility of the medical school is to provide its students with the opportunity to acquire a sound basic education in medicine and also to foster the development of lifelong habits of scholarship and service.

B. A medical school is responsible for the advancement of knowledge through research. In addition to biologically oriented studies, the research carried on in a medical school may include studies related to cultural and behavioral aspects of medicine, methods for the delivery of health care, and the medical education process.

C. Each school is responsible for development of graduate education to produce practitioners, teachers, and investigators, both through clinical residency programs and advanced degree programs in the basic medical sciences.

D. Another important role for the medical school is participation in continuing education aimed at maintaining and improving the competence of those professionals engaged in caring for patients.

In addition, the resources that characterize the modern academic medical center constitute a unique instrument for meeting selected community or regional health needs. As a central intellectual force within the center, the medical school should identify those needs that it might appropriately meet and create programs consistent with its educational objectives and resources to meet them. These efforts can serve as models for students.

Participation by medical schools may contribute to the educational programs of other professions in the health field, such as dentistry, nursing, pharmacy, and the allied health professions.

A medical school should develop a clear definition of its total objectives, appropriate to the needs of the community or geographic area it is designed to serve and the resources at its disposal. When objectives are clearly defined, they should be made familiar to faculty and students alike, so that efforts of all will be directed toward their achievement. Schools should be cautious about overextending themselves in the field of research or service to the detriment of their primary educational mission.

III. Educational Program

The undergraduate period of medical education leading to the M.D. degree is no longer sufficient to prepare a student for independent medical practice without supplementation by a graduate training period which will vary in length depending upon the type of practice the student selects. Further, there is no single curriculum that can be prescribed for the undergraduate period of medical education. Each student should acquire a foundation of knowledge in the basic sciences that will permit the pursuit of any of the several careers that medicine offers. The student should be comfortably familiar with the methods and skills utilized in the practice of clinical medicine. Instruction should be sufficiently comprehensive so as to include the study of both mental and physical disease in patients who are hospitalized as well as ambulatory. At the same time, it should foster and encourage the development of the specific and unique interests of each student by tailoring the program in accordance with the student's preparation, competence, and interests by providing elective time whenever it can be included in the curriculum for this purpose.

Attention should also be given to preventive medicine and public health, and to the social and economic aspects of the systems for delivering medical services. Instruction should stress the physician's concern with the total health and circumstance of patients and not just their diseases. Throughout, the student should be encouraged to develop those basic intellectual attitudes, ethical and moral principles that are essential if the physician is to gain and maintain the trust of patients and colleagues, and the support of the community in which the physician lives.

IV. Administration and Governance

A medical school should be incorporated as a non-profit institution. Whenever possible it should be a part of a university since a university can so well provide the milieu and support required by a medical school. If not a component of a university, a medical school should have a board of trustees composed of public spirited men and women having no financial interest in the operation of the school or its associated hospitals. Trustees should serve for sufficiently long and overlapping terms to permit them to gain an adequate understanding of the programs of the institution and to function in the development of policy in the interest of the institution and the public with continuity and as free of personal and political predilections as possible.

Officers and members of the medical school faculty should be appointed by, or on the authority of, the Board of Trustees of the medical school or its parent university. The chief official of the medical school, who is ordinarily the dean, should have ready access to the university president and such other university officials as are pertinent to the responsibilities of his office. He should have the assistance of a capable business officer and such associate or assistant deans as may be necessary for such areas as student affairs, academic affairs, graduate education, continuing education, hospital matters, and research affairs.

In universities with multiple responsibilities in the health fields, in addition to the school of medicine, as, for example, schools of dentistry, pharmacy, or nursing, it may be useful to have a vice-president for health affairs, or a similarly designated official, who is responsible for the entire program of health-related education at the university. Ordinarily, the deans of the individual health-related schools would report to this individual.

The medical school should be organized so as to facilitate its ability to accomplish its objectives. Ordinarily, this is best effected through the development of a committee structure that is representative of such concerns as admissions, promotions, curriculum, library, and animal care. Names and functions of the committees established should be subject to local determination and needs. Consideration of student representation on all committees is both desirable and useful.

The manner in which the institution is organized, including the responsibilities and privileges of administrative officers, faculty, and students, should be clearly set out in either medical school or university bylaws.

V. Faculty

The faculty must consist of a sufficient number of identifiable representatives from the biological, behavioral, and clinical sciences to implement the objectives that each medical school adopts for itself. The specific fields represented do not have to be reflected in any set pattern of departmental or divisional organization, although the faculty should have professional competence as well as an interest in research and teaching in the fields in which instruction is to be provided. Inasmuch as individual faculty members will vary in the degree of competence and interest they bring to the primary fucntions of the medical school, assignment of responsibility should be made with regard to these variations.

The extent to which the school's educational program may depend on the contributions of physicians who are practicing in the community will vary with many factors, including the size of the community and the availability of qualified teachers in the several medical specialties. The advantage to the student of instruction by such physicians, as well as by those in full-time academic service, should be kept in mind.

Nominations for faculty appointment ordinarily involve participation of both the faculty and the dean, the role of each customarily varying somewhat with the rank of the appointee and the degree to which administrative responsibilities may be involved. Reasonable security and possibility for advancement in salary and rank should be provided.

A small committee of the faculty should work with the dean in setting medical school policy. While such committees have typically consisted of the heads of the major departments, they may be organized in any way that would bring reasonable and appropriate faculty and student influence into the governance of the school. The faculty should meet often enough to provide an opportunity for all to discuss, establish, or otherwise become acquainted with medical school policies and practices.

VI. Students

The number of students that can be supported by the education program of the medical school and its resources, as well as the determination of the qualifications that a student should have to study medicine, are proper responsibilities of the institution. Inasmuch as all medical schools constitute a national resource, and all operate in the public interest, it is desirable for the student body to reflect a wide spectrum of social and economic backgrounds. Decisions regarding admission to medical school should be based not only on satisfactory prior scholastic accomplishments but also on such factors as personal and emotional characteristics, motivation, industry, resourcefulness, and personal health. Information about these factors can be developed through personal interviews, college records of academic and nonacademic activities, admission tests, and letters of recommendation. There should be no discrimination on the basis of sex, creed, race, or national origin.

Ordinarily, at least three years of undergraduate education are required for entrance into medical school, although a number of medical schools have developed programs in which the time spent in college prior to entering medical school has been reduced even further. The medical school should restrict its specified premedical course requirements to courses that are considered essential to enable the student to cope with the medical school curriculum. Students preparing for the study of medicine should have the opportunity to acquire either a broad, liberal education or, if they choose, study a specific field in depth, according to their personal interests and abilities.

Advanced standing may be granted to students for work done prior to admission. The increasing diversity in medical school curricula and the greater integration of the total curriculum require that transfers between medical schools be individually considered so that both school and students will be assured that the courses previously pursued by the students are compatible with the programs they will enter. Otherwise, supplementation of the students' program may be necessary after they have transferred.

There should be a system for keeping student records that summarizes admissions, credentials, grades, and other records of performance in medical school. These records should reflect accurately each student's work and qualifications by including a qualitative evaluation of each student by his instructors.

It is very important that there be available an adequate system of student counselling. Such counselling is especially critical for those students who may require remedial work. Academic programs allowing students to progress at their own pace are desirable.

There should be a program for student health care that provides for periodic medical examination and adequate clinical care for the students.

VII. Finances

The school of medicine should seek its operating support from diverse sources. The support should be sufficient for the school to conduct its programs in a satisfactory manner and it should reflect, as accurately as possible, the educational, research, and service efforts of the faculty.

Special attention must be paid to providing financial aid for students since it is desirable that economic hardship not hinder the acquisition of an education in medicine.

VIII. Facilities

A medical school should have, or enjoy the assured use of, buildings and equipment that are quantitatively and qualitatively adequate to provide an environment that will be conducive to maximum productivity of faculty and students in fulfilling the objectives of the school. Geographic proximity between the preclinical and clinical facilities is desirable, whenever possible. The facilities should include faculty office and research laboratories, student classrooms and laboratories, a hospital of sufficient capacity for the educational programs, ambulatory care facilities, and a library.

The relationship of the medical school to its primary or affiliated hospitals should be such that the medical school has the unquestioned right to appoint, as faculty, that portion of the hospital's attending staff that will participate in the school's teaching program. All affiliation agreements should define clearly the rights of both the medical school and the hospital in the appointment of the attending staff. Hospitals with which the school's association is less intimate may be utilized in the teaching program in a subsidiary way but all arrangements should insure that instruction is conducted under the supervision of the medical school faculty.

A well-maintained and catalogued library, sufficient in size and breadth to support the educational programs that are operated by the institution, is essential to a medical school. The library should receive the leading medical periodicals, the current numbers of which should be readily accessible. The library or other learning resource should also be equipped to allow students to gain experience with newer methods of receiving information as well as with self-instructional devices. A professional library staff should supervise the development and operation of the library.

IX. Accreditation

The American Medical Association through its Council on Medical Education and the Association of American Medical Colleges serve as the recognized accrediting agencies for medical schools. Though retaining their individual identities, both groups work very closely in this activity through the Liaison Committee on Medical Education. To be accredited, a medical school must be approved by the Liaison Committee on Medical Education, by the Council on Medical Education and be offered membership in the Association of American Medical Colleges. This is granted on the finding of a sound educational program as a result of a survey conducted by the Liaison Committee on Medical Education. The Liaison Committee, representing the voluntary professional sector, includes representatives from DHEW and the public, and is recognized by the Council on Postsecondary Accreditation, the United States Commissioner of Education, the U.S. Congress in various health related public laws, and the state licensure boards as providing the official accreditation for medical education leading to the M.D. degree.

It is the intent that newly developing medical schools should be surveyed several times during the initial years of active existence. Provisional accreditation is granted, when the program warrants, for the first years of the curriculum and definitive action is taken during the implementation of the last year of the curriculum.

Existing medical schools are surveyed at regular intervals. Decisions regarding accreditation require assessment of the school's constellation of resources in relation to the total student enrollment. Any significant change in either should be brought to the attention of the Liaison Committee and may occasion review of the accreditation status. Every attempt is made to fulfill requests for interim surveys as a service to the medical schools.

Further information about accreditation can be obtained from the Secretary, Council on Medical Education, American Medical Association, 535 North Dearborn Street, Chicago, Illinois 60610, or from the Director, Division of Accreditation, Association of American Medical Colleges, One Dupont Circle, N.W., Washington, D.C. 20036.

Notes

Prologue

1. President Lyndon Baines Johnson made the quoted statement in *Proceedings of the White House Conference on Health, November 3–4, 1965* (Washington, D.C., USDHEW, 1966), p. 3.

Chapter 1

1. Dr. Marvin Belsky and Leonard Gross, *Beyond the Medical Mystique: How to Choose and Use Your Doctor* (New York: Arbor House, 1975).

Chapter 2

Portions of this chapter are taken from my textbook, *Health Care Delivery in the United States* (New York: Springer Publishing Co., 1977), Chapter 2, "What Is Health Care?" by David Banta, M.D., and Chapter 3, "Data for Health and Health Care," by myself. This material is used with the kind permission of Dr. Banta and the Springer Publishing Co. The Alexandrian physician Herophilus was quoted by Henry Sigerist in his book *Medicine and Human Welfare* (New Haven: Yale University Press, 1941), p. 57. Dr. Harnes' quote appeared in his essay, "Medical Pests," *Journal of the American Medical Association, 235,* 157, 1976. The quote from *Preventive Medicine, U.S.A.* appeared on p. vii of "Theory, Practice and Application of Prevention in Personal Health Services," one of a series of Preventive Medicine, U.S.A. Task Force Reports, sponsored by the Fogarty International Center of the National Institutes of Health and the American College of Preventive Medicine, published by PRODIST, New York, 1976.

1. The Sigerist quote on the Greek Concept of health is from *Medicine and Human Welfare,* p. 57, cited above.
2. Dr. John Gordon Freymann, *The American Health Care System* (Huntington, New York: Krieger Publishing Co., 1977), p. 52.
3. The citations from Kark are found on p. 11 of his book, *Epidemiology and Community Medicine* (New York: Appleton-Century-Crofts, 1974).
4. Quote appeared in Freymann, *The American Health Care System,* p. 52, cited above.
5. The Sigerist quote on disease appears on p. 23 of his book cited above.
6. The quotes from Cassell are from *The Healer's Art* (Philadelphia: Lippincott, 1976), pp. 26, 48.
7. See the *Monthly Vital Statistics Report* for current leading causes of death. MVSR is published by the National Center for Health Statistics (NCHS) of the USDHEW.
8. Data on patient-reported morbidity are from "Current Estimates from the Health Interview Survey: United States—1975." *Vital and Health Statistics,* Series 10, No. 115, March, 1977, Tables 1, 3 and 9, and other publications of *Vital and Health Statistics* cited in the bibliography of Chapter 3 of my textbook. VHS is also published by the NCHS of the USDHEW.
9. Data on hospital discharges are from "Utilization of Short-Stay Hospitals: Annual Summary for the United States, 1975," *Vital and Health Statistics,* Series 13, Number 31, April, 1977, table No. 20.
10. Data from doctors' offices are from the *National Ambulatory Medical Care Survey,* which now appears periodically in *Monthly Vital Statistics Report.*
11. The arguments contained in *Changes in Population Health Levels Over Time* are primarily from Henry Sigerist's *Medicine and Human Welfare,* cited above, esp. pp. 45–52; Thomas McKeown's "A historical appraisal of the medical task," which is Chapter 2 in *Medical History and Medical Care,* edited by Gordon McLachlan and Dr. McKeown (London: Oxford University Press, 1971); and Chapter 1 of *An Introduction to Social Medicine* by Thomas McKeown and C.R. Lowe (Oxford: Blackwell Scientific Publications, 1974). Dr. McKeown more recently has published two books expanding and fortifying his arguments. They are *The Modern Rise of Population* (New York: Academic

Press, 1976); and *The Role of Medicine: Dream, Mirage or Nemesis?* (London: The Nuffield Provincial Hospitals Trust), 1976.

12. The Massachusetts TB data are cited on p. 46 of Sigerist's *Medicine and Human Welfare.*

13. The TB and diarrheal disease (later) death data from New York City are from NYC Department of Health figures cited by Stephen C. Joseph, M.D. in "Worldwide Patterns of Disease," Unit I/2, p. 12, *International Health Course* (Washington, D.C.: Association of American Medical Colleges, 1977).

14. The quote from Leonard Hayflick appeared on p. 1302 of his paper "The Cell Biology of Human Aging," *New England Journal of Medicine, 295,* 1302, 1976.

15. The disease-specific death rates come from table 65 of Robert Grove's and Alice Hetzel's *Vital Statistics Rates in the United States, 1940–1960,* National Center for Health Statistics (Washington, D.C.: USDHEW, 1968); *Monthly Vital Statistics Report,* 25, (8), Oct. 27, 1976, table 6; and the "Annual Summary for the United States, 1975: Births, Deaths, Marriages, and Divorces," *Monthly Vital Statistics Report,* 24 (13), June 30, 1976, table 9.

16. The material from Charles-Edward Amory Winslow, comes from his Editorial, "Who Killed Cock Robin?" which appeared in the *American Journal of Public Health, 34,* 658, 1944.

17. The environmental relationships to cancer are discussed by Dr. Higginson in his paper "A Hazardous Society? Individual versus Community Responsibility in Cancer Prevention," *American Journal of Public Health, 66,* 359, 1976.

18. Dr. Thomas' comments on syphilis appeared in "Notes of a Biology-Watcher: On Meddling," *New England Journal of Medicine, 294,* 599, 1976.

19. The current "state of the art" in prevention is contained in the several volumes of *Preventive Medicine USA,* referred to above.

20. The principal references for Lester Breslow's work are "A Quantitative Approach to the World Health Organization Definition of Health," *International Journal of Epidemiology, 1,* 347, 1972; Belloc, N.B. and Breslow, "Relationship of Physical Health Status and Health Practices," *Preventive Medicine, 1,* 409, 1972; and Belloc, N.B. "Relationship of Health Practices and Mortality," *Preventive Medicine, 2,* 67, 1973.

21. Prof. Fuchs' comment on life-style appears on p. 54 of his *Who Shall Live?* (New York: Basic Books, 1974).

22. Prof. Somers made his statement in "Health and Public Policy," *Inquiry, XII:* 94, 1975.

23. Dean Wildavsky made his comment in his 1976 Michael M. Davis Lecture, "Can Health be Planned?" delivered on April 23, 1976 at the University of Chicago, and subsequently published by The Center for Health Administration Studies, Graduate School of Business, The University of Chicago.

24. The MSSNY statement appeared on p. 3 of the May 1, 1976 issue of their regular newsletter, *News of New York.*

25. Fuchs' last word appears on p. 151 of *Who Shall Live?*

26. The data on advertising expenditures is from the Statistical Abstract of the United States, 1974 (Washington, D.C.: U.S. Department of Commerce, 1974), tables 1302 and 1307.

27. The data on cigarette smoking come from *Adult Use of Tobacco, 1975,* Public Health Service (Washington, D.C.: USDHEW, June, 1976).

28. Milton Terris' paper is "Epidemiology of Cirrhosis of the Liver: National Mortality Data," *American Journal of Public Health, 57,* 2076, 1967.

29. Meenan's paper was "Improving the Public's Health—Some Further Reflections," *New England Journal of Medicine, 294,* 45, 1976.

30. For calculations of commercial insurance company profits see my paper "Issues in National Health Insurance in the United States of America," the *Lancet,* July 20, 1974, p. 413.

Chapter 3

Portions of this chapter, especially the first section containing the lengthy quotes from other works, are taken from Chapter 1, "Introduction," of my textbook, *Health Care Delivery in the United States* and are used with the kind permission of Springer Publishing Co., New York.

1. The *Harper's Magazine* quote appeared on p. 123 of "The Crisis in American Medicine" published in the October, 1960 issue, pp. 123–168.

2. The Battistella and Southby paper appeared in the *Lancet,* March 16, 1968, p. 581.

3. The *Fortune* quote is from p. 9 of *Our Ailing Medical System: It's Time to Operate* by the Editors of *Fortune* (New York: Perennial Library, Harper and Row, 1970).

4. The quote citing Senator Kennedy is from p. xi of Spencer Klaw's *The Great American Medicine Show* (New York: The Viking Press, 1975).

5. Among the other critical studies undertaken in the last 15 years are: J.R. Moskin's "The challenge to our doctors," *Look,* November 3,

1964, p. 26; *Health is a Community Affair* (Cambridge, Mass.: Harvard University Press, 1966); *Rx for Action,* the Report of the Health Task Force of the Urban Coalition, Washington, D.C., 1969; *Business Week's* "The $60-billion crisis over medical care," which appeared in the January 17, 1970 issue; Daniel Schorr's *Don't Get Sick in America* (Nashville, Tenn.: Aurora Publishers, Inc., 1970); *Heal Yourself,* the Report of the Citizens Board of Inquiry into Health Services for Americans, Washington, D.C., 1971; *The American Health Empire: Power, Profits, and Politics,* by John and Barbara Ehrenreich (New York: Vintage Books, 1971); Senator Edward Kennedy's *In Critical Condition* (New York: Simon and Schuster, 1972); and Senator Abraham Ribicoff's *The American Medical Machine,* written with P. Danaceau (New York: Saturday Review Press, 1972).

6. Professor Roemer's list of critical analyses of the U.S. health care delivery system appeared in: "Review Article: The American Health Empire: Power, Profits, and Politics," *International Journal of Health Services, 2,* 119, 1972. He said:

   Every few years, more recently in the last decade, there appears a book analyzing the serious defects of health care in America. In 1927, Harry H. Moore produced *American Medicine and the People's Health,* in the 1930s were the magnificant 27 volumes of the Committee on the Costs of Medical Care, in 1939 there was James Rorty's *American Medicine Mobilizes,* and in 1940 Hugh Cabot's *The Patient Dilemma.* After World War II Carl Malmberg wrote *140 Million Patients* in 1947, Michael Davis wrote *Medical Care for Tommorrow* in 1955, and Richard Carter wrote *The Doctor Business* in 1958. In 1965 there there was Selig Greenberg's excellent *The Troubled Calling: Crisis in the Medical Establishment.* The year after Medicare, 1966, saw two critical outputs: *The American Health Scandal* by Roul Tunley and *The Doctors* by Martin L. Gross. In 1967 there was Fred J. Cook's *Plot Against the Patient* and in 1970 Ed Cray's *In Failing Health.*

7. The statement by the Committee on the Costs of Medical Care comes from p. 2 of its *Medical Care for the American People* (Chicago: University of Chicago Press, 1932, reprinted by the USDHEW, Washington, D.C., 1970).

8. The article quoting Dr. Parrott, entitled "AMA hits federal NHI plans," appeared on p. 1 of the *American Medical News,* November 17, 1975.

9. The material on and from Harry Schwartz's book appeared in the *American Medical News* of October 16, 1972, in an article entitled: "The Case for American Medicine. Chapter II: What Health Crisis? From the New Book by Harry Schwartz."

10. Sections I and II of Dr. Freymann's book, *The American Health Care System* (New York: Medcom Press, 1974) contain his historical analysis of the development of the U.S. health care delivery system.

11. Data on expenditures on sanitation and sewage are projected from Table 422 of the Statistical Abstract of the United States, 1976 (Washington, D.C.: U.S. Department of Commerce, 1976).

12. The data on proportional health expenditures come from "National Health Expenditures, Fiscal Year 1975," by Marjorie Smith Mueller and Robert M. Gibson, *Social Security Bulletin,* February 1976, p. 3, esp. Table 2.

13. The Breslow-Somers estimate of expenditures on prevention is from their paper "The Lifetime Health-Monitoring Program," *New England Journal of Medicine, 296,* 601, 1977.

14. The study by Cooper and Rice entitled "The Economic Cost of Illness Revisited" appeared in the *Social Security Bulletin,* February, 1976, p. 21.

15. The material by Dr. Freymann on the separation of acute care from other health services is in his work cited above.

16. As above, the data on health expenditures come from "National Health Expenditures, Fiscal Year 1975," by Marjorie Smith Mueller and Robert M. Gibson, *Social Security Bulletin,* February 1976, p. 3. See also Chapter 4 of this book, and Chapter 9, "Financing for Health Care," by Carol McCarthy, of *Health Care Delivery* cited above. For additional material on rising costs, see Chapter 5 of this book.

17. The report of the Council on Wage and Price Stability was published by the USGPO in Washington, D.C., 1977. The quotes are from pp. i–iii.

18. The data on geographic maldistribution of physicians come from "Physician Distribution: Solving the Specialty-Location Dilemmas," by E. Martin Egelston and Linda Camp, *Hospitals, J.A.H.A.,* December 16, 1976, p. 101.

19. The study on factors related to physician geographic movement of physicians is contained in "Analysis of the Impact of the Hill-Burton Program on the Distribution of the Supply of General Hospital Beds and Physicians in the United States, 1950–1970," by L.J. Clark and T.L. Koontz, delivered at the Annual Meeting of the American Public Health Association, San Francisco, Calif., November, 1973.

20. The physician-population ratios over time are from Appendix Table 7 of *Physicians for a Growing America,* Report of the Surgeon General's Consultant Group on Medical Education (the Bane Report) (Washington, D.C.: USDHEW, October, 1959) and "False Starts and

Lesser Alternatives," by Milton Terris, *Bulletin of the New York Academy of Medicine, 53,* 129, 1977.

21. I offered my definition of primary care in "Some Thoughts on Primary Care: Problems in Implementation," *International Journal of Health Services, 3,* 177, 1973. Dr. Roemer defined secondary and tertiary care in "A Realistic System: Health Maintenance Organizations in a Regionalized Framework," Chapter 10 in *Planning Urban Services,* edited by Ruth Roemer, et. al. (New York: Springer Publishing Co., 1975), p. 263.

22. The comparative study of surgeons and surgery by Dr. Bunker entitled "Surgical Manpower" appeared in the *New England Journal of Medicine, 282,* 135, 1970.

23. The data on the workload of surgeons come from "Surgeons in the United States: Activities, Output, and Income," by W.W. Hauck, Jr., et al., *Journal of the American Medical Association, 236,* 1864, "Doctors Who Perform Operations," by Rita J. Nickerson, et al., *New England Journal of Medicine, 295,* 921, and an editorial in the *Journal of the American Medical Association, 237,* 267, 1977, "Too Many Surgeons?" by Rudolph H. deJong.

24. For the evidence on quality measurement and control see Chapter 6 below, and "Measurement and Control of the Quality of Health Care" by myself, Chapter 13 in *Health Care Delivery,* cited above.

25. For basic information on health services planning in the U.S., see Chapter 12, "Planning for Health Care" by Carol McCarthy, in *Health Care Delivery,* cited above.

26. The study by Lebow is "Consumer Assessments of the Quality of Medical Care," *Medical Care, 12,* 328, 1974.

27. The Report of the Secretary's Commission was published by the USDHEW (Pub. No. (OS) 73–88) in Washington, D.C., January 16, 1973. The quoted material is from pp. 67–68.

28. The paper by Birch and Wolfe is "Consumers Assess Alternative Kinds of Health Services." It was presented at the Annual Meeting of the American Public Health Association, Chicago, Ill., Nov. 20, 1975.

29. and 30. Marvin Belsky's book was published in 1975 by Arbor House in New York City. The quote on communication appears on p. 22. The quoted material on the Medical Mystique begins on p. 29.

31. The proportional figures for health services utilization are from Dr. White's article, "Life and Death and Medicine," *Scientific American,* Sept. 1973, p. 23. The figure from which the data are drawn is on p. 30.

Chapter 4

Dr. Holden's quote is from *Hospital Week,* the weekly newsletter of the *American Hospital Association,* Vol. 13, No. 5, February 4, 1977. The quoted editorial appeared in the *American Medical News,* the weekly newspaper published by the American Medical Association, December 18, 1972.

1. The material on governmental structure is based on Chapter 10 "Government in the Health Care Delivery System" by myself, David Banta, and Michael Enright, in our textbook, *Health Care Delivery,* some material quoted directly and is used with the kind permission of Dr. Banta, Mr. Enright, and the Springer Publishing Co. There is a great deal of reference material in that chapter.

2. The quotation on the police power is from Frank P. Grad's *Public Health Law Manual* (Washington, D.C.: American Public Health Association, 1975), p. 5.

3. For additional material on health care planning see Chapter 12, "Planning for Health Care" by Carol McCarthy, in *Health Care Delivery.*

4. Basic reference material on health care expenditures can be found in "Financing for Health Care," by Carol McCarthy, Chapter 9 of our textbook, *Health Care Delivery.* Sections of that Chapter have been used, with the permission of the author and Springer Publishing Co. The most important recurring source of health care financing information is the article, "National Health Expenditures," appearing annually in the *Social Security Bulletin,* usually in the February or March issue.

5. For data on private health insurance, see "Private Health Insurance in 1974: A Review of Coverage, Enrollment, and Financial Experience" by Marjorie Smith Mueller and Paula A. Piro, *Social Security Bulletin,* March, 1976, p. 3, and similar articles appearing in the *Bulletin* at about the same time each year.

6. For the estimation of commercial insurance company profits see my paper "Issues in National Health Insurance in the United States of America," the *Lancet,* July 20, 1974, p. 143.

7. For arguments on the fee-for-service method of health care provider reimbursement see "Medical Care as a Right: A Refutation," by R.M. Sade *New England Journal of Medicine, 285,* 1288, 1971, defending it, and Milton Roemer's "On Paying the Doctor and the Implications of Different Methods," *Journal of Health and Human Behavior, 3,* 4, Spring, 1972, and "An Ideal Health Care System for America," *Transaction, 8,* 31, 1971, and Rolf Lium's "Choice, Fees, and Quality," *Harvard Medical Alumni Bulletin, 4,* 1971, attacking it.

Chapter 5

1. Some of the material in the section on hospitals is taken from Chapter 7, "Hospitals" by Michael Enright and myself, of my textbook, *Health Care Delivery in the United States,* cited above. The material is used with the kind permission of Mr. Enright and the Springer Publishing Company of New York City.

2. Sources of data on hospitals. There are two major agencies that count and classify hospitals in the United States: the American Hospital Association (AHA) and the National Center for Health Statistics (NCHS) of the USDHEW. The AHA annually publishes the Guide Issue of its journal *Hospitals,* followed by a companion publication, *Hospital Statistics* (which until 1972 was published as part of the *Guide Issue*). These publications list each hospital registered by the AHA, giving its basic characteristics, as well as much summary data. *Hospitals* also includes "Hospital Indicators," monthly compilations of data on trends in hospital use and financing. The NCHS publishes a volume called *Health Resources Statistics* on an annual or biennial basis, as well as results of the NCHS *Hospital Discharge Survey,* which appear periodically in *Monthly Vital Statistics Report* and *Health and Vital Statistics.* In 1976, a publication somewhat similar to *Health Resources Statistics,* called *Health: United States, 1975,* appeared. It may either supplement or supplant the former. The NCHS defines its terms and counts slightly differently from the AHA. This chapter uses AHA definitions and data except as specifically noted.

3. The definition of community hospital is from the American Hospital Association's *Hospital Statistics,* 1977 edition, p. xviii.

4. The descriptive data on hospitals are taken from *Hospital Statistics,* 1977 edition, Tables 1, 2, and 8 and "Hospital Indicators," *Hospitals, J.A.H.A.,* Feb. 16, 1977, p. 54.

5. The data on hospital discharge diagnoses and surgical operations are from, "Utilization of Short-Stay Hospitals: Annual Summary for the United States, 1975," *Vital and Health Statistics,* Series 13, Number 31, Rockville, Md.; April 1977, tables G and 23.

6. The data on the geographical distribution of hospital beds are from *Health, United States, 1975* (Washington, D.C.: USDHEW Pub. No. (HRA) 76–1232, 1976), table B.II.2.

7. A discussion of how to rationally determine an appropriate bed-population ratio is contained in Sattler and Bennett's *A Statistical Profile of Short-Term Hospitals in the United States as of 1973* (Minneapolis, Minn.: Interstudy, 1975), p. 30. See also the Institute of Medicine's

A Policy Statement: Controlling the Supply of Hospital Beds (Washington, D.C.: National Academy of Sciences), October 1976. The quote on text p. 100 is from p. vii of the Report.

8. Milton Roemer framed his "law" in "Bed Supply and Hospital Utilization: A Natural Experiment," *Hospitals, J.A.H.A.*, November, 1961.

9. The datum on personnel costs as a percentage of total costs is from *Hospital Indicators, Hospitals, J.A.H.A.*, April 16, 1976, table 1.

10. The datum on the proportion of filled bed cost needed to maintain an empty bed was given by Blue Cross/Blue Shield of Greater New York, quoted in an article "Just How Much Hospital Does this City Need?" *New York Times*, August 24, 1976.

11. The estimate of optimum hospital bed occupancy is in the Sattler-Bennett study cited above, pp. 36–39.

12. The quote from Mr. McMahon was contained in an article " 'More Beds Than We Need', AHA admits," *Medical World News*, November 8, 1974, p. 114.

13. The subsequent AHA position was contained in an editorial, "Are There Too Many Hospital Beds?", *Hospitals, J.A.H.A.*, April 1, 1975, p. 17.

14. Sattler and Bennett's estimates on potential savings are worked out on pp. 40–46 of the report cited above.

15. The HRG report was published by Public Citizen in Washington D.C., 1975. An AHA response entitled *A Critique of the Public Citizen Health Research Group Report $8 Billion Hospital Bed Overrun* (Chicago, Ill.: Bureau of Research Services, July, 1975) was published, followed by an HRG reply printed in their newsletter, *Consumers Health Action Network*, January, 1976, p. 7.

16. Additional evidence of the causes and cures of hospital expenditure increases is to be found in *The Rapid Rise of Hospital Costs*, Executive Office of the President: Council on Wage and Price Stability, Washington, D.C.: January, 1977.

17. The Roemer-Schonick study is "HMO Performance: The Recent Evidence," *Health and Society*, *51*, 271, 1973, see esp. pp. 281–291.

18. The studies cited by Ensminger are on pp. 26–28 of his report.

19. The 1976 HMO/Hospitalization study is by C.R. Gaus, et al., "Contrasts in HMO and Fee-for-Service Performance" *Social Security Bulletin*, May, 1976, p. 3.

20. The McCarthy-Widmer study is "Effects of Screening by Consultants on Recommended Elective Surgical Procedures," *New England Journal of Medicine*, *291*, 1331, 1974. The Lewis study is "Variations in the Incidence of Surgery," *New England Journal of Medicine*, *281*,

880, 1969. The Williams book is *How to Avoid Unnecessary Surgery,* Nash Publishing, 1971.

21. The Ensminger estimate of unnecessary deaths is on p. 18 of his report.

22. The *New York Times* piece was "Incompetent Surgery Is Not Found Isolated," January 17, 1976. Part of a five-part piece on the quality of medical care, it aroused considerable controversy. For additional data on unnecessary surgery, see *Cost and Quality of Health Care: Unnecessary Surgery,* Report by the Subcommittee on Oversight and Investigations of the House of Representatives Committee on Interstate and Foreign Commerce, 94th Congress, Washington, D.C., January, 1976.

23. Dr. Moore's response to the *Times'* article was quoted in *"How Much Unnecessary Surgery?" Medical World News,* May 3, 1976, p. 50.

24. The American Medical News position was found in "Unnecessary Surgery," February 9, 1976, p. 4. The issue of the AMN quoted Dr. Todd on p. 15.

25. Dr. Zuidema was quoted in *Medical World News,* May 3, 1976, p. 92.

26. The MWN bibliography on unnecessary surgery appears in "How Much Unnecessary Surgery?" May 3, 1976, p. 66.

27. The suit in which a hospital medical staff won complete control over its own bylaws is discussed in "Few Winners Seen in Huron Affair," *Hospitals, J.A.H.A.,* Nov. 1, 1976, p. 77.

28. The definition of health administration is from p. 139 of C.J. Austin's "Emerging Roles and Responsibilities in Health Administration," which appeared in *Education for Health Administration* Vol. 1, pp. 137–151 (Ann Arbor, Mich.: Health Administration Press, 1975).

29. Portions of the text on private practice and organized ambulatory care are taken from Chapter 6, "Ambulatory Care" by myself and Barbara Rimer, of our textbook, cited above.

30. The data on the distribution of physicians by type of practice are from Cantwell J.R., ed., *Profile of Medical Practice,* 1975–76 Edition (Chicago, Ill.: American Medical Association), table 18.

31. The figure on the proportion of total ambulatory visits made to private doctors' offices is from K.M Danchik's "Physician Visits Volume and Interval Since Last Visit 1971." *Vital and Health Statictics,* Series 10, No. 97 (Washington, D.C.: USDHEW, March, 1975).

32. A useful paper on physicians' patient-referral practices is Steven M. Shortell's "Determinants of Physician Referral Rates: An Exchange Theory Approach." *Medical Care, 12,* 13, 1974.

33. The figures on physician working patterns are from Warner, J. and Aherne, P., *Profile of Medical Practice,* 1974 edition (Chicago, Ill.: American Medical Association), tables 44, 52, 60, 61, 62.

34. The historical data on the growth of hospitals is from Rosemary Stevens' book *American Medicine and The Public Interest,* cited previously, p. 52.

35. The information on the location of the clinics at Johns Hopkins is from Dr. Freymann's book, p. 56. The quote is from p. 200.

36. The quote from Dr. Knowles is to be found on p. 70 of "The Role of the Hospital: The Ambulatory Clinic," *Bulletin of the New York Academy of Medicine,* 41, 68, 2nd series, January, 1965.

37. Dr. Sheps' observation appeared on p. 148 of "Conference Summary and the Road Ahead," *Bulletin of the New York Academy of Medicine, 41,* No. 1, 2nd series, January, 1965, p. 146.

38. Dr. Weinerman's "ultimate solution" is found in Weinerman, E.R. and Edwards, H.R., "Yale Studies in Ambulatory Medical Care I. Changing Patterns in Hospital Emergency Service," *Hospitals, J.A.H.A.,* November 16, 1964.

39. The AMA's definition of group practice is quoted from p. 6 of C. Rufus Rorem's *Private Group Clinics,* Publication No. 8, The Committee on the Costs of Medical Care, Chicago, Ill., 1931 (Reprinted, New York, N.Y.: Milbank Memorial Fund, 1971).

40. For a history of the development of prepaid group practice see W.A. MacColl's *Group Practice and Prepayment of Medical Care* (Washington, D.C.: Public Affairs Press, 1966). For a bibliography on prepaid group practice, and Health Maintenance Organizations, see the appropriate sections of Chapter 6, "Ambulatory Care" by myself and Barbara Rimer, in our textbook. The *Harvard Law Review* definition of PPGP is in "The Role of Prepaid Group Practice in Relieving the Medical Care Crisis," *84,* 887, 1971.

41. The figures on physicians in group practice and PPGP are from the Cantwell/AMA work cited above, tables 1–4, and accompanying text.

42. Dr. Silver's comments on group practice are contained in "Group Practice—What It Is." *Medical Care, 1,* 94, 1963.

43. Dr. Weinerman's paper on PPGP is "Problems and Perspectives of Group Practice," *Bulletin of the New York Academy of Medicine 44,* 2nd Series, 1423, 1968.

44. The 1971 USDHEW statement on HMO's is from its document *Health Maintenance Organizations: The Concept and Structure* (Washington, D.C., 1971). Dr. Elwood and his colleagues laid out their origi-

nal ideas in "Health Maintenance Strategy," *Medical Care, 9,* 291, 1971.

45. The independent-dependent-supporting staff model is similar to that described by Eliot Freidson in *Professional Dominance: The Social Structure of Medical Care* (New York: Atherton Press, 1970), especially Chapter 5.

46. Figures on health manpower supply are from *Health Resources Statistics* (Washington, D.C.: USDHEW, 1974).

47. *The Final Report of the Commission on Medical Education* was published by the Commission itself in New York in 1932. The quotation is from pp. 119–20.

48. The Surgeon General's Consultant Group report, entitled *Physicians for a Growing America,* also known as the Bane Report for the Group's chairman, was published by the USDHEW in October 1957. The quote is from p. 57. The apology for the use of physician-population ratios is on p. 12.

49. In October, 1970, the Carnegie Commission on Higher Education published *Higher Education and the Nation's Health: Policies for Medical and Dental Education* (New York: McGraw-Hill Book Company). The quotation is from p. 2. The 50,000-figure for the dimension of the doctor shortage appears on p. 18.

50. *Progress and Problems in Medical and Dental Education: Federal Support Versus Federal Control* was published in 1976 for the Carnegie Council by Jossey-Bass Publishers of San Francisco. The quote is from p. 3.

51. Dr. Fein's excellent book, still apropós, is *The Doctor Shortage: An Economic Diagnosis,* Washington, D.C.: The Brookings Institution. The quotes are from pp. 21 and 141.

52. An excellent paper on the need for rational task analysis is Anthony Robbin's "Allied Health Manpower Solution or Problem?" *New England Journal of Medicine, 286,* 918, 1972.

Chapter 6

Dr. Fineberg's statement appeared in his November 1976 Report to the House of Delegates of the Medical Society of the State of New York, which was excerpted in the MSSNY's *News of New York,* Jan. 15, 1977, p. 3. Piet Hein's poem appeared on p. 42 of the *Harvard Medical Alumni Bulletin,* Nov./Dec., 1976. In this and following sections there are certain excerpts from Chapter 13, "Measurement and Control of the Quality of Health Care" written by myself, in *Health Care Delivery in the United States.* The material is used with the permission of the Springer Publishing Co., New York, N. Y.

1. For an excellent layman's guide to the medical examination, see Chapters 2 and 4 of Marvin Belsky's *Beyond the Medical Mystique: How to Choose and Use Your Doctor,* cited above.

2. Dr. Lister's note on Dr. Clifton appeared in Dr. Lister's regular column in the *New England Journal of Medicine,* "By the London Post," on Feb. 24, 1977, *296,* 436.

3. The quotes from Dr. Codman appeared on p. 84 of "Medical Care Evaluation: An Old New Idea," by Tom Christoffel, *Journal of Medical Education, 51,* 83, 1976. The additional information on Codman's work is also from Dr. Christoffel's paper.

4. The quote from Dr. Donabedian appears on p. 3 of his classic work, *A Guide to Medical Care Administration, Volume II: Medical Care Appraisal —Quality and Utilization* (New York: American Public Health Association, 1969).

5. The quote from Dr. Christoffel was contained in a letter from him to me dated March 15, 1976.

6. The basic information on individual licensing is derived from: Richard H. Shryock's *Medical Licensing in America, 1650–1965* (Baltimore, Md.: The Johns Hopkins Press, 1967); *The Report of the National Advisory Commission on Health Manpower* (Washington, D.C.: USGPO, November 1967), Volume II, Appendix VII; *State Licensing of Health Occupations,* by M. Y. Pennell and P. A. Stewart (Washington, D.C.: USDHEW, 1968); Robert C. Derbyshire's *Medical Licensure and Discipline in the United States* (Baltimore, Md.: The Johns Hopkins Press, 1969); The Secretary's *Report on Licensure and Related Health Personnel Credentialing* (Washington, D.C.: USDHEW, June, 1971); and *Developments in Health Manpower Licensure* (Washington, D.C.: USDHEW, June, 1973), by Harris S. Cohen and Lawrence H. Miike.

7. Data on institutional licensure is taken from G. Hollis' *State Licensing of Health Facilities* (Washington, D.C.: National Center for Health Statistics, USDHEW, 1968).

8. The JCAH's PEP is thoroughly described in *Measuring the Quality of Patient Care: The Rationale for Outcome Audit,* by Charles M. Jacobs, Tom H. Christoffel, and Nancy Dixon (Cambridge, Mass.: Ballinger Publishing Co., 1976).

9. The *PSRO Program Manual* is published by the Office of Professional Standards Review (Washington, D.C.: USDHEW). The quote is from p. 7.

10. The AMA lashed out at PSROs in *PSRO Deleterious Effects: Information Kit* (Chicago, 1974). Cooler heads have prevailed since then, and the AMA, although still condemning "government interference,"

has become cautiously cooperative. Some state and county medical societies remain aggressively uncooperative, however.

11. The quote from the *American Homeopath,* written by one George W. Winterburn, appeared on p. 144 of Martin Kaufman's *American Medical Education* (Westport, Conn.: Greenwood Press, 1976).

12. Dr. Roth's statement on quality was quoted in an article "Peers' Role stressed by AMA President" which appeared in the *American Medical News,* December 10, 1973, p. 3.

13. The quote from Lee and Jones is from p. 6 of their book *The Fundamentals of Good Medical Care* (Chicago: The University of Chicago Press, 1933).

14. The Weinerman quote is in his paper "The Quality of Medical Care," which appeared in *The Annals of the American Academy of Political and Social Science,* January 7, 1951, p. 185.

15. The quote from Kessner, et al., appeared in their paper "Assessing Health Quality—The Case for Tracers," *New England Journal of Medicine, 288,* 189, 1973.

16. The quote from Brook appeared in his paper "Critical Issues in the Assessment of Quality of Care and their Relationship to HMO's," *Journal of Medical Education, 48,* 114, April 1973, Part 2.

17. The literature in quality assessment is enormous. There is a bibliography of moderate length attached to my chapter "Measure and Control of the Quality of Health Care" in *Health Care Delivery,* cited above. Interested readers may also wish to consult bibliographies and literature reviews in the following works: Dr. Avedis Donabedian's *A Guide to Medical Care Administration,* II: Medical Care Appraisal—Quality and Utilization (New York: American Public Health Association, 1969). Dr. Robert Brook's *Quality of Care Assessment: A Comparison of Five Methods of Peer Review* (Washington, D.C., USDHEW, 1973), esp. Chapter 3. Tom Christoffel's "Selected Bibliography" which appeared in *Measuring the Quality of Patient Care: The Rationale for Outcome Audit* by C. M. Jacobs, et al. (Cambridge, Mass.: Ballinger Publishing Co., 1976).

18. Dr. Peterson's study, done with colleagues, was "An Analytical Study of North Carolina General Practice," *The Journal of Medical Education, 31,* December, 1956, Part 2.

19. Lembcke's classic work was "Medical Auditing by Scientific Methods," *Journal of the American Medical Association, 162,* 646, 1956.

20. The Columbia/Teamsters studies were reported in: Trussell, R. E., et al., *The Quantity, Quality and Costs of Medical and Hospital Care Secured by a Sample of Teamster Families in the New York Area* (New York: Columbia University School of Public Health and Administrative Medi-

cine, 1962) and Morehead, M. A., et al., *A Study of the Qaulity of Hospital Care Secured by a Sample of Teamster Family Members in New York City* (New York: Columbia University School of Public Health and Administrative Medicine, 1964).

21. The study by Kessner, et al., was reported in *Contrasts in Health Status, 2: A Strategy for Evaluating Health Services* (Washington, D.C.: Institute of Medicine, 1974). The quotes are from p. 4.

22. The Brook study, done with Francis A. Appel, appeared in the *New England Journal of Medicine, 288,* 1323, as "Quality-of-Care Assessment: Choosing a Method for Peer Review."

23. The Kelley-Manlon study appeared as "Ambulatory Medical Care Quality: Determination by Diagnostic Outcome," *Journal of the American Medical Association, 227,* 1155, 1974.

24. The results of the antibiotic therapy test were reported by Dr. Harold C. Neu and Sara P. Howsey in "Testing the Physician's Knowledge of Antibiotic Use," *New England Journal of Medicine, 293,* 1291, 1975.

25. The Wiener-Nathanson study was reported in "Physical Examination: Frequently Observed Errors," *Journal of the American Medical Association, 236,* 852, 1976.

26. The Forgotson-Roemer-Newman study is entitled "Legal Regulation of Health Personnel in the United States." It appeared as Appendix VII, Volume II of the *Report of the National Advisory Commission on Health Manpower* (Washington, D.C.: USGPO, November, 1967). The quote is from p. 290.

27. Important papers in the history of medical licensure are those of Henry Sigerist, "The History of Medical Licensure," *Journal of the American Medical Association, 104,* 1057, 1935, and Sidney Shindell, "A Survey of the Law of Medical Practice," *Journal of the American Medical Association, 193,* 601, 1965.

28. The quote from the original charter of the Royal College of Medicine is from Rosemary Stevens' *Medical Practice in Modern England* (New Haven: Yale University Press, 1966), p. 11.

29. Dr. Derbyshire's book was cited above. The quote is from p. 2.

30. Dr. Shryock's book is cited above. The quote is from p. 5. The bulk of the history I give is from the work of Drs. Derbyshire and Shryock.

31. The material on the medical license as a privilege is from pp. 13–15 of Dr. Derbyshire's book.

32. Mr. Vodicka's statement on the medical license as a property right appeared in "Medical Discipline: Part VI. The Offenses," *Journal of the American Medical Association, 235,* 302, 1976.

33. *State Licensing of Health Occupations* by Maryland Y. Pennell and Paula A. Stewart (Washington, D.C.: USDHEW, 1965) is a very useful source on the composition, powers, and functioning of state licensing boards. The book covers licensing of all health professions.

34. The Derbyshire quote on the typical physician Medical Board member is from p. 44 of his book, cited above.

35. The phenomenon of lay appointments to Boards of Medicine is described in "MD-public meeting favorable, so far," *American Medical News,* January 19, 1976, p. 13

36. The *New York Times* figures appeared in an article entitled "Few Doctors Ever Report Colleagues' Incompetence," published on January 29, 1976.

37. The story of the physician who gained in Michigan what he lost in New York appeared in "L. I. Doctor Who Lost License Got Backing," by Boyce Rensberger, *New York Times,* April 15, 1977.

Chapter 7

The major source of material for this chapter is *American Medical Education: The Formative Years, 1765–1910,* by Martin Kaufman (Westport, Conn.: Greenwood Press, 1976). Additional material is drawn from Dr. Freymann's *The American Health Care System,* esp. Chapters 3 and 4, and Dr. Stevens' *American Medicine and the Public Interest,* esp. Part I. Both books are referenced in earlier chapters.

1. State requirements for licensure are from Professor Shryock's *Medical Licensing in America,* referenced in the previous chapter, pp. 23–27.

2. The data on the number of medical schools in the 19th century are from p. 6 of the Flexner Report, *Medical Education in the United States and Canada* (New York: The Carnegie Foundation for the Advancement of Teaching, Bulletin Number Four, 1910; Reproduced, Washington, D.C.: Science and Health Publications, 1960).

3. The quote from Kaufman is from p. 45 of his book.

4. The section "Early Attempts at Reform" is largely based on Chapters 5 and 6 of Mr. Kaufman's book.

5. "Reform Begins" draws on Chapters 8–10 of Mr. Kaufman's book.

6. The description of the Johns Hopkins is based on pp. 147–50 of Mr. Kaufman's book and pp. 53–59 of Dr. Freymann's.

7. The material on the AAMC in the 1890s is based largely on Chapter 10 of Mr. Kaufman's book.

8. For the details of the AMA's internal structure, some rather murky, and of its various reorganizations from 1847 to 1901, see James G.

Burrow's excellent account, *AMA: Voice of American Medicine* (Baltimore: The Johns Hopkins Press, 1963), pp. 14–20, 27–33.

9. The figures on doctors, medical schools and medical schools graduates are from tables 60 and 104 of *Final Report of the Commission on Medical Education* (New York: Association of American Medical Colleges, 1932).

10. The material on the AMA and its Council on Medical Education is largely from Chapter 10 of Mr. Kaufman's book, and pp. 58–66 of Dr. Stevens' book.

11. The Kaufman quote is from p. 159 of his book.

12. The Stevens quote on CME standards is from p. 65 of her book, cited above.

13. The Kaufman quote on the 1907 CME Report is from p. 160 of his book.

14. The Stevens quotes on the AMA link to the state medical boards are from pp. 65–66 of her book.

Chapter 8

The biographical material on Abraham Flexner is primarily from "Abraham Flexner—A Reappraisal" by H. David Banta, *Social Science and Medicine, 5,* 655, 1971. I also used material from Chapter 11 of the Kaufman book, cited in the previous chapter. Another useful paper, analyzing the whole socioeconomic setting of the "Flexnerian Reforms" is "Doctors in Crisis: A Study of the Use of Medical Education Reform to Establish Modern Professional Elitism in Medicine," *American Quarterly, 25,* 83, 1973, by G.E. Markowitz and D.K. Rosner. The quote from Dr. Philbrick is from the *Journal of the American Medical Association,* June 15, 1901, p. 1700.

1. A proponent of spread-out medical schools is Dr. Edmund D. Pellegrino: "The Regionalization of Academic Medicine: The Metamorphosis of a Concept," *Journal of Medical Education, 48,* 119, 1973.

2. The quote on the content of the first two years is from p. 61 of the *Report.*

3. Flexner's prescription for the distribution of clinical work is to be found on pp. 95 and 96 of the *Report.*

4. The quote on the place of research is from pp. 58–59 of the *Report.*

5. The information on the CME ranking system and its effect on the proprietary schools is from Kaufman's book, pp. 176–77.

6. Howard Berliner's paper is "A Larger Perspective on the Flexner Report," *International Journal of Health Services, 5,* 573, 1975.

7. The views of Dr. Pritchett are to be found on pp. x–xii of Flexner's *Report.*

8. Stevens' data on foundation support of medical education are to be found on p. 69 of her book.

9. For examples of modern misinterpretation of Flexner, see D.W. Seldin's "The Intimate Coupling of Biomedical Science and Physician Education," *Clinical Research, 23,* 280, December, 1975, and The Carnegie Commission on Higher Education, *Higher Education and the Nation's Health* (New York: McGraw-Hill Book Company, 1970), p. 25.

Chapter 9

1. The data on the 1945 physician/population ratio and the proportion of primary care physicians in 1931 and 1945 are from Surgeon General's Consultant Group on Medical Education, *Physicians for a Growing America* (Washington, D.C.: USDHEW, 1959), Appendix, tables 6 and 7.

2. The 1925 entrance requirements and the material on the formation of the NBME are from Kaufman, pp. 179 and 178, respectively.

3. The material on foundation support is from Freymann's book, cited above, p. 58.

4. and 5. The material on the Osler-Mall controversy is based on Freymann, pp. 57–58, and the Osler quote is from Freymann, p. 57.

6. and 7. The material on the AAMC and the FSMB is from pp. 165–67 of Association of American Medical Colleges, *Final Report of the Commission on Medical Education,* New York, 1932.

8. The quote from the Commission's Report is to be found on pp. 23–24.

9. For an excellent description and analysis of the current situation in medical board certification, see Herbert J. Lerner's *Manpower Issues and Voluntary Regulation in the Medical Specialty System,* (New York: Prodist, 1974).

10. and 11. The material from Freymann on specialization, including the quote from Herodotus is found on p. 61 of his book.

12. The material on regulation of specialty boards and residencies is based in part on Chapter X, "Specialization and the Specialty Boards," of *A Half-Century of American Medical Education: 1920–1970,* by Vernon W. Lippard (New York: Josiah Macy, Jr. Foundation, 1974).

13. The description of the LCGME (not the analysis) is from Augustus Swanson's "The Genesis of the Coordinating Council on Medical Education and The Liaison Committee on Graduate Medical Education," *Bulletin of the New York Academy of Medicine, 50,* 1216, 1974.

14. The data on physician incomes during the Great Depression are from Elton Rayack's *Professional Power and American Medicine: The Economics of the American Medical Association* (Cleveland: The World Publishing Co., 1967), table 23.

15. The data on the number of medical schools and graduates 1930–1945 are from Rayack, table 20. The material on AMA influence on medical school enrollment is from Rayack, pp. 72–79, and tables 20 and 24.

Chapter 10

1. The section, "Building the Research Base," is based in part upon the work of Stevens, Freymann, Lippard, Rayack, and Burrow, all previously cited, and Stephen P. Strickland's *Politics, Science, and Dread Disease* (Cambridge, Mass.: Harvard University Press, 1972).

2. The quote from Dr. Allen is on p. 133 of his book *Medical Education and the Changing Order* (New York: The Commonwealth Fund, 1946).

3. The Lasker and Gregg quotes are from Strickland, p. 250.

4. The data on doctor-population ratios are from Rayack, table 21, and Appendix, table 1 of *Physicians for the Future,* Report of the Macy Commission (New York: Macy Foundation, 1976).

5. The details on 1949 legislative proposals are from Stevens, p. 356.

6. The AAMC position on aid to medical education is quoted from Ryack, p. 83.

7. Freymann's figures on medical school faculty size are on p. 87 of his book.

8. The material on NIH growth and development is primarily from Freymann, pp. 83–93, and Stevens pp. 357–62. For a fascinating "outsider's view" of the NIH, see Strickland's book. For a fascinating "insider's view" see "Federal Support of Biomedical Sciences: Development and Academic Impact," *Journal of Medical Education,* Vol. 51, No. 7, July 1976, Part 2 by James A. Shannon, director of the NIH during its halcyon years, 1955–68. Some of my figures are from Dr. Shannon's tables.

9. Rayack's thought on the effects of aid to research and aid to education is on p. 99 of his book.

10. The section "Distortions" is based in part on Freymann, pp. 87–93.

11. For a brief but cogent description of the work of Rep. Fountain see Stevens, pp. 367–70.
12. The data on medical schools and graduates are from Rayack, table 20, the Macy Commission Report, Appendix, table 12, and the 1975 AMA report, "Medical Education in the United States, 1974–75," *Journal of the American Medical Association, 234,* Dec. 29, 1975, table 9.
13. The Bayne-Jones Report was formally entitled *The Advancement of Medical Research and Education through the Department of Health, Education, and Welfare,* Final Report of the Secretary's Consultants on Medical Research and Education (Washington, D.C.: USDHEW, 1958). The Bane Report was formally entitled *Physicians for a Growing America,* Report of the Surgeon General's Consultant Group on Medical Education (Washington, D.C.: USDHEW, 1959).
14. On Sheppard-Towner, see Burrow, pp. 157–58, 160–64.
15. The legislative history of federal aid to medical education in the 60's is from Rayack, pp. 94–101, and Stevens, pp. 362–67.
16. The NIH figures are from Shannon, tables 6 and 14.
17. The 1970 Carnegie Commission Report was published by McGraw-Hill Book Company, New York, 1970.
18. The quote on *health care delivery* medical schools is from the 1970 Report, p. 4.
19. For Dr. Seldin's views, see his paper "The Medical Model: Biomedical Science as the Basis of Medicine," in *Beyond Tomorrow* (New York, N.Y.: The Rockefeller University, 1977), p. 31.
20. The figures on FMGs are from the Macy Commission Report, Appendix, table 18.
21. The 1976 Carnegie Council *Report* is published by Jossey-Bass, San Francisco, Calif., 1976.
22. The quote from the Carnegie Council is on p. 3 of their *Report.*

Chapter 11

Dr. Jason's quote appeared in his paper "The Relevance of Medical Education to Medical Practice," *Journal of the American Medical Association, 212,* 2092, 1970. The Petersdorf quote is from his "Presidential Address to the Convocation of the American College of Physicians." Philadelphia, Pa., April 5, 1976. Anne Sexton's poem "Doctors" was reprinted in the *Harvard Medical Alumni Bulletin,* Nov/Dec, 1976, p. 12.

1. Data on the number of medical schools are from pp. 2957–78, and Appendix II, table 1, of the *76th Annual Report, Medical Education in the*

United States: 1975–76, JAMA, December 27, 1976, hereinafter referred to as the *Annual Report.*

2. The datum on the proportion of private schools receiving aid from their respective governments is from p. 3 of *Medical Education: Institutions, Characteristics and Programs,* a useful Background Paper from the AAMC, Washington, D.C., 1977.
3. Data on medical school faculty are from the *Annual Report.* pp. 2959–60.
4. The IOM cost study is *Costs of Education in the Health Professions: Report of Study Parts I and II,* Julius B. Richmond, M.D., Chairman, Ruth Hanft, Study Director (Washington, D.C.: National Academy of Sciences, 1974).
5. The data on medical students are from the *Annual Report,* pp. 2960–64 and the Datagram in the February, 1977 number of the *Journal of Medical Education.*
6. The data on state of origin of medical students are the *Annual Report,* Appendix II, tables 5 and 6.
7. The data and the quote on female enrollment are from the *Annual Report,* pp. 2960–61, and the JME *Datagram* for August, 1976, pp. 691–93.
8. The material on minority student enrollment is taken from the AAMC Datagram, "Medical Student Enrollment, 1972–73 through 1976 77," *JME,* February, 1977, pp. 161–66.
9. The quote from Grace Ziem is found in "Medical Education Since Flexner," *Health/PAC Bulletin,* May/June, 1977, p. 8.
10. Barbara Caress' article is "Medical School Sweepstakes," *Health-/PAC Bulletin,* May/June, 1977, p. 2.
11. A very useful review of the medical school admissions process is *The Medical School Admissions Process. A Review of the Literature, 1955–76,* by J.M. Cuca, et al., Health Resources Administration (Rockville, Md.: USDHEW, October, 1976, reproduced by the National Technical Information Service: U.S. Department of Commerce, Publ. No. PB–263 962). I am not citing this as a reference, but calling the attention of interested readers to its existence.
12. On the relationship between MCAT scores and future physician performance see for example "The Medical College Admission Test as Related to Achievement Tests in Medicine and to Supervisory Evaluations of Clinical Physicians," by Margaret A. Howell and John W. Vincent, *Journal of Medical Education, 42,* 1037, 1967.

13. Data on numbers of applicants come from the Datagram "Applicants for 1976–77 First-Year Medical School Class," *JME,* September 1977, pp. 780–82, table 1, and the *Annual Report,* pp. 2960–64.

14. Data on curriculae are from the *Annual Report,* p. 2964, and the *1976–77 AAMC Curriculum Directory* (Washington, D.C.: Association of American Medical Colleges, 1976).

15. Dr. Koran's paper, "The Reliability of Clinical Methods, Data, and Judgments," appeared in the *NEJM, 293,* 642, 695, 1975.

16. The editorial "Goals and Objectives in Medical Education," appeared in the *Lancet,* May 7, 1977, p. 985.

17. The work by Creditor is "Urbana-Champaign: A Prospective View of Paradigm Change," a paper that was unpublished as of June, 1977. It is cited by permission of the author.

18. Problem-orientation in medical records and practice is described in Dr. Weed's *Medical Records, Medical Education and Patient Care* (Cleveland, Ohio: Case Western Rserve University Press, 1969) and *The Problem-Oriented System,* by J. Willis Hurst and H. Kenneth Walker (New York: Medcom, Inc., 1972).

19. Dr. Weed's paper on medical education is "A New Paradigm for Medical Education" which appeared in Purcell, E.F., editor, *Recent Trends in Medical Education* (New York: Macy Foundation, 1976). The quotes are from p. 56 and pp. 79–82.

20. The data on grading systems is from the 1976–77 AAMC *Curriculum Directory,* p. 283.

21. The Wingard/Williamson paper is "Grades as Predictors of Physicians' Career Performance: An Evaluative Literature Review," *Journal of Medical Education, 48,* 311, 1973.

22. The quote by Dr. Weed on teaching and measuring retention of bodies of knowledge is from p. 58 of his paper cited above.

23. The quotes by Dr. Weed on present and proposed systems of behavior are from pp. 86, 87, 81, and 88, consecutively.

24. Dr. Rezler's paper appeared in the *Journal of of Medical Education, 49,* 1023, 1974. Readers who are especially interested in this subject are advised to refer to Dr. Rezler's paper, and the very important studies she describes.

25. The Hogness-Akin paper is "Administration of Education Programs in Academic Health Centers," *New England Journal of Medicine, 296,* 656, 1977.

26. The cost and source of funds figures for 1974–75 are from the *Annual Report,* table 30.

27. The *IOM–NAS Report* on the costs of health sciences education is presently available from the National Technical Information Service of the U.S. Department of Commerce, publication number PB–238 328.

28. The quote on what is included in health sciences education costs is from p. 25 of the *IOM–NAS Report.*

29. Unless otherwise noted the cited data on the costs of medical education are from Chapter 5 of the *IOM–NAS Report.*

30. The data on distribution of educational costs between instruction, research, and patient care are from p. 35 of the *IOM–NAS Report.*

31. The data on instructional faculty/student ratios are from p. 36 of the *IOM–NAS Report.*

32. The quote on faculty time distribution is from p. 69 of the *IOM–NAS Report.*

33. The quotes from "Functions and Structure of a Medical School" are from pp. 3, 4, and 5 respectively.

34. The Coggeshall Committee's statement on the quality of American medical education is to be found on p. 33 of *Planning for Medical Progress Through Education* (Evanston, Ill.: Association of American Medical Colleges, 1965).

35. Flexner's position on state regulation of medical education is clearly stated on p. 154 of his *Report.* See Appendix I.e. of this book.

36. The quotes from the *Final Report* of the Commission on Medical Education are from pp. 383 and 3, respectively.

37. The quotes from the Coggeshall *Report* are from pp. 33 and 34 respectively.

Chapter 12

The Petersdorf quote is from his "Presidential Address to the Convocation of the American College of Physicians," Philadelphia, Pa., April 5, 1976. The Palmer quote is from an undated form letter on AMA stationery addressed "Dear Doctor" which I received sometime in November, 1976. The Kennedy quote is from a letter of his published in the *New York Times* on March 21, 1976.

1. The quote from Dr. Berliner appeared in "Sharp debate emerging on need for specialty in care of the aging," *American Medical News,* Nov. 1, 1976, p. 10.

2. For the AAMC position on health manpower act provisions affecting geographic maldistribution of physicians see the AAMC *Weekly Report* of September 13, 1976, and AAMC *Memorandum* #76–46, "The

Health Professions Educational Assistance Act of 1976 (P.L. 94-484)."

3. Dr. Palmer's statement was made during a debate on national health insurance with Senator Edward Kennedy, held in the Eisenhower Theatre of the Kennedy Center, Washington, D.C., May 18, 1977.
4. The Mellinkoff statement from his guest editorial "Medical discovery and medical education," *New England Journal of Medicine, 279,* 659, 1968, was quoted by Dr. Freymann in his book, p. 187.
5. The Russell Baker column was "Light in Dark Corners," *New York Times,* June 21, 1977.
6. Dr. Winslow's editorial, "The Place of Preventive Medicine in the Medical Curriculum" appeared in the *American Journal of Public Health, 34,* 1285, 1944.
7. The study on factors affecting geographic movement of physicians is "Analysis of the Impact of the Hill-Burton Program on the Distribution of the Supply of General Hospital Beds and Physicians in the United States, 1950–1970," by L.J. Clark and T.L. Koontz. The paper was delivered at the Annual Meeting of the American Public Health Association, November, 1973, San Francisco, Calif.
8. The quote from Dr. Berliner is to be found in his paper "Medical Education and Scholarly Inquiry," in *Beyond Tomorrow* (New York, N.Y.: Rockefeller University, 1977), pp. 41–42.
9. See *Notes* for Chapter 3 for the citation of Klaw's book.
10. Dr. Ingelfinger's "anti-doctor book" editorial appeared in *The New England Journal of Medicine, 294,* 442, 1976.
11. This quote from Dr. Ingelfinger comes from his editorial "The Physician Contribution to the Health System," *New England Journal of Medicine, 295,* 565, 1976.
12. Dr. Golden discusses his work in *An Inventory for Primary Health Care Practice* (Cambridge, Mass.: Ballinger Publishing Co., 1976). Another useful paper on the subject is Anthony Robbins' "Allied Health Manpower-Solution or Problem?" *New England Journal of Medicine, 286,* 918, 1972.
13. Dr. Kane refers to his work, largely limited to physician tasks, in Kane, R., et al., "Toward Defining the End Product of Medical Education." *Journal of Medical Education, 48,* 615, 1973.
14. For an excellent review of some of the principal examples of resistance to change in medicine over the centuries see Chapter 9 of *Society and Medical Progress,* Bernhard J. Stern (Princeton: Princeton University Press, 1941).
15. The "leave us alone" and "it's all life style" position is taken by

Berliner, Ingelfinger, Fuchs, Palmer, all previously quoted, and many others.

16. The AMA position paper appears in *Informational Papers* (Chicago, Ill.: American Medical Association). The publication as a whole is undated, but this particular paper is dated January, 1971.

17. The first Virchow quote, which appeared in the first issue of his journal *Die medizinische Reform,* is cited by Henry Sigerist on p. 93 of *Medicine and Human Welfare* (New Haven: Yale University Press, 1941).

18. The second Virchow quote, which also appeared in the first issue of *Die medizinische Reform,* is cited by Bernhard Stern in his book *Society and Medical Progress* (Princeton, N.J.: Princeton University Press, 1941), p. 133.

19. The Rutstein quote is from "Measuring the Quality of Medical Care. *New England Journal of Medicine, 294,* 582, 1976, p. 586, by David D. Rutstein, et al.

20. For a description of Herman Biggs' Health Center program see C.-E.A. Winslow's *The Life of Hermann Biggs* (Philadelphia: Lea and Febiger, 1929), Chapter XVII and Appendix V.

21. Studies on the quality of the work of nurse practitioners and physicians' assistants in primary care include: Voltmann, J.D. "Jamestown Medical Clinic System," *Journal of the American Medical Association, 234,* 303, 1975; Spector, R., et al., "Medical Care by Nurses in an Internal Medicine Clinic," *Journal of the American Medical Association, 232,* 1234, 1975; Yankauer, A., et al., "The Outcomes and Service Impact of a Pediatric Nurse Practitioner Training Program—Nurse Practitioner Training Outcomes," *American Journal of Public Health,* March, 1972, p. 347; Spitzer, W.O., et al., "The Burlington Randomized Trial of the Nurse Practitioner" *New England Journal of Medicine, 290,* 251, 1974; Kane, R.L., et al., "Medex and the Physician Preceptors: Quality of Care." *Journal of the American Medical Association, 236,* 2509, 1976; Komaroff, A.L. "Protocols for Physician Assistants." *New England Journal of Medicine, 290,* 307, 1974; and Charles, C. "Physician's [sic] Assistants and Clinical Algorithms in Health Care Delivery." *Annals of Internal Medicine, 81,* 733, 1974.

Chapter 13

Dr. Peabody's quotes are taken from his classic paper "The Care of the Patient," *The Journal of the American Medical Association, 88,* 877, 1927. The quote from Dr. Creditor is the Abstract of his paper "The Process of Medical Education: Its

Contribution to the Problems of Medical Care" (Urbana, Ill., 1976). Unpublished as of mid–1977. Used with the permission of the author.

1. Dr. Harnack's remark was quoted by Dr. Stephen Abrahamson is an editorial, "Changing Curriculum in the Medical School," *Journal of Medical Education, 52,* 778, 1977.
2. The Breslow-Somers paper is "The Lifetime Health-Monitoring Program," *New England Journal of Medicine, 296,* 601, 1977.
3. The Neufeld-Barrows paper is "The 'McMaster Philosophy': An Approach to Medical Education," *JME, 49,* 1040, 1974. The quote is from pp. 1040–41.
4. The quote on "biomedical problem-solving" is from the Neufeld-Barrows paper, p. 1043.
5. The Barrows-Tamblyn quote is from their *Guide to the Development of Skills in Problem Based Learning and Clinical (Diagnostic) Reasoning* (Hamilton, Ontario: Project for Learning Resources Design, Monograph No. 1, McMaster University Faculty of Health Sciences, 1976). See also, *Problem Based Learning in Medicine,* by Howard Barrows, Hamilton (Ontario: Education Monograph 4, M.D. Programme, Faculty of Medicine, McMaster University, June, 1973).
6. The quotes by Dr. Weed are from pp. 81–82 of his paper "A New Paradigm for Medical Education" which appeared in Purcell, E.F., editor, *Recent Trends in Medical Education* (New York: Macy Foundation, 1976).
7. The definition of "pedagogy" is from p. 698 of *The Living Webster Encyclopedic Dictionary of the English Language* (Chicago, Ill.: The English Language Institute of America, 1975).
8. The statement by Lambert is from the "Report of the Committee on Social Insurance of the AMA," *Journal of the American Medical Association, 68,* 1721, 1917; cited by John Gordon Freymann in his paper "Leadership in American Medicine," *New England Journal of Medicine, 270,* 710, 1964.
9. Dr. Coggeshall's warning is given on p. 13 of *Planning for Medical Progress Through Education* (Evanston, Ill.: Association of American Medical Colleges, 1965).

Bibliography

The following is a selected list of books in medical history, politics, and economics which were particularly helpful in the preparation of this book:

Belsky, Marvin and Gross, Leonard. *Beyond the Medical Mystique: How to Choose and Use Your Doctor.* New York: Arbor House, 1975.

Burrow, James. *AMA: Voice of American Medicine.* Baltimore: The Johns Hopkins Press, 1963.

Cassell, Eric J. *The Healer's Art.* New York: J. P. Lippincott Co., 1976.

Committee on the Costs of Medical Care, The. *Final Report: Medical Care for the American People.* Chicago: The University of Chicago Press, 1932. Reprinted, Washington, D. C.: U.S. Department of Health, Education and Welfare, 1970.

Commission on Medical Education, The. *Final Report. New York, 1932.*

Flexner, Abraham. *Medical Education in the United States and Canada.* New York: The Carnegie Foundation for the Advancement of Teaching, 1910. Reprinted, Washington, D.C.: Science and Health Publications, 1960.

Friedson, Eliot. *Profession of Medicine.* New York: Dodd, Mead, and Co., 1975.

Freymann, John Gordon. *The American Health Care System: Its Genesis and Trajectory.* New York: Medcom Press, 1974.

Fuchs, Victor R. *Who Shall Live?* New York: Basic Books, 1974.

Kaufman, Martin. *American Medical Education: The Formative Years,* 1765–1910. Westport, Conn.: Greenwood Press, 1976.

Klaw, Spencer. *The Great American Medicine Show.* New York. The Viking Press, 1975.

McKeown, Thomas. *The Role of Medicine: Dream, Mirage or Nemesis?* London: The Nuffield Provincial Hospitals Trust, 1976.

Rayack, Elton. *Professional Power and American Medicine.* Cleveland: The World Publishing Co., 1967.

Rosen, George. *A History of Public Health.* New York: MD Publications, 1958.

Sigerist, Henry. *Medicine and Human Welfare.* New Haven: Yale University Press, 1941.

Stern, Bernhard J. *Society and Medical Progress.* Princeton: Princeton University Press, 1941.

Stevens, Rosemary. *American Medicine and the Public Interest.* New Haven: Yale University Press, 1971.

Strickland, Stephen. *Politics, Science, and Dread Disease.* Cambridge, Mass.: Harvard University Press, 1972.

Index